AMOGS
Handbook on Practical Aspects of
Infertility

AMOGS
Handbook on Practical Aspects of Infertility

Editors

Nandita Palshetkar
MD FICOG FCPS FRCOG (UK)
President, ISAR
Past President
FOGSI, IAGE, AMOGS, MOGS
FOGSI Representative to FIGO

Chaitanya Shembekar
MD FICOG FICMCH Diploma in Pelviscopy
Chairman and Managing Director
Omega Hospitals, Unit of Shembekar
Hospitals Pvt Ltd, Nagpur
Past President, Nagpur Obstetric and
Gynaecological Society
Nagpur, Maharashtra, India
Chairman, Infertility Committee, AMOGS
Librarian, Maharashtra Chapter, ISAR
Member, PCPNDT Committee
Nagpur Municipal Corporation

Co-Editors

Nilesh Balkawade
MBBS MS DNB
Clinical Head and Fertility Specialist
Oasis Fertility
Pune, Maharashtra, India

Rohan Palshetkar
MBBS MD
IVF Consultant
Bloom IVF and DY Patil Medical College
Mumbai, Maharashtra, India

Parul Saoji
MD DNB MNAMS
Executive Director, Omega Group of Hospitals, Nagpur
Endoscopic Surgeon and Aesthetic Gynecologist
Omega Hospitals, Unit of Shembekar Hospitals Pvt Ltd
Nagpur, Maharashtra, India

Forewords
Hrishikesh Pai
Rajendra Singh Pardeshi

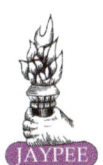

JAYPEE BROTHERS MEDICAL PUBLISHERS
The Health Sciences Publisher
New Delhi | London

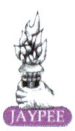 **Jaypee Brothers Medical Publishers (P) Ltd**

Headquarters
Jaypee Brothers Medical Publishers (P) Ltd
EMCA House, 23/23-B
Ansari Road, Daryaganj
New Delhi 110 002, India
Landline: +91-11-23272143, +91-11-23272703
+91-11-23282021, +91-11-23245672
Email: jaypee@jaypeebrothers.com

Corporate Office
Jaypee Brothers Medical Publishers (P) Ltd
4838/24, Ansari Road, Daryaganj
New Delhi 110 002, India
Phone: +91-11-43574357
Fax: +91-11-43574314
Email: jaypee@jaypeebrothers.com

Overseas Office
JP Medical Ltd
83 Victoria Street, London
SW1H 0HW (UK)
Phone: +44 20 3170 8910
Fax: +44 (0)20 3008 6180
Email: info@jpmedpub.com

Website: www.jaypeebrothers.com
Website: www.jaypeedigital.com

© 2023, Jaypee Brothers Medical Publishers

The views and opinions expressed in this book are solely those of the original contributor(s)/author(s) and do not necessarily represent those of editor(s) or publisher of the book.

All rights reserved. No part of this publication may be reproduced, stored or transmitted in any form or by any means, electronic, mechanical, photocopying, recording or otherwise, without the prior permission in writing of the publishers.

All brand names and product names used in this book are trade names, service marks, trademarks or registered trademarks of their respective owners. The publisher is not associated with any product or vendor mentioned in this book.

Medical knowledge and practice change constantly. This book is designed to provide accurate, authoritative information about the subject matter in question. However, readers are advised to check the most current information available on procedures included and check information from the manufacturer of each product to be administered, to verify the recommended dose, formula, method and duration of administration, adverse effects and contraindications. It is the responsibility of the practitioner to take all appropriate safety precautions. Neither the publisher nor the author(s)/editor(s) assume any liability for any injury and/or damage to persons or property arising from or related to use of material in this book.

This book is sold on the understanding that the publisher is not engaged in providing professional medical services. If such advice or services are required, the services of a competent medical professional should be sought.

Every effort has been made where necessary to contact holders of copyright to obtain permission to reproduce copyright material. If any have been inadvertently overlooked, the publisher will be pleased to make the necessary arrangements at the first opportunity.

Inquiries for bulk sales may be solicited at: jaypee@jaypeebrothers.com

AMOGS Handbook on Practical Aspects of Infertility

First Edition: 2023

ISBN: 978-93-5465-555-5

Contributors

Aditi Tandon MS
Consultant Gynecologist
Dr Sudha Tandon Gynaec Endoscopy
and Infertility Centre
Mumbai, Maharashtra, India

Aditya Khurd MBBS
Laparoscopic and Fertility Specialist
Consultant Gyne Endoscopic Surgeon
Khurd Hospital
Pune, Maharashtra, India

Ameet Patki
MD DGO DNB FICOG FCPS FRCOG (UK)
Medical Director
Fertility Associates
Mumbai, Maharashtra, India
Vice President-ISAR

Amiti Agrawal MS MBBS
Reproductive Endocrinologist
(Infertility)
SAS Hospital
Mumbai, Maharashtra, India

Amit Patankar MBBS DNB
Managing Director
Patankar Fertility Solutions Pvt Ltd
Pune, Maharashtra, India

Amrita Tandon
MS DNB (OBGY) MRM (London) FMAS
Consultant Gynec Endoscopic Surgeon
Fertility and IVF Specialist
Dr Sudha Tandon Fertility IVF
Endoscopy and Maternity Centre
Mumbai, Maharashtra, India

Anil Bendre MBBS
Consultant
Bendre Hospital and
Maternity Home
Ahmednagar, Maharashtra, India

Anil Chittake MBBS DNB
Infertility Specialist
Embrio IVF Centre
Pune, Maharashtra, India

Anjali Bhirud MD
IVF Specialist
Chandrama Hospital and
Durga Test Tube Baby Centre
Jalgaon, Maharashtra, India

Ashish Kale MD DNB
Director
Ashakiran Hospital, Pune
Director
Arunachal IVF Center
Pune, Maharashtra, India

Ashish Zarariya MBBS MD
Associate Professor
Government Medical Collage
Nagpur, Maharashtra, India

Ashutosh Thole MBBS DNB DGO
Gynecologist
Janki Hospital
Artillery Center Road
Nashik, Maharashtra, India

Contributors

Ashwini Yelikar Kale
MBBS DGO DNB FICMCH
Director
Ashakiran Hospitals and
Asha IVF Centre
Pune, Maharashtra, India
Ex-Assistant Professor
BJ Medical College
Ahmedabad, Gujarat, India
Hon'ble Consultant
Kamla Nehru Hospital
New Delhi, India
Executive Committee Member, ISAR
Managing Committee Member, MSR
Past Secretary, Pune Obstetric and
Gynecological Society

Balasaheb Khadbade
MD (Obstetrics and Gynecology)
Consultant IVF and Infertility Specialist
Yashoda Fertility and IVF Centre
Navi Mumbai
Director
FOGSI Recognised Advanced Infertility
Training Centre for Gynaecologist
Director
Postgraduate Institute for Obstetrics
and Gynaecology
Yashoda Hospital
Navi Mumbai, Maharashtra, India

Bansi Shinde MBBS DNB
Director
Shinde Hospital, Ahmednagar
Consultant Infertologist and
Laparoscopic Surgeon
Shinde Hospital and
Ankur Infertility Centre
Ahmednagar, Maharashtra, India

Bindu Chimote MS MPhill
Chief Clinical Embryologist
Vaunshdhara Clinic and
Assisted Conception Centre
Nagpur, Maharashtra, India

Chaitanya Shembekar
MD FICOG FICMCH Dip Pelviscopy (Germany)
Chairman and MD
Omega Hospitals, Unit of Shembekar
Hospitals Pvt Ltd, Nagpur
Past President, Nagpur Obstetric and
Gynaecological Society
Nagpur, Maharashtra, India
Chairman, Infertility Committee
AMOGS
Librarian, Maharashtra Chapter, ISAR
Member, PCPNDT Committee
Nagpur Municipal Corporation

Duru Shah
MD FRCOG FCPS FICS FICOG DGO DFP FICMCH
Director
Gynaecworld—The Center for
Women's Health and Fertility
Mumbai, Maharashtra, India
Consultant Obstetrician and
Gynecologist
Breach Candy Hospital/
Jaslok Hospital
Mumbai, Maharashtra, India

Firuza R Parikh MD PhD
Director
FertilTree-Jaslok International
Fertility Centre
Department of Assisted
Reproduction and Genetics
Jaslok Hospital and
Research Centre
Mumbai, Maharashtra, India

Garima Sharma MBBS DGO MS
Infertility Specialist
Gunjan IVF World
New Delhi, India

Gayatri Wadekar MD
Director
Nanded Test Tube Baby Centre
Nanded, Maharashtra, India

Contributors

Girish Godbole MBBS MD
Honorary Consultant
Deenanath Mangeshkar Hospital and Research Center
Pune, Maharashtra, India

Gouri Sultane Gupta
MBBS DNB (Obstetrics and Gynecology)
DGO FCPS (Mid and Gyne)
Director
DZIRE IVF
Mumbai, Maharashtra, India

Hemangi Abhyankar DA
Consultant
Omega Hospitals
Nagpur, Maharashtra, India

Indrajeet Mulik MBBS DNB
Senior Consultant
Mulik Hospital and Research Centre
Nagpur, Maharashtra, India

Jatin Shah MBBS MD
Infertility Specialist
Mumbai Fertility Clinic and IVF Centre
Mumbai, Maharashtra, India

Jhelam Deshmukh MBBS DGO
Gynecologist
Deshmukh Multi Speciality Hospital
Akola, Maharashtra, India

Jyotsana Daule MBBS DGO
Consultant for Obstetrics
Gynecology and Infertility Specialist
Daule Hospital and Matrutwa Test Tube Baby Centre
Ahmednagar, Maharashtra, India

Kalpana Jetha DNB
Vice President
Omega Hospital
Nagpur, Maharashtra, India

Kalyan Baramade
MBBS DNB DGO FCPS DFP
Surgeon
Barmade Hospital and
LIFE Advanced
Test Tube Baby Center
Mumbai, Maharashtra, India

Kanchan Ghuse Kelwade MD
Consultant
Omega Hospitals
Nagpur, Maharashtra, India

Kedar N Ganla
MD DNB DGO DFP FCPS
Consultant Fertility Physician
Ankoor Fertility Clinic
Mumbai, Maharashtra, India
Hon'ble Secretary, ISAR

Laxmi Shrikhande
MBBS MD FICOG FICMU FICMCH
Consultant
Shrikhande Hospital and
Research Centre Pvt Ltd
Nagpur, Maharashtra, India

Leena Patankar
MD (Obstetrics and Gynecology) MSc
Lab Director
Patankar Fertility Solutions Pvt. Ltd.
Pune, Maharashtra, India

Manisha Barmade MBBS DGO
Gynecologist
Barmade Hospital and
LIFE Advanced
Test Tube Baby Center
Latur, Maharashtra, India

Manisha Shembekar MD DGO
Consultant
Joint MD Omega Hospital
Nagpur, Maharashtra, India

Contributors

Manjiri Valsangkar
MS (Obstetrics and Gynecology) Dip Endoscopy (Germany)
Director
Bhide Hospital IVF Centre
Nagpur, Maharashtra, India
Clinical Secretary, POGS
Life Member, ISAR and IFS

Meenal Chidgupkar MBBS DNB
Gynecologist
Dr Chidgupkar Hospital Pvt Ltd
Solapur, Maharashtra, India

Meghashree Deshmukh MBBS DGO
Infertility Consultant and Endoscopist
Sushrusha Hospital
Nanded, Maharashtra, India

Milind Patil MD DNB
Director
Shobha Nursing Home and Infertility Centre
Solapur, Maharashtra, India

Milind R Shah MD DGO DFP FICOG FIAOG
Consultant
Department of Obstetrics and Gynecology
Naval Maternity, Endoscopy and Infertility Center
Mumbai, Maharashtra, India
Past Vice President, FOGSI
Professor and Head
Department of Obstetrics and Gynecology
Gandhi Natha HM College
Solapur, Maharashtra, India
Secretary General, FAOPS
Past Committee Chairperson, Aesthetic and Cosmetic Gynecology, AMOGS

Mohan Raut MD DGO
Gynecologist
Dr Raut's Maternity and Surgical Nursing Home
Mumbai, Maharashtra, India

Mugdha Raut MD DGO
Gynecologist
Dr Raut's Centre for Reproductive Immunology
Mumbai, Maharashtra, India

Nagadeepti Naik
MBBS DNB (Obstetrics and Gynecology) FRM (ICOG)
Consultant Gynecologist and Reproductive Medicine Specialist
Indira IVF Hospital
New Delhi, India
Committee Member, PCOS Youth Brigade

Nandita Palshetkar
MD FICOG FCPS FRCOG (UK)
President, ISAR
Past President
FOGSI, IAGE, AMOGS, MOGS
FOGSI Representative to FIGO

Neelam Bhise
MS (Obstetrics and Gynecology)
Infertility Consultant and Reproductive Endocrinologist
ACME FERTILITY
Mumbai, Maharashtra, India

Nilesh Balkawade MBBS MS DNB
Clinical Head and Fertility Specialist
Oasis Fertility
Pune, Maharashtra, India

Nisha Nikheel Pansare
MBBS DGO DNB MNAMS
Fertility Specialist and Consultant
Nova IVF Fertility
Pune, Maharashtra, India

Parag Hitnalikar MBBS MD
IVF Consultant
Director and Infertility Consultant
Orion Hospital and IVF Centre
Pune, Maharashtra, India

Contributors ix

Paresh Gandecha MBBS DGO
Obstetrician and Gynecologist
Infertility Specialist
Laparoscopic Surgeon and Sonologist
Kamala Nursing Home
Yavatmal, Maharashtra, India

Parul Saoji MD DNB MNAMS
Executive Director
Omega Group of Hospitals, Nagpur
Endoscopic Surgeon and
Aesthetic Gynecologist
Omega Hospitals
Unit of Shembekar Hospitals Pvt Ltd
Nagpur, Maharashtra, India

Parzan Mistry MS DNB
Consultant Obstetrician Gynecologist
and IVF Specialist
Wockhardt Hospitals Ltd
Mumbai, Maharashtra, India

Priyanka Harshavardhan Vora
MBBS DGO FCPS DFP BIMIE Masters in
Reproductive Medicine and IVF (UK)
Diploma in Reproductive
Medicine and IVF (Germany)
Associate Consultant
Ankoor Fertility Clinic
Mumbai, Maharashtra, India

Rahul Patil MBBS MS
Assistant IVF Consultant
Embryo IVF
Pune, Maharashtra, India

Rajeev Dabade MBBS MD
Director
Krishna Mai Hospital
Solapur, Maharashtra, India

Rajvi Mehta PhD
Clinical Embryologist
Academic Consultant
Origio India and Trivector Biomed
Mumbai, Maharashtra, India

Rana Choudhary MBBS DNB
Fertility Specialist
Ankoor Fertility Clinic and
Wockhardt Hospital
Mumbai, Maharashtra, India

Revati Rane MBBS DNB
Fertility Specialist
Akluj Fertility Centre
Akluj, Maharashtra, India

Rishma Dhillon Pai
MD FRCOG DNB FCPS DGO FICOG
Consultant Gynecologist and
Infertility Specialist
Lilavati, Jaslok and
Hinduja Hospitals
Mumbai, Maharashtra, India
Treasurer
International Federation of Fertility
Societies (IFFS)
Former President
FOGSI, ISAR, IAGE, MOGS

Ritu Hinduja
MD MRM (UK) DRM (Germany) FICOG
Fellowship in Reproductive Medicine (India,
Spain, Israel) Certificate in Genetic Counselling
Senior Consultant Fertility Specialist
Nova IVF Fertility
Mumbai, Maharashtra, India
Member
Managing Committee, Indian Society
of Assisted Reproduction
Member
Managing Committee
Maharashtra Chapter of Indian Society
of Assisted Reproduction

Rohan Palshetkar MBBS MD
IVF Consultant
Bloom IVF and
DY Patil Medical College
Mumbai, Maharashtra, India

Rooprekha Waghmare PG DMLT
Embryologist
Omega Hospitals
Nagpur, Maharashtra, India

Contributors

Sachin Jadhav MBBS DNB
IVF Consultant
Gupte Hospital
Pune, Maharashtra, India

Sachin Kulkarni MBBS
Chief IVF Consultant
Jehangir Hospital
Pune, Maharashtra, India

Sadhana Desai MS
Senior IVF Consultant
Fertility Clinic and IVF Centre
Mumbai
Breach Candy Hospital
Mumbai, Maharashtra, India

Sadhana Khurd MBBS MD
Consultant IVF Specialist
Khurd Hospital
Pune, Maharashtra, India

Sandip Nikhade MD
IVF Consultant and Endoscopic Surgeon
Lifesprings Hospital
Nagpur, Maharashtra, India

Sangeeta Tajpuriya
MBBS MD FICOG FICMCH
Consultant and Director
Vedansha Hospital
Nagpur, Maharashtra, India

Sanjay Gupte MD
Consultant
Gupte Hospital
Pune, Maharashtra, India

Sanjeev Madhav Khurd MD FICOG
Director
Dr Khurd's Gynaec
Endoscopic Surgery
Fertility and IVF Centre
Pune, Maharashtra, India
Past President, POGS

Sarika Zunjare MBBS MS
Consultant
Obstetrician and Gynecologist
Ankur Hospital
Nanded, Maharashtra, India

Satish Patki
MD (Obstetrics and Gynecology)
IVF Consultant
Patki Hospital
Kolhapur, Maharashtra, India

Shalaka Mamidwar MD
IVF Consultant
Manomay Hospital
Chandrapur, Maharashtra, India

Shashikant Raghuwanshi MBBS MS
Laparoscopic Surgeon
Raghuwanshi Hospital
Nagpur, Maharashtra, India

Shashikant Umbardand MBBS
Director
Mangalya Nursing Home and
Atharva Fertility Centre
Solapur, Maharashtra, India

Sheetal Sawankar MBBS DNB
Director
Surya Fertility Clinics
Mumbai, Maharashtra, India

Shilpa Bhendarkar Joshi DGO
Consultant Gynecologist
Omega Hospitals
Nagpur, Maharashtra, India

Shilpi Sood MD DNB
IVF Consultant
Safal Hospital
Nagpur, Maharashtra, India

Shravani Welekar MSC PhD
Embryologist
Shembekar Hospital Pvt Ltd
Nagpur, Maharashtra, India

Contributors xi

Sonali Tawde
MS DNB MNAMS PGDMLS MRM
(Masters in Reproductive Medicine, UK)
Consultant, Gynecologist and
Fertility Specialist
Aveta Fertility Clinic, Fortis Hospital
Hira Mongi Hospital
Bapat Urology Centre
Currae Hospital
Mumbai, Maharashtra, India

Soumya Ramesh MBBS MD
IVF Consultant
Millan IVF
Mumbai, Maharashtra, India

Sudha Tandon MS DGO
Consultant Gynecologist
Dr Sudha Tandon Gynaec Endoscopy
and Infertility Centre
Mumbai, Maharashtra, India

Sunita Tandulwadkar
MD FICS FICOG
Consulting Gynecologist and
Obstetrician
ART Consultant and Endoscopist
Head of Department and Chief
IVF and Endoscopy Centre
Rubyhall Clinic, Pune
Adviser and Consultant
Dr DY Patil IVF and
Endoscopy Centre, Pune
Founder and Medical Director
Solo Clinic IVF—A Centre of Excellence
in Infertility, Pune
Founder and Medical Director
Solo Stemcells—A Stem Cell Research
and Application Centre
Pune, Maharashtra, India

Sushma Deshmukh MD DGO
Infertility and IVF Specialist and
Hysteroscopist
Director
Central India Test Tube Baby Centre
Nagpur
Head
Department of Obstetrics and
Gynecology
Getwell Multispeciality Hospital, Nagpur
In-Charge
Deshmukh Hospital
Latur, Maharashtra, India

Swati Sarda MBBS DNB
Consultant Gynecologist
Child Urology and Child Surgery Center
Nagpur, Maharashtra, India

Umesh Sawarkar MBBS MS
IVF Consultant
Sawarkar Hospital
Amravati, Maharashtra, India

Unnati Mamtora DNB
Fertility Consultant
Nova IVF
Mumbai, Maharashtra, India

Vaishali Mundhe Akarte
MBBS DGO Fetal Medicine Fellowship
(Bengaluru)
Senior Fetal Medicine Consultant
Omega Hospital and Safal Hospital
Nagpur, Maharashtra, India

Vijay Mangoli PhD
Clinical Embryologist and
Lab Director
Fertility Clinic
Mumbai, Maharashtra, India

Foreword

"Today a reader...Tomorrow a leader"
Arise! Awake! And Stop not until the Goal is Reached!

—Swami Vivekananda

AMOGS Handbook on Practical Aspects of Infertility gives the similar vibes!!

Infertility affects one in six couples in India forming a significant number of patients in any gynecologist's outpatient department (OPD). There are many national and international publications in infertility. But to make a practically usable "Handbook of Infertility" was important.

This book has carefully selected topics with experienced authors in this subject.

The editors have given great thought in the careful designing of the book and making it more and more user-friendly!

A complete and well-written manual that covers a large range of topics from basic physiology and primary management of infertility to the very latest in implantation and embryo selection and screening. The chapters are authored by the acknowledged consultants in the field of infertility.

This edition of *AMOGS Handbook on Practical Aspects of Infertility* has been fully revised to provide clinicians with the latest advances in the diagnosis and management of infertility. Divided into seven sections, the book provides step-by-step guidance on each stage of the process, from initial examination and identifying the causes of infertility in both females and males, to ovarian stimulation and assisted reproductive techniques. The comprehensive text is enhanced by case studies, clinical photographs, diagrams, flowcharts, and tables.

The book covers the different aspects of infertility from basic to advanced levels, including diagnoses, management, treatment modalities, complications, and fertility in a concise manner.

I congratulate the editors Dr Nandita Palshetkar and Dr Chaitanya Shembekar for this Herculean task. They have done justice to this book. The Co-editors Dr Nilesh Balkawade, Dr Rohan Palshetkar, and Dr Parul Saoji have done justice to their job.

I never dreamed about success, I worked for it!
Hard work pays off. I wish all the readers a very Happy Reading.

Hrishikesh Pai
MD FCPS FRCOG (UK) MSc
President, FOGSI 2022–23
Past President, IAGE, ISAR, MOGS
Board Member, IFFS

Foreword

Why is it important to learn about infertility?

It is essential for every doctor to understand what normal fertility is, what the risk factors for infertility are, and the proper time to seek help if needed. If your patients are not able to get pregnant, this is the book *AMOGS Handbook on Practical Aspects of Infertility*, you should consider this book as a right approach for the management of infertility.

The purpose of the book is to make readers aware of the newer technology to solve the problem of male and female infertility, and to continue to arm readers with scientific information that will prevent them from undergoing needless and useless conventional therapy.

This handbook also gives sensitive information and advice on the feasibility and legality of egg donation, and of gestational surrogate approaches, which are increasing as older women now are trying desperately to have a child. With each chapter, you will come to know the insights of infertility.

Contributors have given information of about intrauterine insemination (IUI), intracytoplasmic sperm injection (ICSI), egg donation, and all procedures in a lucid manner...

Congratulation to Drs Nandita Palshetkar, Chaitanya Shembekar, Nilesh Balkawade, Rohan Palshetkar, and Parul Saoji for editing such an academic handbook.

Rajendra Singh Pardeshi
President, AMOGS 2022-24

Preface

Dear AMOGSians,

The Association of Maharashtra Obstetric and Gynaecological Societies (AMOGS) has always been a leader in women's health. Through various academic and social programs AMOGS aims to uplift the quality of care that is given to every woman who comes to us.

Infertility affects millions of people of reproductive age worldwide—and has an impact on their families and communities. Estimates suggest that between 48 million couples and 186 million individuals live with infertility globally. This book on practical tips in infertility has been created to give you quick tricks to manage your patients on a daily basis. The book has updated knowledge by all the experts in Maharashtra and I really hope that all the readers benefit from this boom. I would like to thank Chaitanya Shembekar, Nilesh Balkawade, Dr Rohan Palshetkar and Dr Parul Saoji for creating this wonderful book to update all our readers. I would also like to thank all contributors for taking out time and compiling this wonderful book for all our readers to enjoy.

Happy Reading!

Nandita Palshetkar
President
AMOGS 2020–2022
President
ISAR 2022

Preface

*"Live as if you were to die tomorrow
Learn as if you were to live forever."*
—**Mahatma Gandhi**

The Association of Maharashtra Obstetric and Gynaecological Societies (AMOGS) is a strong organization of all gynecologists from Maharashtra, India. When Dr Nandita Palshetkar took over as a President of this prestigious organization in February 2019, no one was aware of the unprecedented COVID wave and its serious effects. However, Dr Nandita Palshetkar along with Dr Rajendra Singh Pardeshi, Dr Arun Nayak and her team, took the organization to great heights. I was fortunate to work under her leadership in the capacity of Chairperson, Infertility Committee. *In the month of April, we came with CHANGE, a booklet on "Infertility Practices during COVID era".* This book got a tremendous response among infertility practitioners not only in Maharashtra but all over India.

World Health Organization (WHO) has declared infertility as a disease. While organizing webinars and conducting workshops, we realized that a *AMOGS Handbook on Practical Aspects of Infertility* is the need of the hour as infertility is on the rise with each passing day. Every gynecologist even in remote areas must have basic knowledge of infertility. The book has to be precise, updated, and practical, which every gynecologist would like to keep on their desk as a ready reckoner. With this concept in mind, under the able guidance of Dr Nandita Palshetkar, we started working on it. Without a team of young and enthusiastic friends, this task would have been impossible. I must appreciate the efforts of Co-editors, Dr Nilesh Balkawade, Dr Rohan Palshetkar, and Dr Parul Saoji, who made this mammoth task easy.

The book is meticulously planned, starting from an approach toward infertile couple; it includes advanced treatment options like role of Artificial Intelligence in Infertility.

Whenever it comes to publishers, M/s Jaypee Brothers Medical Publishers (P) Ltd, New Delhi, India is undoubtedly the leader in the field of medical publications. The support and cooperation of Jaypee Brothers is worth appreciating.

This Herculean task would not have been possible without the experienced infertility specialists who contributed chapters from basic to advanced topics in infertility.

We are fortunate to have Dr Hrishikesh Pai and Dr Rajendra Singh Pardeshi as our leaders and mentors. The forewords by the two stalwarts are the highlights of the book.

This book will no doubt prove invaluable for assisted reproductive technology (ART) consultants as well as gynecologists doing basic infertility work and for the fellows and residents who are future ART consultants. We are sure that this book would be an integral part of day-to-day infertility practice for not only gynecologists practicing in Maharashtra but also for the practitioners all over India.

"Knowledge is power.
Information is liberating.
Education is the premise of progress in every society."

—**Kofi Annan**

Happy Reading!

Chaitanya Shembekar
Chairperson, Infertility Committee, AMOGS 2020–2022
Librarian Maharashtra Chapter of ISAR
Past President, Nagpur Obstetric and Gynaecological Society

Contents

1. **Evaluation of Infertile Couple** 1
   Sachin Kulkarni, Meghashree Deshmukh
   - Physical Examination of Infertile Female 2
   - Diagnostic Investigations 2
   - History Taking 3
   - Primary Investigations 4
   - Secondary Investigations 4
   - Evaluation of Ovaries 4
   - Evaluation of Fallopian Tubes 6
   - Evaluation of Uterus 7
   - Evaluation of Male Infertility 8
   - Evaluation of Retrograde Ejaculation 12

2. **Evaluation of Male Partner** 15
   Gayatri Wadekar, Soumya Ramesh
   - Evaluation of the Male Partner 16

3. **Semen Analysis and Beyond Role of Sperm Function Tests** 20
   Gouri Sultane Gupta, Firuza R Parikh
   - Semen Analysis 20
   - Antisperm Antibodies 21
   - Hormonal Evaluation 21
   - Sperm DNA Fragmentation Index 22
   - Sperm Fluorescent In Situ Hybridization 22
   - Genetic Testing 23

4. **Ovarian Reserve Tests** 26
   Swati Sarda, Kanchan Ghuse Kelwade
   - Age 26
   - Menstrual Cycle Pattern 27
   - Ovarian Volume 29
   - Ovarian Doppler 29
   - Ovarian Biopsy 29
   - Key Notes (The American Society for Reproductive Medicine Committee Opinion, 2020) 30

5. **Ultrasound in Infertility** 33
   Ritu Hinduja, Vaishali Mundhe Akarte
   - Male Infertility—Workup *34*

6. **Hysterolaparoscopy in Infertility** 45
   Parul Saoji, Chaitanya Shembekar
   - Polycystic Ovary Syndrome *45*
   - Ectopic Pregnancy *46*
   - Endometriosis *46*
   - Pelvic Adhesions *47*
   - Ovarian Cysts *47*
   - Tubal Block *48*
   - Fibroids *48*
   - Low Ovarian Reserve *49*
   - Hysteroscopy in Infertility *49*
   - Tubal Cornual Occlusion *50*

7. **Evaluation and Management of Tubal Factors** 55
   Anjali Bhirud, Sarika Zunjare, Ashish Zarariya
   - Causes for Tubal Infertility *55*
   - Hull and Rutherford 2002 Classification of Tubal Damage *56*
   - Tubal Assessment Tests *56*
   - The Royal College of Obstetricians and Gynaecologists Guidelines for Tubal Evaluation *59*
   - Tuberculosis and Tubal Factor Infertility *60*
   - Management of Tubal Factor Infertility *60*

8. **Evaluation and Management of Uterine Factors in Infertility** 63
   Amrita Tandon, Sudha Tandon
   - Evaluation and Management of Congenital Uterine Factors *63*
   - Septate Uterus *65*
   - Unicornuate Uterus *67*
   - Bicornuate Uterus *67*
   - Uterine Didelphys *68*
   - Management of Other Complex Müllerian Anomalies *68*
   - Acquired Uterine Pathologies *68*

9. **Evaluation of the Male Infertility Factors** 74
   Rishma Dhillon Pai, Balasaheb Khadbade
   - Interpretation of Semen Analysis: Macroscopic Parameters *76*
   - Interpretation of Semen Analysis: Microscopic Parameters *78*
   - Male Hypogonadism *81*
   - Azoospermia: Evaluation *83*
   - Anejaculation *86*

10. Evaluation and Management of Azoospermia 90
Sheetal Sawankar, Satish Patki
- Definition *90*
- Evaluation of an Azoospermic Male *91*
- Management of Cases of Azoospermia *94*

11. Step by Step Management of Infertility in Polycystic Ovary Syndrome 99
Girish Godbole, Manjiri Valsangkar
- Management of PCOS—OI in PCOS-Fertil-Steril 2008 *100*
- Strategies to Improve Pregnancy Rates in IVF in PCOS *104*

12. Thyroid Disorders and Hyperprolactinemia in Infertility 106
Milind R Shah, Jhelam Deshmukh
- Thyroid Disorders and Female Infertility *106*
- Hyperprolactinemia *111*

13. Endometriosis and Infertility 117
Ashish Kale, Ashwini Yelikar Kale
- Proposed Biological Mechanisms to Explain Infertility in Endometriosis *117*
- Impaired Endocrine Function, Folliculogenesis and Ovulatory Functions in Endometriosis *118*
- Endometriosis Fertility Index *124*

14. Fibroids and Fertility 127
Chaitanya Shembekar, Parul Saoji
- Fibroids—Evaluation and Classification *127*
- Recommendations *128*
- Classification of ESGE/FIGO PALM-COEIN *128*
- Mechanisms of Infertility *129*
- Does the Presence of Uterine Fibroids Reduce Implantation Rates? *131*
- What About the Fibroids that do not Cause Distortion of a Cavity? *131*
- To Remove or not to Remove? That is the Question *131*
- What is the Pragmatic Approach to Management? *132*
- Does the Medical Treatment have any Role in the Management of Fibroids with Infertility? *134*
- Surgical Treatment *134*

15. Infections in Infertility 140
Jyotsana Daule, Anil Bendre
- Infections Causing Infertility in Male and Female *140*
- Investigations *143*
- Treatment *145*
- Male Infertility *147*

16. **Unexplained Infertility** 149
    Chaitanya Shembekar, Parul Saoji
    - Laparoscopic Surgery in Unexplained Infertility *150*

17. **Step by Step Management of Infertility** 155
    Aditi Tandon, Sadhana Desai
    - Epidemiology of Infertility *155*
    - Evaluation and Workup for Infertile Couples *156*
    - Sperm Chromosome Aneuploidy *168*
    - Unexplained Infertility *168*

18. **Intrauterine Insemination: Indications and Protocol** 174
    Unnati Mamtora, Parzan Mistry
    - Indications of Intrauterine Insemination *174*
    - Factors Influencing IUI Success Rates *174*
    - Prerequisite for Intrauterine Insemination *174*
    - Protocol for Intrauterine Insemination *175*
    - Timing of Intrauterine Insemination *176*
    - Role of Double Intrauterine Insemination *177*
    - Gonadotropins and Intrauterine Insemination *177*
    - Adjuvants in Ovulation Induction *179*

19. **Ovulation Induction** 181
    Parag Hitnalikar, Anil Chittake, Rahul Patil
    - Hyperprolactinemia *181*

20. **Adjuvants in Polycystic Ovarian Syndrome** 190
    Rajeev Dabade, Meenal Chidgupkar
    - Rationale for Use of Adjuvants *190*
    - Adjuvants *192*

21. **Adjuvants in Diminished Ovarian Reserve** 198
    Shilpi Sood, Chaitanya Shembekar, Laxmi Shrikhande
    - Management of Diminished Ovarian Reserve *199*
    - Role of Adjuvants in Diminished Ovarian Reserve *199*
    - Managing Diminished Ovarian Reserve Patients Based on the POSEIDON Criteria *205*

22. **Diagnosis of Diminished Ovarian Reserve** 208
    Ameet Patki, Garima Sharma
    - Diagnosis *208*
    - The Bologna Criteria *208*
    - Limitations of the Existing POR Criteria *209*
    - POSEIDON (Patient-oriented Strategies Encompassing Individualized Oocyte Number) Classification *210*

23. **Pre-In Vitro Fertilization Evaluation** 213
    Sangeeta Tajpuriya, Umesh Sawarkar
    - General Evaluation *213*
    - Reproductive System Evaluation *214*

Contents

24. **Ovarian Stimulation in Normal Responders** 217
    Sanjeev Madhav Khurd, Aditya Khurd, Sadhana Khurd
    - Desired and Optimum Response to Ovarian Stimulation 217
    - Factors Affecting Ovarian Response 218
    - Drugs for Ovarian Stimulation 219
    - Superovulation for Intrauterine Insemination Cycle 220
    - Controlled Ovarian Stimulation for IVF/ICSI with GnRH Antagonist Protocol 221
    - Controlled Ovarian Stimulation for IVF/ICSI with Long GnRH Agonist Protocol 222

25. **Preinduction Adjuvants** 224
    Paresh Gandecha, Shalaka Mamidwar
    - Metformin 224
    - Myoinositol 225
    - Dehydroepiandrosterone 226
    - Testosterone 226
    - Growth Hormones 227
    - Antioxidants 227
    - Folic Acid 228
    - Aspirin 228
    - Low-Molecular-Weight Heparin 228
    - Corticosteroids 229
    - Estrogen 229

26. **Various Ovarian Stimulation Protocols and their Clinical Significance** 231
    Sanjay Gupte, Sachin Jadhav
    - Ovarian Stimulation Protocols 232
    - Pre-In Vitro Fertilization Priming 234
    - Which Gonadotropin? 235
    - Decision Making on Type of Protocol to Use 236
    - Newer Protocols 236
    - Our Experience and Clinical Evidence 238

27. **Complications of Ovarian Stimulation** 241
    Kedar N Ganla, Priyanka Harshavardhan Vora, Rana Choudhary
    - Ovarian Hyperstimulation Syndrome 241
    - Multiple Gestation 242
    - Ectopic (Tubal) Pregnancies 245
    - Adnexal Torsion (Ovarian Twisting) 246
    - Cancer 247
    - Limited or Overall Body Reactions 248

28. **Controlled Ovarian Hyperstimulation and Management of Polycystic Ovaries in In Vitro Fertilization** 249
    Nagadeepti Naik, Duru Shah
    - Pathogenesis 249
    - Indications 252
    - Cryopreservation of Embryos (Freeze-All Strategy) 253
    - Complications 253

29. **Management in Diminished Ovarian Reserve and Controlled Ovarian Hyperstimulation** 257
    Jatin Shah, Amiti Agrawal
    - Newer Advances *260*

30. **Trigger in In Vitro Fertilization** 262
    Sonali Tawde, Revati Rane, Milind Patil
    - Physiology of Trigger *262*
    - Prerequisites of Trigger *268*
    - Choice of Trigger *269*
    - Empty Follicle Syndrome *270*

31. **Luteal Phase Support** 272
    Nisha Nikheel Pansare, Chaitanya Shembekar
    - Luteal Phase Defect Mechanism *272*
    - Duration of Luteal Phase Support *272*
    - Drugs Used in Luteal Phase Support *273*
    - Luteal Phase Support in Intrauterine Insemination and Ovulation Induction Cycle *276*

32. **Managing Quality Control and Quality Management of IVF Laboratory** 279
    Kalyan Baramade, Manisha Barmade
    - What are the Standard Quality Indicators? *280*
    - Quality Management in ART Laboratory *282*
    - Sterility and Infection Control in the Sterile Zone *285*
    - Maintenance of Essential Pieces of Equipment and Checkpoints in an IVF Laboratory *286*
    - Disposables and Consumables *286*
    - Monitoring of Laboratory Environment *288*
    - Record Keeping and Documentation *289*
    - Laboratory Staffing *290*
    - Occupational Training *290*
    - Code of Practice *291*

33. **Ovarian Hyperstimulation Syndrome** 293
    Bansi Shinde, Shashikant Umbardand
    - Incidence *293*
    - Pathophysiology *293*
    - Clinical Diagnosis *294*
    - Classification *294*
    - Prevention *296*
    - Prognosis *298*
    - Management *299*

34. **Recurrent Implantation Failure** 304
    Mohan Raut, Mugdha Raut
    - Incidence *304*
    - Definitions *304*

- Causes *305*
- Investigations *305*
- Treatment *310*
- Prognosis *313*
- Guidelines *314*

35. Thin Endometrium *316*

Nandita Palshetkar, Rohan Palshetkar

- Causes *316*
- Diagnosis *318*
- Management *319*
- Platelet-rich Plasma *321*
- Endometrial Scratching *322*
- Stem Cell Therapy *322*

36. Recurrent Pregnancy Loss *325*

Sushma Deshmukh, Ashutosh Thole, Shashikant Raghuwanshi

- Spectrum and Definition *325*
- Etiology *325*
- Endocrine Etiologies *333*
- Idiopathic Factors *334*
- Complete Evaluation and Counseling *334*

37. Application of Stem Cells in Infertility..*337*

Sunita Tandulwadkar, Nilesh Balkawade

- Introduction: What are Stem Cells? *337*
- Characteristics of Mesenchymal Stem Cell *337*
- Stem Cell Harvest and Infusion *337*
- Azoospermia *339*
- Refractory Endometrium *339*
- Premature Ovarian Failure *340*
- Regulation of Research in India *342*
- Ethical Concerns *342*

38. Algorithms for Artificial Intelligence in Reproductive Medicine..*345*

Leena Patankar, Amit Patankar

- Role of Artificial Intelligence in Reproductive Medicine *345*
- Workflow of Artificial Intelligence in Reproductive Medicine *346*

39. Sperm Selection Technique *355*

Shilpa Bhendarkar Joshi, Indrajeet Mulik, Sandip Nikhade, Rajvi Mehta

- Need of Sperm Preparation *355*
- Sperm Preparation Techniques *355*
- Microfluidics for Sperm Sorting (Future Prospects) *362*

40. Selecting Best Embryo for Transfer..*364*

Vijay Mangoli, Neelam Bhise

- Criteria for Embryo Selection based on Morphology *364*

41. What is New in In Vitro Fertilization? 375
Bindu Chimote, Kalpana Jetha, Shravani Welekar, Rooprekha Waghmare
- Laboratory Culture Conditions (Culture Media) 375
- Newer Culture Media Options 376
- New Advances in Fertilization Techniques 376
- Time-lapse Technology 377
- Assisted Embryo Hatching 378
- Safety Concerns Associated with Laser Application 378
- Preimplantation Genetic Testing 379

42. Anesthesia for Laparoscopy 381
Manisha Shembekar, Hemangi Abhyankar
- Physiological Effects of Pneumoperitoneum 382
- Physiological Effects of Positioning 382
- Management of Anesthesia 382

43. Anesthesia for Oocyte Retrieval 386
Manisha Shembekar
- Types of Anesthesia 386

44. Anesthetic Considerations for Operative Hysteroscopy 389
Manisha Shembekar
- Anesthesia for Hysteroscopic Procedures 390
- Tips and Tricks to Reduce Fluid Absorption 392

Index 395

CHAPTER 1: Evaluation of Infertile Couple

Sachin Kulkarni, Meghashree Deshmukh

INTRODUCTION

According to WHO, "infertility" is defined as an inability to conceive after 12 months of unprotected intercourse.

- Incidence is 16%. Wherein 40% are female causes, 40% constitute male causes, and 20% are unexplained causes.
- Investigation to be started after 12 months if the couple is having regular intercourse without contraception.
- Start investigations after 6 months in situations such as:
  - Irregular cycles
  - Oligomenorrhea
  - Grade III or grade VI endometriosis
  - Previous ovarian surgeries
  - Age >35 years
  - Male subfertility

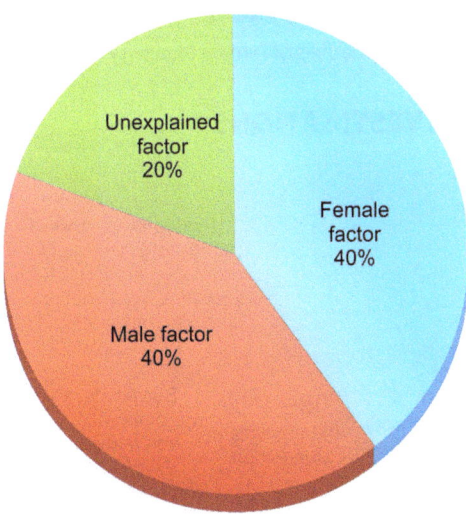

General causes of infertility.

PHYSICAL EXAMINATION OF INFERTILE FEMALE

- Body mass index (BMI)
- Blood pressure and pulse:
  - Thyroid examination
  - Breast examination
  - Signs of androgen excess
  - Vaginal or cervical abnormality or discharge
  - Uterine size, shape, and mobility
- Any adnexal masses or tenderness, nodularity at pouch of Douglas

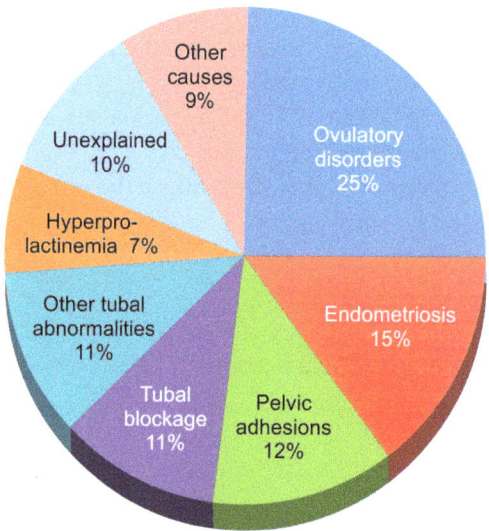

Causes of female infertility.

DIAGNOSTIC INVESTIGATIONS

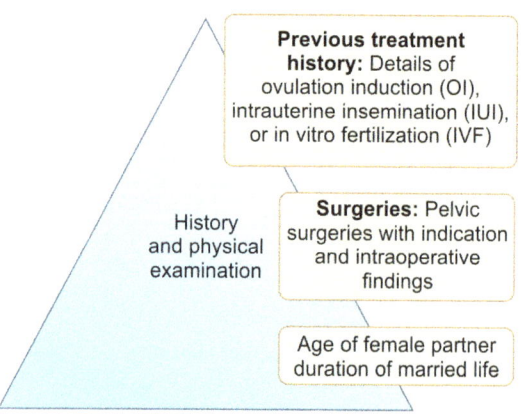

Evaluation of Infertile Couple

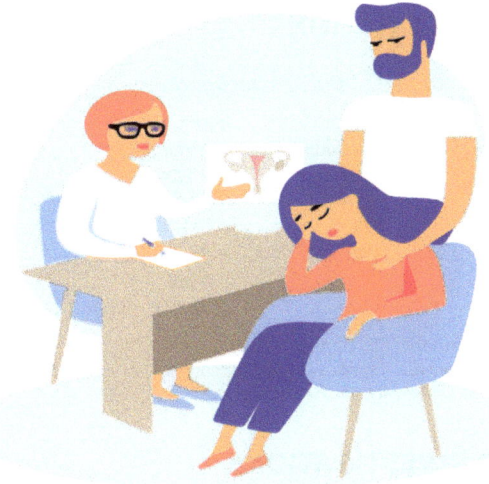

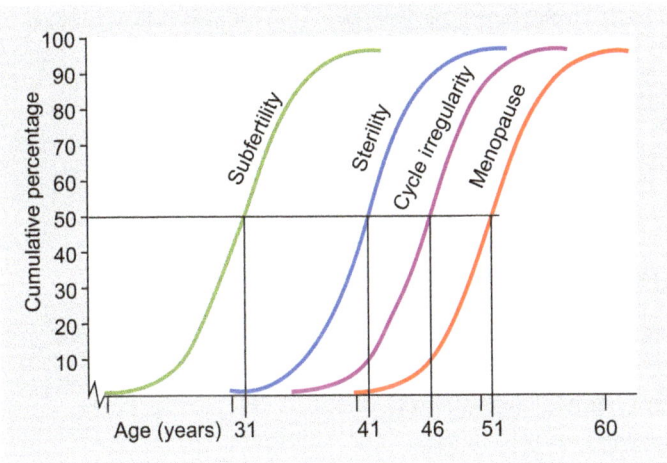

HISTORY TAKING

History					
General health history:	*Sexual history:*	*Family history:*	*Drug history:*	*Medical history:*	*Menstrual history:*
• BMI • Smoking • Alcohol • Age • Occupation • Stress	• Sexual dysfunction • Frequency of coitus	• Birth defect • Genetic mutation • Premature ovarian failure	• Immunosuppressant • NSAID • Phenothiazine • Metoclopramide	• PID/CKD/DM • Hirsutism • Surgery in pelvic region • Chemo-/radiotherapy • PCT	• Oligoamenorrhea • Amenorrhea

(BMI: body mass index; CKD: chronic kidney disease; DM: diabetes mellitus; NSAID: nonsteroidal anti-inflammatory drug; PCT: perfusion computed tomography; PID: pelvic inflammatory disease)

PRIMARY INVESTIGATIONS

Blood investigations

General blood investigations:
- Total blood count (TC)
- Hemoglobin (HB)
- Random blood sugar (RBS)
- Serum plasma
- Lipid test

Serological investigations:
- HIV
- HBSAG
- VDRL
- HCV

Hormonal investigations:
- T3, T4, TSH
- AMH
- FSH, LH
- Serum prolactin
- Estrogen
- Mid-luteal serum P4

Other investigations:
- Ovarian reserve test
- Antral follicular count
- CC challenge test

(AMH: anti-Müllerian hormone; CC: clomiphene citrate; FSH: follicle-stimulating hormone; HBsAG: hepatitis B surface antigen; HCV: hepatitis C virus; HIV: human immunodeficiency virus; LH: luteinizing hormone; VDRL: Venereal Disease Research Laboratory)

SECONDARY INVESTIGATIONS

Secondary investigations

- *Cervical factor:* Chronic cervicitis and cervical cancer
- *Uterine factor:* Fibroids septate, and uterus
- *Tubal factor:* Blockage of both Fallopian tube
- *Ovarian factor:* PCOS, ovarian tumors
- *Peritoneal factor:* Endometriosis
- Genital tuberculosis

- Ultrasonography/transvaginal screening
- Hysterosalpingography
- Hysteroscopy
- MRI
- Laparoscopy

(PCOS: polycystic ovary syndrome)

EVALUATION OF OVARIES

Ovarian reserve test specifically
- Women over 35 years of age
- Family history of early menopause
- Single ovary or ovarian surgery or radiotherapy
- Unexplained infertility

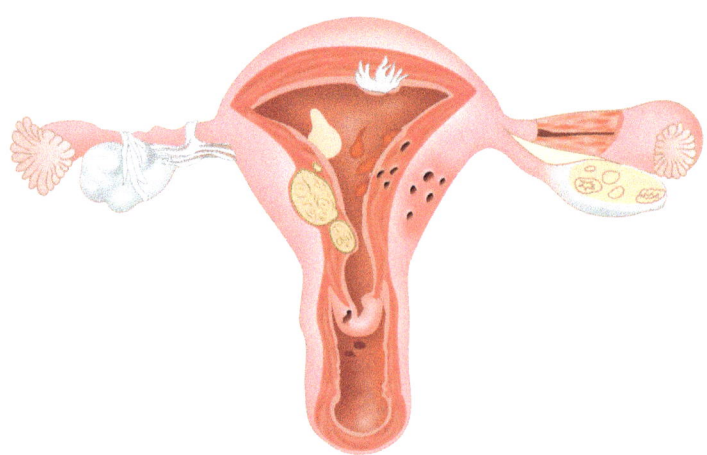

Evaluation of Infertile Couple

Ovarian Reserve Test

- Antral follicle count (AFC):
  - 2–10 mm in mean diameter in two-dimensional plane
  - Measured in 2–5 days in menstrual cycle
    - Low AFC <5–7
    - High AFC >12
- Anti-Müllerian hormone (AMH)

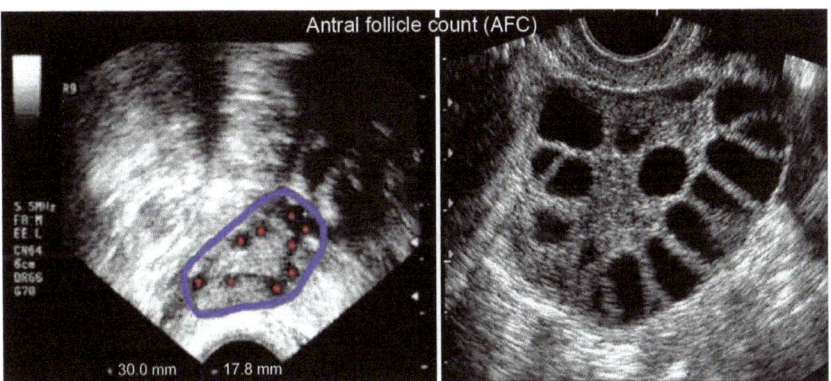

Normal – 6 to 10 antral follicles   Abnormal (increased 20–30 antral) follicles in a PCOS ovary

(PCOS: polycystic ovary syndrome)

- Serum AMH:
  - Low serum AMH levels (<0.5 ng/mL)
  - Higher serum AMH levels (>3.5 ng/mL) PCOS
  - Helps in fertility procedure by oocyte or embryo freezing prior to chemo- or radiotherapy
- Serum follicle-stimulating hormone (FSH): >10–20 IU/mL
  - Serum estradiol >60–80 ng/mL

POSEIDON Group 1

- Young patients <35 years with adequate ovarian reserve parameters (AFC ≥5; AMH >1.2 ng/mL) and with and unexpected poor or suboptimal ovarian response
- Subgroup 1a: <4 oocytes
- Subgroup 1b: 4–9 oocytes retrieved
- After standard ovarian stimulation

POSEIDON Group 2

- Older patients >35 years with adequate ovarian reserve parameters (AFC >5; AMH >1.2 ng/mL) and with an unexpected poor or suboptimal ovarian response
- Subgroup 2a: <4 oocytes
- Subgroup 2b: 4–9 oocytes retrieved
- After standard ovarian stimulation

POSEIDON Group 3
- Young patients (35 years) with poor ovarian reserve prestimulation parameters
- (AFC <5; AMH <1.2 ng/mL)

POSEIDON Group 4
- Older patients (>35 years) with poor ovarian reserve prestimulation parameters (AFC <5; AMH <1.2 ng/mL)

EVALUATION OF FALLOPIAN TUBES

- Hysterosalpingography (HSG):
    - Sensitivity is 65%.
    - Specificity is 83%.
- *Hysterosalpingography:* It involves infusion of saline or contrast media under ultrasound guidance to look tubal patency.

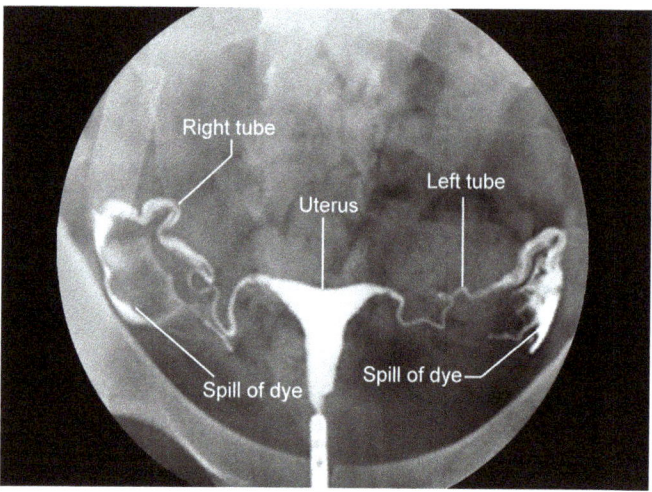

Hysterosalpingography-Contrast Sonography

- Tubal patency is demonstrated with ultrasound sonography (USG) by visualizing intratubal flow of hyperechogenic contrast medium.
- As compared to saline infusion sonography (SIS), hysterosalpingography-contrast sonography (HyCoSy) with contrast is more efficient.
- Both HSG and HyCoSy have comparable result with gold-standard laparoscopy.
- The color-coded 3D power Doppler imaging (PDI) with surface rendering allows the flow of contrast through the entire tube and the free spill from the fimbrial ends can be appreciated easily.

EVALUATION OF UTERUS

- *Hysterosalpingography:*
  - It can be used to determine the shape and size of the uterine cavity.
  - It helps to diagnose various congenital anomalies such as unicornuate, septate, bicornuate uterus, or acquired abnormalities in the uterine cavity like endometrial polyps, submucous fibroids, or synechiae.
  - Hysterosalpingography has relatively lower sensitivity (50%) and low positive predictive value (30%) as compared to hysteroscopy.
  - Evaluation with pelvic MRI or 3D-USG may help to differentiate between septate and bicornuate uterus.
- *Sonohysterography:*
  - It is a procedure in which normal saline is instilled into the uterine cavity during transvaginal USG.
  - Sonohysterography can diagnose various intrauterine pathology like endometrial polyps, submucous fibroids, and intrauterine synechiae with 90% accuracy.

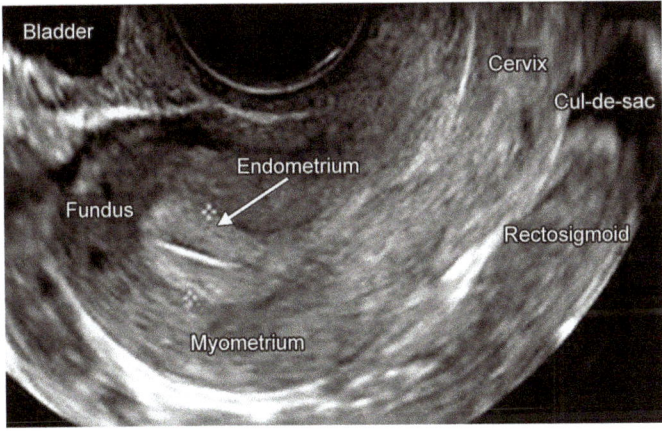

Three-dimensional Ultrasound and Magnetic Resonance Imaging

These can be used for further assessment of the findings of suspected pathology in TVS or HSG.

- *Hysteroscopy:*
  - It is the gold standard to diagnose and treat intrauterine pathologies.
  - Biopsy can be taken at the same sitting for endometrial culture and gene report for TB.
  - Hysteroscopy can be combined with SIS to be seen for tubal patency.
  - Abnormal hysteroscopy findings are seen in 10–35% in normal HSG and 13.5% patients with normal USG.

- There is very low-quality evidence suggesting that routine pre-IVF hysteroscopy increases live birth rate (relative risk: 1.48) and moderate quality evidence that it increases pregnancy rate (RR: 1.45) in infertile women without any intrauterine abnormalities.
- *Cervical factor:* Chronic cervicitis/cervical cancer can be detected by Pap smear and cryocauterization for erosion uterine factor.
- *Peritoneal factors:*
  - Pelvic or adnexal adhesions and endometriosis are peritoneal causes leading to infertility.
  - Laparoscopy is not recommended as routine during evaluation of an infertile woman; unless history or physical examination findings may raise suspicion of pelvic pathology or USG/HSG has revealed pelvic pathology such as an endometrioma or tubal disease.
  - Diagnostic laparoscopy will be of value in young infertile women with long duration (>3 years) of infertility without any identifiable causative factor.

Laparoscopy

- A dilute solution of indigo carmine or methylene blue is introduced transcervically and tubal patency is looked for, as evidenced by spillage of the dye from the tubes.
- In the same sitting, corrective procedures such as peritubal adhesiolysis, opening fimbrial phimosis, and hysteroscopic tubal cannulation under laparoscopic under guidance can be done, which is not possible with HSG.
- It is regarded as the gold standard to look for tubal patency, and in addition to the above-mentioned examinations, confirmation of hydrosalpinx can also be done.
- Tubal cannulation can be done either by fluoroscopy or hysteroscopy if proximal tubal occlusion is detected either or HSG or laparoscopy with chromopertubation.
- A set of specialized catheters are used to cannulate the fallopian tubes transcervically.

EVALUATION OF MALE INFERTILITY (FLOWCHART 1)

- About 30–50% couples are infertile due to male factor.
- To identify potentially correctable conditions.
- To identify irreversible condition that may be amenable to assisted reproduction.

Infertile Male History

- History of fever, illness, cancer, and infection
- Reproductive history should include:

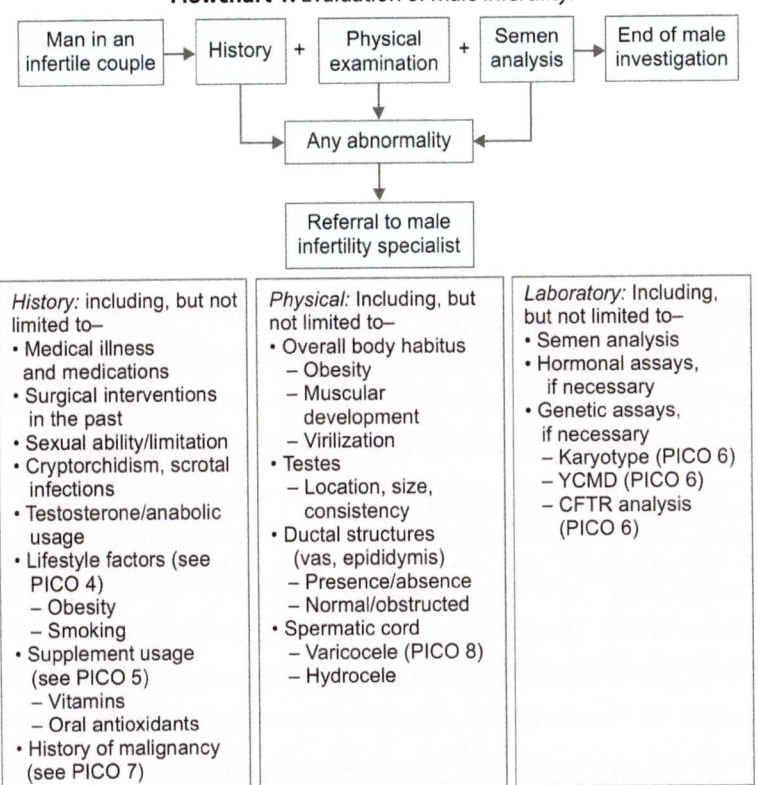

Flowchart 1: Evaluation of male infertility.

(CFTR: CF transmembrane conductance regulator; PICO: patient/problem, intervention, comparison and outcome; YCMD: Y chromosome microdeletion)

- Duration of infertility
- Age of partners
- Previous fertility with same or different partner
- Previous evaluation and treatment for infertility
- Knowledge of reproductive cycle
- Coital frequency and timing
- Use of contraceptive and lubricants
- Sexual dysfunction, nature, and volume of ejaculate
■ Medical history should include:
    - Congenital anomalies, cryptorchidism *(50% of men with unilateral and with bilateral cryptorchidism are subfertile)*
    - Chronic bronchitis *(maybe related to young's or Kartagener syndrome or motility disorders)*
    - Onset of puberty *(precocious in congenital adrenal hyperplasia and delayed in Kallmann and Klinefelter syndromes)*

Physical Examination

- Examination of testes:
  - Small soft testes indicate poor spermatogenesis.
  - Small hard testes suggest postorchitis or post-torsion atrophy or Klinefelter syndrome.
  - Focal irregularities in consistency raise the suspicion of malignancy.
  - Mobile small hard bodies, corpora amylacea, may be palpated floating within the tunica vaginalis.

Examination of Epididymis

- The normal epididymis is soft and barely palpable and is posterolateral to the testes.
- Epididymal pathology is often associated with irregularities or modularity.

Examination of Varicoceles

- Subclinical or questionable varicoceles are of limited clinical interest.
- Examination should be done in standing position.

Examination of Prostate

In patient with azoospermia, digital rectal examination is recommended to confirm the size and consistency of the prostate, midline prostatic cyst, irregularities, tenderness, and palpable seminal vesicle, and it is noted.

When should the Male be Evaluated?

- Evaluation of the male should occur simultaneously with that of the female partner when there is no pregnancy after 1 year of regular unprotected intercourse. This should be included in both primary and secondary infertility.
- Known male risk factor for infertility like cryptorchidism
- Female risk factor for infertility such as age >35 years

Diagnosis of Male Infertility

- Semen analysis:
  - At least two semen samples must be obtained, preferably about a month apart with a 3–5 days abstinence period prior to each sample.
  - In the 3 months period prior to the sample, the patient should ideally have been free from any febrile or systemic illness and should not have been on medications known to affect spermatogenesis, particularly steroids, androgens, and antibiotics.
  - Febrile illness may even result in azoospermia in an otherwise fertile male.

- A man reporting difficulty in semen collection who produces "yellow" or scanty ejaculate should be asked to provide a semen sample by vibratory stimulation.
- 5% of Indian men have difficulty in collecting a semen sample by masturbation.
- Sample must be examined within 1 hour of collection.

Classification Based on Semen Analysis

Based on semen analysis, patient should be classified into the following:
- *Oligoasthenoteratozoospermia (OAT):* Most semen analysis will lead to a diagnosis of this abnormality.

  Abnormalities may be present in only parameter.

  However, two or more of the following parameters—sperm density, motility, and morphology are usually abnormal leading to the diagnosis of OAT.
- *Azoospermia:* Complete absence of sperm in the ejaculate sample refers to azoospermia.

  The semen specimen must be centrifuged at 3,000 g for at least 15 minutes and the pellet examined for sperms.

  Azoospermia should be confirmed in a second semen analysis.

  The azoospermia can be categorized into three etiological conditions.

World Health Organization semen analysis, 2010.		
Parameter	*1992*	*Lower reference limit 2010*
Semen volume	2 mL	1.5 mL
Sperm concentration	20 M	15×10^6/mL
Total sperm number		39×10^6/ejaculate
Progressive motility	>50%	32% A
Total motility		40% A + B
Vitality (live sperms)		58%
Sperm morphology	>15%	4%
pH	≥7.2	≥7.2
Leukocyte	<1 M	$<1 \times 10^6$/mL
MAR/Immunobead test	<10%	<50%

(MAR: mixed agglutinin reaction)

Sperm DNA Fragmentation and Its Diagnostic Value

- Viable fertile prospects are independently associated with sperm DNA damage.

- These include defective fertilization, slow early embryo development, reduced implantation, and miscarriage, also birth defect in the offspring were noticed in animal studies.
- The oxidative damaged to sperm DNA due to paternal smoking has also been associated with childhood cancer.
- DNA fragmentation is proven to be a helpful technique in predicting the outcomes of couples undergoing IVF/ICSI.

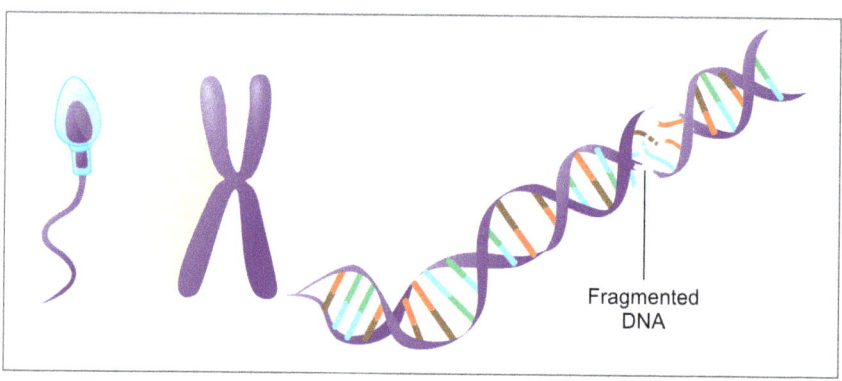

Fragmented DNA

EVALUATION OF RETROGRADE EJACULATION

- Postejaculate urine examination:
  - The presence of sperm in the postejaculate urine sample of a man with azoospermia or aspermia signifies retrograde ejaculation.
  - Low-volume ejaculate <1 mL associated with positive orgasm may be clue for retrograde ejaculation.
  - During low-volume azoospermia or absent ejaculation postejaculate urine should be checked for sperms in men.
  - In men suspected to have partial retrograde ejaculation (low-volume ejaculate with OAT), the urine should be collected in two containers.
  - If the second sample has a large number of sperm then this indicates partial retrograde flow of the ejaculate.

Reactive Oxygen Species Estimation
Hormonal Evaluation

Clinical diagnosis based on hormonal status.			
Clinical status	*FSH*	*LH*	*Testosterone*
Normal men or obstruction	Normal	Normal	Normal
Isolated spermatogenic failure	↑	Normal	Normal
Testicular failure	↑	↑	Normal or ↓
Hypogonadotropic hypogonadism	↓	↓	↓

(FSH: follicle-stimulating hormone; LH: luteinizing hormone)

Genetic Testing

Recommendations for genetic testing and counseling.	
If complete AZFA or AZFB microdeletion is detected, micro-TESE should not be performed because it is extremely unlikely that any sperm will be found	A
If a man with Yq microdeletion and his partner wish to proceed with ICSI, they should be advised that microdeletion will be passed to sons, but not to daughters	A
When a man has structural abnormalities of the vas deferens A (unilateral or bilateral absence), he and his partner should be tested for CF gene mutations	A

(AZFA: azoospermia factor A; AZFB: azoospermia factor B; CF: cystic fibrosis; ICSI: intracytoplasmic sperm injection; TESE: testicular sperm extraction)

Role of Imaging in the Evaluation of Male Infertility

- *Detection of varicoceles:*
  - Doppler ultrasound should be asked for only to confirm a clinical suspicion or in men with a short, scarred, or indurated scrotum that is difficult to evaluate.
  - Doppler may also be used to detect subclinical varicoceles on the right side of a patient with clinical left-sided varicoceles that is planned for surgical correction.
- *Scrotal ultrasound and Doppler:* Doppler may be done to confirm a clinical diagnosis of varicoceles and to evaluate the opposite side when there is unilateral clinical varicocele.
- *Abdominal ultrasound:* In men with congenital bilateral absence of the vas deferens (CBAVD) have a higher incidence of congenital renal anomalies, hence, abdominal ultrasound should be done, particularly for the kidneys.

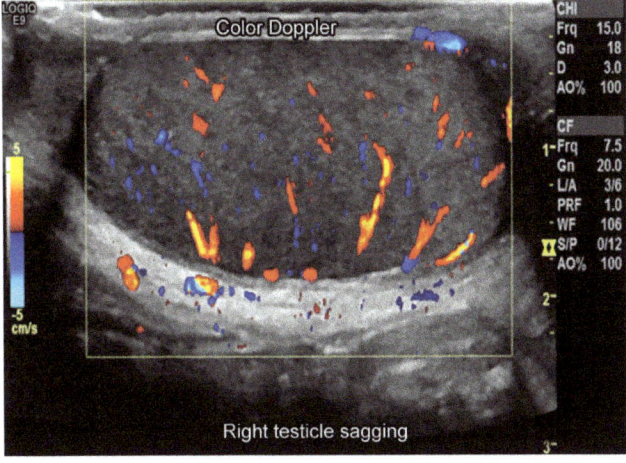

Transrectal Ultrasound

- *Transrectal ultrasonography:*
  - The transrectal ultrasonography (TRUS) is indicated in men with low volume ejaculate and palpable vas deferens. It may show ejaculatory duct obstruction (EDO) as the etiology.
  - Seminal vesicles may be normally present or present but hypofunctional in a subset of men with absent vas deferens.

Invasive Imaging Technique

- *Testicular biopsy:*
  - Before diagnosing obstructive azoospermia in men with a normal ejaculate volume, testicular biopsy is usually essential.
  - In men with small testis and FSH raised above two times normal, testicular biopsy is done only to assess the presence of focal spermatogenesis prior to ICSI.

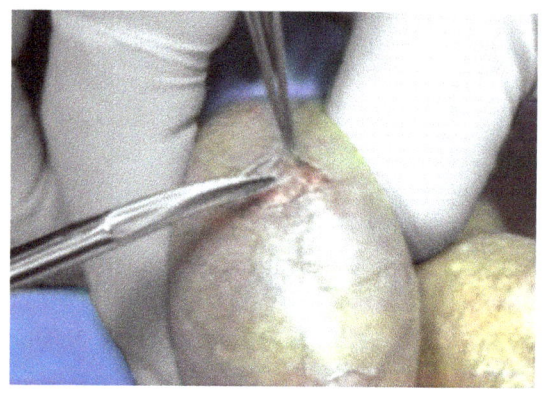

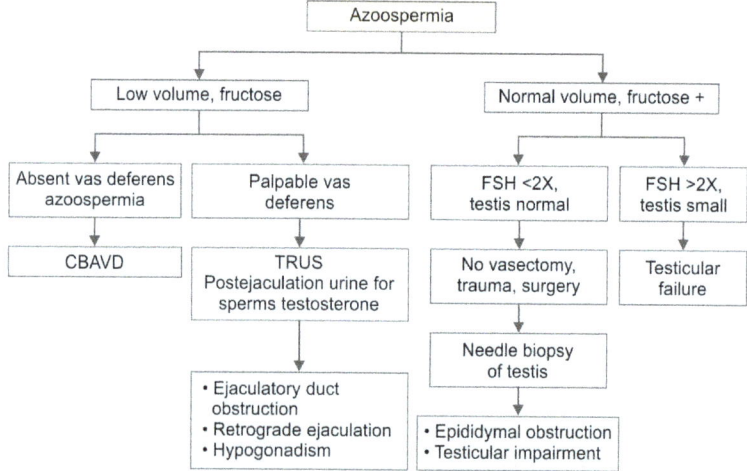

(CBAVD: congenital bilateral absence of the vas deferens; FSH: follicle-stimulating hormone; TRUS: transrectal ultrasonography)

CHAPTER 2: Evaluation of Male Partner

Gayatri Wadekar, Soumya Ramesh

INTRODUCTION

Infertility is defined as failure to achieve a clinical pregnancy after 12 months or more of regular unprotected sexual intercourse.

According to the Indian Society of Assisted Reproduction, infertility currently affects about 10-14% of the Indian population with higher rates in urban areas where one out of six couples is impacted. Nearly 27.5 million couples actively trying to conceive suffer from infertility in India.[1]

A male factor alone is responsible in about 20-30% of infertile couples and contributory in another 30-40%.

A couple seeking treatment for infertility should be evaluated if pregnancy fails to occur within 1 year of regular unprotected intercourse. An evaluation should be done before 1 year if the female partner's age is over 35 years or has other risk factors for infertility like genital tuberculosis (TB), endometriosis or if the male partner has a known history of risk factors such as bilateral cryptorchidism, trauma, etc.

Male infertility can be attributed to different conditions:[2]
- Congenital or acquired urogenital abnormalities
- Malignancies
- Urogenital tract infections
- Increased scrotal temperature (e.g., as a consequence of varicocele, tight underclothes)
- Endocrine disturbances
- Genetic abnormalities
- Immunological factors
- Idiopathic

Evaluation of the male partner can help in identification and treatment of correctable conditions. Occasionally serious underlying medical conditions like malignancies may be diagnosed in the course of the evaluation. Sometimes genetic abnormalities are detected and appropriate genetic counseling with regard to the health of the offspring can be provided to the couple.

EVALUATION OF THE MALE PARTNER

The initial screening should include detailed medical and reproductive history and a reliable semen analysis.[3]

History

- Age
- Duration of infertility
- Previous pregnancy
- Childhood illnesses like mumps and developmental history like age of puberty, cryptorchidism
- Systemic medical illnesses (such as diabetes mellitus and history of recurrent upper respiratory diseases)
- Previous surgery (hernia, hydrocele, and vasectomy)
- Medications (chemotherapy and anabolic steroids)
- Sexual history (frequency of coitus and erectile dysfunction)
- Environmental exposures to chemical toxins, heat, and radiation
- History of trauma to groin
- Smoking, alcohol, and recreational drugs

Semen Analysis

Semen analysis remains the cornerstone of male partner evaluation. Male infertility factor is almost always associated with an abnormal semen analysis; however, other male factors may cause infertility even with a normal semen analysis. Rarely patients with normal semen analyses have sperms that do not function in a manner which is necessary for fertility.[4]

Collection

Semen specimen is obtained by masturbation into a sterile wide-mouth container after 2–5 days of abstinence and should be analyzed within 1 hour of collection. The collection should be ideally done at the laboratory. If the sample is collected at home, the sample should be transported at room temperature to the laboratory within 1 hour of collection.

The semen analysis provides information on semen volume as well as sperm concentration, motility, and morphology.

World Health Organization (WHO) criteria is used as reference values and has a high sensitivity with a low specificity to detect true semen abnormality.[5]

A single abnormal semen analysis should be followed up with a repeat analysis. Ideally, the second analysis should be scheduled at 3 months' time from the first abnormal one to allow a cycle of spermatogenesis. To prevent delay induced undue anxiety the test can be repeated in 6–8 weeks' time. If first analysis shows azoospermia, the second analysis should be performed in 2–4 weeks.[6] Men who have two abnormal semen analyses may need further, more detailed assessment.

TABLE 1: World Health Organization (WHO) semen analysis, 2010.

Parameter	1992	Lower range limit 2010
Semen volume	2 mL	1.5 mL
Sperm concentration in 10^6/mL	20	15
Total sperms 10^6 per ejaculate		39
Progressive motility	>50%	32% A
Total motility		40% (A + B)
Vitality (live sperms)		58%
Sperm morphology	>15%	4%
pH	≥7.2	≥7.2
Leukocyte 10^6/mL	<1.0	<1.0
MAR%	<10	<50

A normal first semen analysis need not be repeated.

Semen analysis: Please refer **Table 1** for more details.

The parameters assessed:
- Physical:
  - Appearance grayish white
  - Volume ≥1.5 mL
  - *Viscosity:* Normally the semen liquefies in 30 minutes. Increased viscosity is diagnosed if liquefaction does not occur in 60 minutes.
  - *pH:* ≥ 7.2. Low volume, pH < 7 and absent sperms would raise suspicion of distal male genital tract obstruction.
- Microscopic:
  - *Sperm count:* Normal count 15 million/mL.
  - *Motility:* Rapid progressive (A) is fast and forward movement in a straight line.
    - Slow progressive (B) Forward movement in a curved or crooked manner
    - Nonprogressive. Only tail movements.
  - *Viability:* The number of live sperms
- *Morphology:* Kruger strict criteria is applied.[7] Men with severe teratozoospermia have better chance of fertilization with intracytoplasmic sperm injection (ICSI).[8] In isolation, however, low morphology does not have a great predictive value for fertilization or pregnancy.
  - Presence of nonsperm cells such as leukocytes and round cells. Presence of pus cells will need further evaluation to rule out infections.
- *Immunological:* More infertile males will show antisperm antibodies as compared to fertile men. As per the WHO criteria when >50% of motile sperms are bound to these antibodies, it results in poor sperm penetration

in cervical mucus and impaired in vivo fertilization and is therefore considered pathological threshold.[9]
  - SpermMar test
  - Immunobead test
- *Biochemical:* Fructose.

Abnormalities in one or more parameters can affect fertility. Certain conditions such as azoospermia and total globozoospermia (all abnormal round-headed sperms with absent acrosome) correlate with infertility by themselves. However, individual sperm parameters by themselves such as concentration, morphology, and motility are not highly predictive of fertility or diagnostic of infertility. The odds ratio for infertility increases as the number of abnormal parameters increases.[10]

Physical Examination

A complete examination from a urologist is sought in case of abnormal semen analysis or abnormal male reproductive history.

General Examination

Obesity, secondary sexual characteristics such as hair distribution, and breast development.

Local Examination

- Examination of the penis and location of urethral meatus
- *Testis:* Location, size, and consistency.
- Presence and consistency of vas deferens, and epididymis
- Presence of varicocele

Other Tests

Further evaluation may be indicated in certain situations.
- *Endocrine tests:* Evaluation of the hypothalamic-pituitary-testicular axis through hormonal tests such as follicle-stimulating hormone (FSH), luteinizing hormone (LH), testosterone, and prolactin. Indicated in oligospermia, sexual dysfunction or other clinical findings suggestive of a specific endocrinopathy.
- *Imaging:* Routine sonography is not recommended in male factor evaluation. Scrotal USG can pick up varicocele, hydrocele, and epididymal cyst. Transrectal sonography is advised in cases of suspected obstructive azoospermia.
- *Genetic tests:* Genetic abnormalities may be associated with severe oligospermia and azoospermia. Karyotype and genetic counseling should be offered in such situations.

- *Sperm function tests:* Sperm function tests assess functional characteristics of the sperm like sperm motility, hyperactivation, mucous penetration, zona interaction, and acrosomal reaction.
- *DNA fragmentation:* TUNEL test to test DNA integrity.
- *Testicular biopsy:* Generally combined with surgical sperm retrieval.

A stepwise but detailed male evaluation gives a better understanding of the cause of a couple's infertility. It is only when the evaluation is comprehensive and thorough that the right treatment options can be offered which could range from lifestyle modifications to specific treatments to assisted reproductive technologies or even donor insemination or adoption.

REFERENCES

1. Shah D. Expanding IVF treatment in India .... need of the day!! J Hum Reprod Sci. 2017;10(2):69-70.
2. Rowe PJ, Comhaire FH, Hargreave TB, Mellows HJ. WHO, Sexual and Reproductive Health. WHO Manual for the Standardized Investigation and Diagnosis of the Infertile Couple. 2000, Cambridge University. World Health Organization. 1993;92.
3. Practice Committee of the American Society for Reproductive Medicine. Diagnostic evaluation of the infertile male: a committee opinion. Fertil Steril. 2015;103(3):e18-25.
4. Jarow J, Sigman M, Kolettis PN, Lipshultz LR, McClure R, Nangia AK, et al. Optimal Evaluation of the Infertile Male. Am Urol Assoc. 2011.
5. Skakkebaek NE. Normal reference ranges for semen quality and their relations to fecundity. Asian J Androl. 2010;12:95-8.
6. National Collaborating Centre for Women's and Children's Health (UK). Fertility: assessment and treatment for people with fertility problems. London: RCOG press; 2004.
7. Kruger TF, Acosta AA, Simmons KF, Swanson RJ, Matta JF, Oehninger S. Predictive value of abnormal sperm morphology in in-vitro fertilization. Fertil Steril. 1988;49:112-7.
8. Pisarska MD, Casson PR, Cisneros PL, Lamb DJ, Lipshultz LI, Buster JE, et al. Fertilization after standard in vitro fertilization versus intracytoplasmic sperm injection in subfertile males using sibling oocytes. Fertil Steril. 1999;71:627-32.
9. Lotti F, Baldi E, Corona G, Lombardo F, Maseroli E, Degl'Innocenti S, et al. Epididymal more than testicular abnormalities are associated with the occurrence of antisperm antibodies as evaluated by the MAR test. Hum Reprod. 2018;33:1417-29.
10. Guzick DS, Overstreet JW, Factor-Litvak P, Brazil CK, Nakajima ST, Coutifaris C, et al. Sperm morphology, motility, and concentration in fertile and infertile men. N Engl J Med. 2001;345:1388-93.

CHAPTER 3

Semen Analysis and Beyond Role of Sperm Function Tests

Gouri Sultane Gupta, Firuza R Parikh

INTRODUCTION

Assessment of male partner forms the foundation of evaluation of an infertile couple. But, it has been seen that even though there are a battery of tests to detect female fertility, the male has been essentially neglected. Apart from semen analysis and antisperm antibodies, most assisted reproductive techniques (ARTs) programs do not offer anything more. Though semen analysis is enough to stamp a male as normal, this test alone is insufficient to evaluate a subfertile male.[1,2]

SEMEN ANALYSIS

The first-line laboratory investigation for male fertility includes semen analysis. Semen should be ideally collected by masturbation after 2–5 days of abstinence.

The lower limit of reference values for semen parameters [the World Health Organization (WHO) 2010] are as follows[3] **(Table 1)**.

TABLE 1: Macroscopic and microscopic analysis of semen.

Parameters	Reference values
Ejaculate volume	1.5 mL
pH	7.2
Sperm concentration	15×10^6 spermatozoa/mL
Total sperm count	39×10^6 spermatozoa/ejaculate
Motility	40%
Forward progression	32%
Normal morphology	4%
Sperm agglutination	Absent
Viscosity	<2 cm thread after liquefaction
Vitality	58%

Aspermia

It is the absence of sperms.

Causes: This could be due to retrograde ejaculation due to psychological/neurological factors.

Low Semen Volume

Causes: Blockade of seminal vesicles or ejaculatory ducts in prostrate.

pH <7 with low volume and azoospermia—signifies ejaculatory duct obstruction or congenital bilateral absence of the vas deferens (CBAVD).

Low/Absent Fructose

Due to ejaculatory duct obstruction and seminal vesicle agenesis/dysfunction.

Oligoasthenoteratozoospermia

Causes: Varicoceles, hormonal abnormalities, infection, and genetic aberrations.

Azoospermia

It can be categorized into:
- *Pretesticular:* Hypogonadotropic—correctable. Uncommon.
- *Testicular:* Have poor/absent spermatogenesis. Need ART.
- *Post-testicular:* Due to ductal obstruction/agenesis. Correctable.

ANTISPERM ANTIBODIES[4]

Antisperm antibodies (ASA) are suspected when:
- There is disruption of blood epithelial barrier as in vasectomy, hernia repair, testicular trauma, torsion, and orchitis.
- Isolated asthenospermia
- Agglutination of sperms in semen analysis

Tests

Immunobead or mixed antiglobulin reaction (MAR)—gold standard to assay ASA.

But, the clinical utility of ASA test is uncertain. ASA should not be part of routine male factor evaluation.

HORMONAL EVALUATION

An endocrine evaluation should be performed when **(Table 2)**:
- Sperm concentration is below 10 million/mL.
- When there is male sexual dysfunction like low semen volume or decreased libido.
- Clinical signs of specific endocrinopathy.

TABLE 2: Endocrine evaluation.

	Semen volume	Total testosterone	Serum follicle-stimulating hormone
Hypogonadotropic hypogonadism	N/decreased	Decreased	Decreased
Primary testicular failure	N	Decreased	Increased
Obstructive azoospermia	N/decreased	N	N
Germinal aplasia	N	N	Elevated

The findings of hormonal analysis should be interpreted according to **Table 2**.

SPERM DNA FRAGMENTATION INDEX[5,6]

Sperm chromatin quality or integrity can be measured by DNA fragmentation assays.

There are two types of assays:
1. Direct
    - Terminal deoxynucleotidyl transferase (TdT) dUTP nick-end labeling (TUNEL) method
    - Comet assay
2. Indirect
    - Sperm chromatin structure assay (SCSA)
    - Sperm chromatin dispersion (SCD) test

Threshold values used to define abnormal tests:
- For SCSA (>25–27%)
- TUNEL assay (>36%)

High-sperm DNA fragmentation index (DFI) corresponds to low pregnancy outcomes in in vitro fertilization (IVF) and high risk of spontaneous recurrent miscarriages.

SPERM FLUORESCENT IN SITU HYBRIDIZATION[7]

Fluorescent in situ hybridization (FISH) allows the analysis of numerical chromosomal abnormalities of spermatozoa. This is performed using different chromosome specific DNA probes.

Advantages: It can be applied on a large number of nonmotile/dysmorphic sperms.

Disadvantages: Only numerical abnormalities of specific chromosomes can be ascertained and no information about other chromosomes can be obtained.

GENETIC TESTING[8]

Infertility associated with severe oligoasthenoteratozoospermia (OAT) and azoospermia are mostly genetic in origin.

Such couples mandate genetic tests like:
- Analysis of karyotype in peripheral lymphocytes
- Detection of Y chrome microdeletions
- Analysis of cystic fibrosis transmembrane conductance regulator (CFTR) gene in which the male partner has CBAVD.

Nonobstructive azoospermia (NOA) and severe oligozoospermia (<5 million/mL): Karyotype analysis and Y chromosome microdeletion are recommended in these conditions before performing intracytoplasmic sperm injection (ICSI).

Karyotype Analysis[9]

Klienfelter's syndrome is the most common abnormality in severe oligospermia cases. If karyotype is abnormal, there is increased risk of aneuploidy. Therefore, preimplantation genetic testing for monogenic (PGT-M) should be discussed with the couple prior to ART.

Y Chromosome Microdeletions[10,11]

The long arm of the Y chromosome (Yq) is important for spermatogenesis. There are three specific regions in the long arm of the Y chromosome (Yq)—(1) Azoospermia factor (AZF) a, (2) AZFb, and (3) AZFc.

Azoospermia factor cis the most common microdeletion—60%. It is associated in >50% of the times with sperm recovery for ICSI on testicular sperm extraction. However, vertical transmission of the microdeletions and infertility in the male offspring is inevitable. Therefore, genetic counseling should be offered to patients.

Azoospermia factor a deletion is seen in Sertoli cell only syndrome, while AZF b deletion is seen in maturation arrest. Therefore, sperm retrieval rate in both these conditions is 0%. Therefore, sperm retrieval is not recommended in these two microdeletions.

It is, therefore, important to determine which microdeletion is present before attempting sperm extraction and ICSI.

Obstructive Azoospermia (Flowchart 1)

Cystic Fibrosis Transmembrane Conductance Regulator Gene Mutation[12,13]

Congenital bilateral absence of the vas deferens is a common cause of obstructive azoospermia (OA). There is a strong association between *CBAVD* and *CFTR* gene. Cystic fibrosis is a serious autosomal recessive condition.

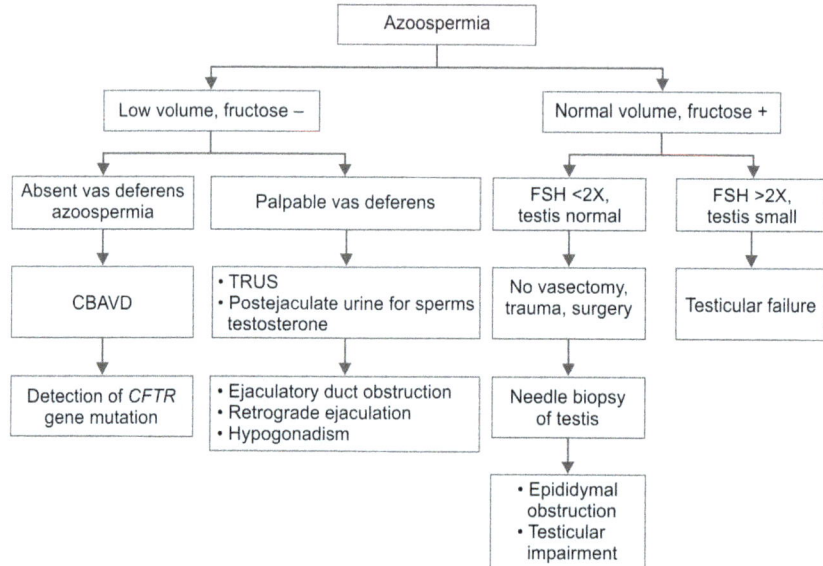

Flowchart 1: Diagnostic algorithm for azoospermia.

(CBAVD: congenital bilateral absence of the vas deferens; CFTR: cystic fibrosis transmembrane conductance regulator; FSH: follicle-stimulating hormone; TRUS: transrectal ultrasound scan)

It is imperative to check for *CFTR* gene in the female partner of a male with CBAVD before undergoing ICSI.

If found present in both the partners, PGT-M should be offered to prevent a child to be born with CF.

CONCLUSION[14,15]

Male factor infertility is the sole reason in 20% of the couples and contributory factor in 30–40% of the couples. Investigations should be based on clinical findings keeping the provisional diagnosis in mind. In case of severe male infertility, good clinical practice requires genetic evaluation before, during, and after ART and proper counseling of the couple. The aim is to inform patients about possible risks, to improve the success rate of ART treatment, and to avoid the birth of children with severe genetic disease.

REFERENCES

1. Practice committee of American society for Reproductive medicine. Diagnostic evaluation of the infertile male: A committee opinion. Fertil Steril. 2015;103(3):e18-25.
2. Male Infertility Best Practice Policy Committee of the American Society of Reproductive Medicine; Practice Committee of the American Society for Reproductive Medicine. Report on optimal evaluation of the infertile male. Fertil Steril. 2006; 86(5 Suppl 1):S202-9.

3. World Health Organization. (2010). WHO Laboratory Manual for the Examination and Processing of Human Semen, 5th edition. [online] Available from https://apps.who.int/iris/handle/10665/44261 [Last accessed April, 2022].
4. Francavilla F, Santucci R, Barbonetti A, Francavilla S. Naturally occurring antisperm antibodies in men: interference with fertility and clinical implications: An update. Front Biosci. 2007;12:2890-911.
5. Sakkas D, Alvarez JG. Sperm DNA fragmentation: Mechanism of origin, impact on reproductive outcome, and analysis. Fertil Steril. 2010;93(4):1027-36.
6. Collins JA, Barnhart KT, Schlegel PN. Do sperm integrity tests predict pregnancy with in vitro fertilisation? Fertil Steril. 2008;89(4):823-31.
7. Moosani N, Pattison HA, Carter MD, Cox DM, Rademaker AW, Martin RH. Chromosomal analysis of sperm from men with idiopathic infertility using sperm karyotyping and fluorescent in situ hybridization. Fertil Steril. 1995;64:811-7.
8. Griffin DK, Finch KA. The genetic and cytogenetic basis of male infertility. Hum Fertil. 2005;8(1):19-26.
9. Kim SY, Lee BY, Oh AR, Park SY, Lee HS, Seo JT. Clinical, hormonal, and genetic evaluation of idiopathic nonobstructive azoospermia and Klinefelter's syndrome patients. Cytogenet Genome Res. 2017;153(4):190-7.
10. Vogt PH, Edelmann A, Kirsch S, Henegariu O, Hirschmann P, Kiesewetter F, et al. Human Y chromosome azoospermia factors (AZF) mapped to different sub regions in Yq11. Hum Mol Genet. 1996;5(7):933-43.
11. Hopps CV, Mielnik A, Goldstein M, Palermo GD, Rosenwaks Z, Schlegel PN. Detection of sperm in men with Y chrome micro deletions of AZFa, AZFb, AZFc regions. Hum Reprod. 2003;18(8):1660-5.
12. Lissens W, Mercier B, Tournaye H, Bonduelle M, Férec C, Seneca S, et al. Cystic fibrosis and infertility caused by congenital absence of vas deferens and related clinical entities. Hum Reprod. 1996;11(Suppl 4):55-78; discussion 79-80.
13. Gajbhiye R, Kadam K, Khole A, Gaikwad A, Kadam S, Shah R, et al. Cystic fibrosis transmembrane conductance regulator (CFTR) gene abnormalities in Indian males with CBAVD and renal anomalies. Indian J Med Res. 2016;143(5):616-23.
14. Jungwirth A, Diemer T, Dohle GR, Giwercman A, Kopa Z. (2015). Guidelines on Male Infertility. European Association of Urology Guideline, 2013 Edition. 61. [online] Available from https://www.researchgate.net/publication/288264436_Guidelines_on_Male_Infertility [Last accessed April, 2022].
15. American Urological Association. (2011). Optimal Evaluation of the Infertile Male. [online] Available from https://www.auanet.org/guidelines/archived-documents/male-infertility-optimal-evaluation-best-practice-statement [Last accessed April, 2021].

CHAPTER 4: Ovarian Reserve Tests

Swati Sarda, Kanchan Ghuse Kelwade

INTRODUCTION

Ovarian reserve is defined as the number of oocytes (oocyte quantity) remaining in the ovary. Ovarian reserve tests (ORTs) are hormone levels and sonographically measured features of ovary. ORTs help to predict the ovarian response to stimulation and not pregnancy. Ovarian response is defined as the actual oocyte yield after ovarian stimulation.

Diminishing ovarian reserve is a phenomenon noted in women during mid to late 30s and at times earlier, reflecting the declining follicular pool and oocyte quality.[1]

An ideal ORT should be easy to perform, reproducible, and easy to interpret for decision making regarding further treatment of the subfertile woman.

Available ORTs are divided into biological, biochemical, biophysical, and histological tests and have been shown in **Flowchart 1**.

AGE

Ovarian reserve correlates inversely with age, but there is considerable variation in ovarian reserve among women of the same chronologic age.[2]

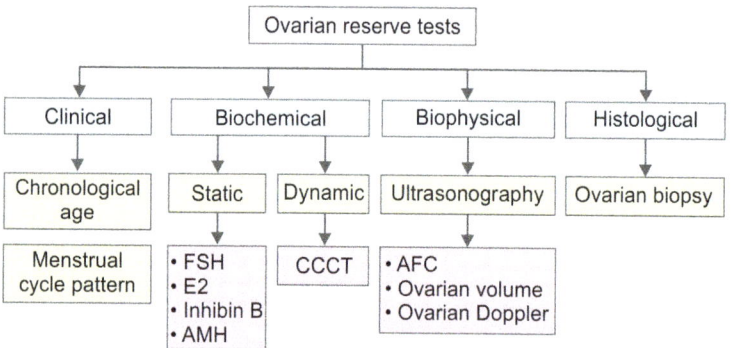

Flowchart 1: Ovarian reserve tests.

(AFC: antral follicle count; AMH: anti-Müllerian hormone; CCCT: clomiphene citrate challenge test; FSH: follicle-stimulating hormone)

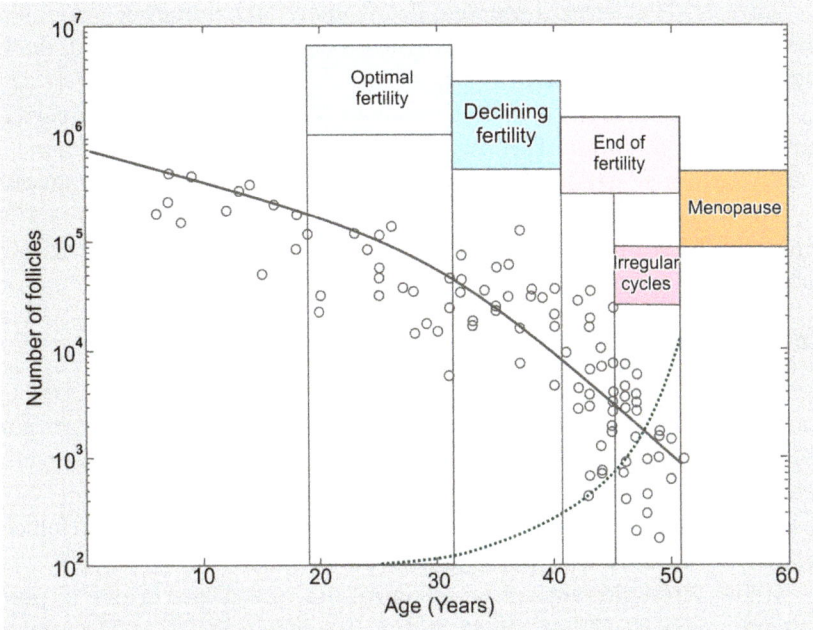

Fig. 1: Quantitative (solid line) and qualitative (dotted line) decline of the ovarian follicle pool, which is assumed to dictate the onset of the important reproductive events.[10]

Fecundity in both natural and stimulated ovarian cycles declines with maternal age, beginning in the late 20s and becoming more abrupt in the late 30s **(Fig. 1)**.

Age is known to be the most important factor determining the pregnancy potential in regularly cycling women.[3-5] However, chronological age alone has a limited value in predicting individual ovarian responses.[6-9]

MENSTRUAL CYCLE PATTERN

Women with normal ovarian reserve have regular predictable menstrual pattern. Women with diminished ovarian reserve (DOR) show altered menstrual pattern with short cycles and reduced menstrual flow.

In DOR, the earlier increase in follicle-stimulating hormone (FSH) levels stimulates an earlier onset of new follicular growth and an increase in estradiol (E2) concentrations, ultimately decreasing the length of the follicular phase and the overall cycle.

Follicle-stimulating Hormone and E2

Basal serum FSH levels are elevated on days 2-4 of the menstrual cycle in women with DOR. Elevated FSH is a specific, but not sensitive, test for DOR.[11] There is no universally accepted cut-off with a wide range in threshold value up to 25 IU/L is used to identify poor response.

However, FSH levels have significant inter- and intracycle variability that limits the reliability of a single measurement, high intercycle variability suggests more advanced DOR.[12,13]

Basal E2 alone is not a reliable predictor of DOR. It has a role in correct interpretation of normal FSH. An early rise in serum E2 concentrations is a classic characteristic of reproductive aging and can lower an otherwise elevated basal FSH level into the normal range. When the basal FSH concentration is normal but the E2 level is elevated (>60–80 pg/mL), this may indicate DOR.[14]

Anti-Müllerian Hormone

Anti-Müllerian hormone (AMH) is a dimeric glycoprotein, produced by granulosa cells of preantral and small antral follicles which are gonadotropin independent. Therefore, AMH levels remain relatively consistent within and between menstrual cycles in both normal and subfertile women.[15-18]

Anti-Müllerian hormone levels strongly correlate with basal antral follicle count (AFC) measured by transvaginal ultrasonography.[19]

Various threshold values, 0.2–1.26 ng/mL, have been used to identify poor responders with 80–87% sensitivity and 64–93% specificity.[20-22] AMH is known to have the ability to predict a hyper-response as well.[19,23]

It is considered that at levels 0.5–1.26 ng/mL, AMH indicates perimenopausal transition within 3–5 years.[24] Levels within this range still suggest favorable results with assisted reproductive technology (ART).

Anti-Müllerian hormone levels may be decreased in women currently using hormonal contraceptives and, therefore, should be interpreted with caution in those patients.[25]

Anti-Müllerian hormone is a more sensitive marker of ovarian reserve than FSH and tends to decline before FSH rises.[26] For this reason, AMH has largely replaced basal FSH and E2 level testing as a biomarker of ovarian reserve.

Anti-Müllerian hormone has a unique place among ORTs as it may be applicable as a screening test in a general subfertile population.[24]

Inhibin B

Inhibin B is a glycoprotein hormone produced by preantral follicles and therefore indicates the follicular pool. As the number of ovarian follicles declines with age, early-follicular-phase inhibin B concentrations decline.

Reduced inhibin B levels lower the level of central negative feedback, causing late-luteal and early-follicular rise in FSH concentrations.

Inhibin B alone is not a reliable predictor of ovarian reserve.[27,28]

Clomiphene Citrate Challenge Test

Clomiphene citrate challenge test (CCCT) is a dynamic test for ovarian reserve involving the administration of 100 mg of clomiphene citrate from the

5th day of the cycle for 5 days. Basal FSH on day 3 of the cycle and stimulated FSH on day 10 is measured.

However, a meta-analysis has shown that CCCT is no better than non-dynamic tests in predicting DOR or pregnancy and should be abandoned.[11]

Antral Follicle Count

Antral follicle count is the sum of number of antral follicles (2–10 mm) in both ovaries measured by transvaginal ultrasonography in the early follicular phase. A count of 8–10 is considered as a predictor of a normal response. It is found that the number of AFs 2–6 mm in size declines with age, correlates with other markers, and appears to be more reliable marker of ovarian reserve.[29]

Antral follicle count is considered to have the best discriminating potential for a poor ovarian response compared to the total ovarian volume and basal serum levels of FSH, E2, and inhibin B on day 3 of the cycle but lacks the sensitivity and specificity to predict the nonoccurrence of pregnancy.[30,31] AFC has low intercycle variability and high interobserver reliability in experienced centers.[32,33]

More than 14 AFs are considered to be a good predictor of hyper-response.[34] Three-dimensional (3D) ultrasound does not have any advantage over two-dimensional (2D) ultrasound in the assessment of ovarian reserve.[35]

OVARIAN VOLUME

The ovarian volume is measured by transvaginal ultrasonography applying the formula for an ellipsoid ($D1 \times D2 \times D3 \times \pi/6$).

The ovarian volume remains unchanged till the perimenopausal period and does not add to the predictive value of AFC.[31,34]

OVARIAN DOPPLER

The observation of the ovarian Doppler flow during ovarian stimulation has been studied in in vitro fertilization (IVF) cycles. The increase in the Doppler flow noted during stimulation is considered not to provide additional information to AFC.[36]

OVARIAN BIOPSY

Ovarian biopsy done at laparoscopy or laparotomy has shown that the follicular density reduces with age.[37] Also, women with unexplained infertility have fewer follicles. However, the distribution of follicles is not uniform within the ovary and, hence, the biopsy may not represent the true follicular density.[38]

It is understood that an invasive ovarian biopsy does not add to the information available through noninvasive modalities and it is not recommended to be used as an ORT.[39]

KEY NOTES (THE AMERICAN SOCIETY FOR REPRODUCTIVE MEDICINE COMMITTEE OPINION, 2020)[40]

- Dynamic tests such as the CCCT do not improve test accuracy for predicting poor ovarian response, pregnancy after IVF, or unassisted conception over basal markers and, therefore, should be abandoned.
- Currently, AMH and AFC are the most sensitive and reliable markers of ovarian reserve.
- Combined ORT models do not consistently improve predictive ability over that of single ovarian reserve tests.
- Markers of ovarian reserve do not predict current reproductive potential among women with unproven fertility.
- Results of ovarian reserve tests are neither useful in predicting the likelihood of unassisted pregnancy in women with infertility nor do they offer clinically meaningful improvements over already established pregnancy prediction models.
- Markers of ovarian reserve do not appear to predict pregnancy after ovarian stimulation (OS)/intrauterine insemination (IUI) for unexplained infertility.
- The ability of AMH and AFC to predict oocyte yield as well as poor and excessive ovarian responsiveness in IVF has been well demonstrated.
- Extremely low AMH values should not be used to refuse treatment in IVF.
- Anti-Müllerian hormone and AFC have only a weak association with qualitative outcomes such as oocyte quality, clinical pregnancy rates, and live birth rates.
- Poor ovarian response to maximal stimulation during IVF procedures reflects DOR, and further ovarian reserve testing is unnecessary.

REFERENCES

1. Scott RT, Hofmann GE. Prognostic assessment of ovarian reserve. Fertil Steril. 1995;63:1-11.
2. Hansen KR, Knowlton NS, Thyer AC, Charleston JS, Soules MR, Klein NA. A new model of reproductive aging: the decline in ovarian nongrowing follicle number from birth to menopause. Hum Reprod. 2008;23:699-708.
3. Padilla SL, Garcia JE. Effect of maternal age and number of in vitro fertilization procedures on pregnancy outcome. Fertil Steril. 1989;52:270-3.
4. Seibel MM, Kearnan M, Kiessling A. Parameters that predict success for natural cycle in vitro fertilization-embryo transfer. Fertil Steril. 1995;63:1251-4.
5. van Rooij IA, Broekmans FJ, Hunault CC, Scheffer GJ, Eijkemans MJ, de Jong FH, et al. Use of ovarian reserve tests for the prediction of ongoing pregnancy in couples with unexplained or mild male infertility. Reprod Biomed Online. 2006;12:182-90.
6. Scott RT, Toner JP, Muasher SJ, Oehninger S, Robinson S, Rosenwaks Z. Follicle-stimulating hormone levels on cycle day 3 are predictive of in vitro fertilization outcome. Fertil Steril. 1989;51:651-4.

7. Toner JP, Philput CB, Jones GS, Muasher SJ. Basal follicle stimulating hormone level is a better predictor of in vitro fertilization performance than age. Fertil Steril. 1991;55:784-91.
8. Sharif K, Elgendy M, Lashen H, Afnan M. Age and basal follicle stimulating hormone as predictors of in vitro fertilization outcome. Br J Obstet Gynaecol. 1998;105:107-12.
9. Erdem M, Erdem A, Gursoy R, Biberoglu K. Comparison of basal and clomiphene citrate induced FSH and inhibin B, ovarian volume and antral follicle counts as ovarian reserve tests and predictors of poor ovarian response in IVF. J Assist Reprod Genet. 2004;21:37-45.
10. de Bruin JP, teVelde ER. Female reproductive ageing: Concepts and consequences. In: Tulandi T, Gosden RG (Eds). Preservation of Fertility. London, UK: Taylor and Francis; 2004. p. 3.
11. Jain T, Soules MR, Collins JA. Comparison of basal follicle-stimulating hormone versus the clomiphene citrate challenge test for ovarian reserve screening. Fertil Steril. 2004;82:180-5.
12. Jayaprakasan K, Campbell B, Hopkisson J, Clewes J, Johnson I, Raine Fenning N. Establishing the intercycle variability of three-dimensional ultrasonographic predictors of ovarian reserve. Fertil Steril. 2008;90:2126-32.
13. Kwee J, Schats R, McDonnell J, Lambalk CB, Schoemaker J. Intercycle variability of ovarian reserve tests: results of a prospective randomized study. Hum Reprod. 2004;19:590-5.
14. Evers JL, Slaats P, Land JA, Dumoulin JC, Dunselman GA. Elevated levels of basal estradiol-17b predict poor response in patients with normal basal levels of follicle-stimulating hormone undergoing in vitro fertilization. Fertil Steril. 1998;69:1010-4.
15. Fanchin R, Taieb J, Lozano DH, Ducot B, Frydman R, Bouyer J. High reproducibility of serum anti-Mullerian hormone measurements suggests a multi-staged follicular secretion and strengthens its role in the assessment of ovarian follicular status. Hum Reprod. 2005;20:923-7.
16. Tsepelidis S, Devreker F, Demeestere I, Flahaut A, Gervy C, Englert Y. Stable serum levels of anti-Müllerian hormone during the menstrual cycle: a prospective study in normo-ovulatory women. Hum Reprod. 2007;22:1837-40.
17. La Marca A, Stabile G, Artenisio AC, Volpe A. Serum anti-Müllerian hormone throughout the human menstrual cycle. Hum Reprod. 2006;21:3103-7.
18. Hehenkamp WJ, Looman CW, Themmen AP, de Jong FH, te Velde ER, Broekmans FJ. Anti-Müllerian hormone levels in the spontaneous menstrual cycle do not show substantial fluctuation. J Clin Endocrinol Metab. 2006;91:4057-63.
19. Broer SL, Dólleman M, Opmeer BC, Fauser BC, Mol BW, Broekmans FJ. AMH and AFC as predictors of excessive response in controlled ovarian hyperstimulation: a meta-analysis. Hum Reprod Update. 2011;17:46-54.
20. Muttukrishna S, McGarrigle H, Wakim R, Khadum I, Ranieri DM, Serhal P. Antral follicle count, anti-Mullerian hormone and inhibin B: predictors of ovarian response in assisted reproductive technology? BJOG. 2005;112:1384-90.
21. Tremellen KP, Kolo M, Gilmore A, Lekamge DN. Anti-Müllerian hormone as a marker of ovarian reserve. Aust N Z J Obstet Gynaecol. 2005;45:20-4.
22. La Marca A, Giulini S, Tirelli A, Bertucci E, Marsella T, Xella S, et al. Anti-Müllerian hormone measurement on any day of the menstrual cycle strongly predicts ovarian response in assisted reproductive technology. Hum Reprod. 2007;22:766-71.
23. Nelson SM, Yates RW, Lyall H, Jamieson M, Traynor I, Gaudoin M, et al. Anti-Müllerian hormone-based approach to controlled ovarian stimulation for assisted conception. Hum Reprod. 2009;24:867-75.
24. Gnoth C, Schuring AN, Friol K, Tigges J, Mallmann P, Godehardt E. Relevance of anti-Müllerian hormone measurement in a routine IVF program. Hum Reprod. 2005;23:1359-65.

25. van den Berg MH, van Dulmen-den Broeder E, Overbeek A, Twisk JW, Schats R, van Leeuwen FE, et al. Comparison of ovarian function markers in users of hormonal contraceptives during the hormone-free interval and subsequent natural early follicular phases. Hum Reprod. 2010;25:1520-7.
26. de Vet A, Laven JS, de Jong FH, Themmen AP, Fauser BC. Anti-Müllerian hormone serum levels: a putative marker for ovarian aging. Fertil Steril. 2002;77:357-62.
27. Corson SL, Gutmann J, Batzer FR, Wallace H, Klein N, Soules MR. Inhibin-B as a test of ovarian reserve for infertile women. Hum Reprod. 1999;14:2818-21.
28. Hall JE, Welt CK, Cramer DW. Inhibin A and inhibin B reflect ovarian function in assisted reproduction but are less useful at predicting outcome. Hum Reprod. 1999;14:409-15.
29. Haadsma MA, Bukman A, Groen H, Roeloffzen EM, Groenewoud ER, Heineman MJ, et al. The number of small antral follicles (2–6 mm) determines the outcome of endocrine ovarian reserve tests in a subfertile population. Hum Reprod. 2007;22:1932-41.
30. Maheshwari A, Fowler P, Bhattacharya S. Assessment of ovarian reserve should we perform tests of ovarian reserve routinely? Hum Reprod. 2006;21:2729-35.
31. Hendriks DJ, Kwee J, Mol BW, teVelde ER, Broekmans FJ. Ultrasonography as a tool for the prediction of outcome in IVF patients: A comparative meta-analysis of ovarian volume and antral follicle count. Fertil Steril. 2007;87:764-75.
32. Eldar-Geva T, Ben-Chetrit A, Spitz IM, Rabinowitz R, Markowitz E, Mimoni T, et al. Dynamic assays of inhibin B, anti-Müllerian hormone and estradiol following FSH stimulation and ovarian ultrasonography as predictors of IVF outcome. Hum Reprod. 2005;20:3178-83.
33. Kwee J, Schats R, McDonnell J, Themmen A, de Jong F, Lambalk C. Evaluation of anti-mullerian hormone as a test for the prediction of ovarian reserve. Fertil Steril. 2008;90:737-43.
34. Kwee J, Elting ME, Schats R, McDonnell J, Lambalk CB. Ovarian volume and antral follicle count for the prediction of low and hyper responders with in vitro fertilization. Reprod Biol Endocrinol. 2007;5:9.
35. Jayaprakasan K, Hilwah N, Kendall NR, Hopkisson JF, Campbell BK, JohnsonI R, et al. Does 3D ultrasound offer any advantage in the pretreatment assessment of ovarian reserve and prediction of outcome after assisted reproduction treatment? Hum Reprod. 2007;22:1925-31.
36. Järvelä IY, Sladkevicius P, Kelly S, Ojha K, Campbell S, Nargund G. Quantification of ovarian power Doppler signal with three-dimensional ultrasonography to predict response during in vitro fertilization. Obstet Gynecol. 2003;102:816-22.
37. Lass A, Silye R, Abrams DC, Krausz T, Hovatta O, Margara R, et al. Follicular density in ovarian biopsy of infertile women: a novel method to assess ovarian reserve. Hum Reprod. 1997;12:1028-31.
38. Schmidt KL, Byskov AG, Andersen AN, Müller J, Andersen CY. Density and distribution of primordial follicles in single pieces of cortex from 21 patients and in individual pieces of cortex from three entire human ovaries. Hum Reprod. 2003;18:1158-64.
39. Sharara FI, Scott RT. Assessment of ovarian reserve. Is there still a role for ovarian biopsy? First do no harm! Hum Reprod. 2004;19:470-1.
40. Practice Committee of the American Society for Reproductive Medicine. Testing and interpreting measures of ovarian reserve: a committee opinion. Fertil Steril. 2020;114:1151-7.

CHAPTER 5: Ultrasound in Infertility

Ritu Hinduja, Vaishali Mundhe Akarte

INTRODUCTION

The modality of ultrasound is a useful and a first-line investigation which enables the gynecologist to assess the cause of female infertility and to monitor the progress during treatment. It is safe, noninvasive, inexpensive, radiation free, easily accessible, easy to get trained in, and is repeatable. It has revolutionized the management of infertility and is the most widely method of imaging.[1,2] The recognition as well as evaluation by ultrasound is half the battle done when it comes to the treatment of infertility.

Nevertheless, ultrasound does have its limitations, it is operator dependent, and the diagnosis is only as good as the person who is doing the ultrasound. It does have technical limitations as well like interference due to obesity and failure to visualize Fallopian tubes, broad ligaments, inability to delineate small ovaries, and its inability to obtain images in surgical plane.[1,3] However, the advent of three-dimensional (3D) ultrasonography works like a visual endoscopy and does give us a reliable insight into the pathology that we are dealing with **(Flowchart 1)**.[4]

Flowchart 1: Ultrasound monitoring during treatment.[4]

```
                Ultrasound monitoring
                  during treatment
                    /          \
              Endometrium[4]    Ovary
               /       \           \
      Endometrial   Vascularity   Monitoring of
    thickness/pattern   zone      ovarian response
```

- Trilaminar morphology
- Thickness between 8 and 12 mm

Applebaum scoring
- Zone 1 – Myometrium surrounding the endometrium
- Zone 2 – Hyperechoic endometrial edge
- Zone 3 – Internal endometrial hypoechoic zone
- Zone 4 – Endometrial cavity

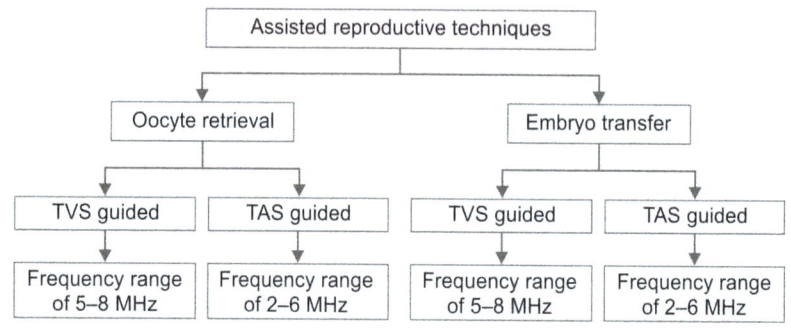

(TAS: transabdominal sonography; TVS: transvaginal sonography)

The field of infertility relies on the access to ultrasound to such a large extent that not only the diagnosis and evaluation is dependent on it but also most of our treatment modalities like oocyte retrieval and embryo transfer are also done under ultrasound guidance **(Flowchart 2)**.[5]

MALE INFERTILITY—WORKUP[6]

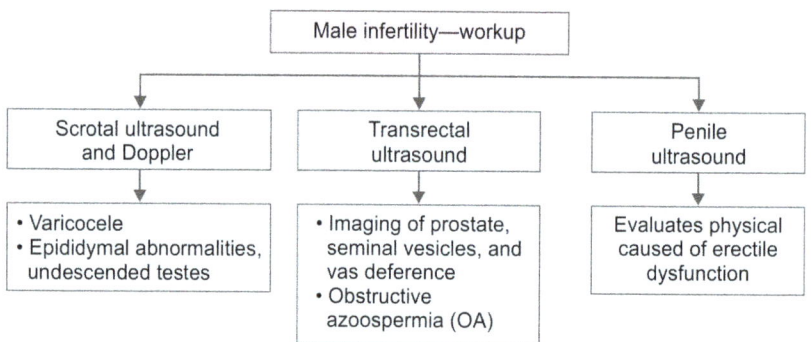

Ultrasound of Ovary

Evaluation of Ovarian Reserve

Antral follicle count: The number of visible ovarian follicles (2–8 mm) on cycle day 2–3 **(Table 1)**.

Follicular Monitoring

Serial ultrasounds done on day 2, 7, and 11 up until the follicle size is 18–20 mm. Follicle grows 2–3 mm/day **(Box 1)**.

Ultrasound in Infertility

TABLE 1: Evaluation of ovarian reserve.

Normal morphology: 2.5–5 cm long, 1.5–3 cm wide, and 0.6–1.5 cm **(Fig. 1)**

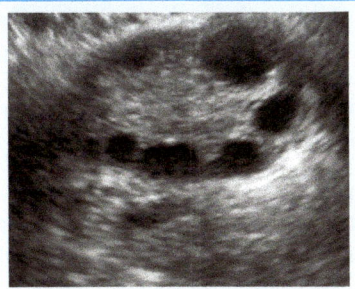

Fig. 1: Normal morphology.

Polycystic morphology:
- Using ultrasound transducers with a frequency >8 MHz, the threshold for PCOM should be a follicle number per ovary ≥18 and/or an ovarian volume >10 mL **(Fig. 2)**
- If using lower resolution ultrasound transducers with a frequency <8 MHz, the threshold for PCOM should be a follicle number per ovary ≥12 and/or an ovarian volume >10 mLl[7]

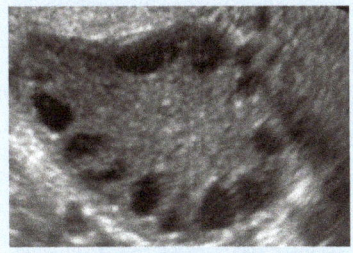

Fig. 2: Polycystic morphology.

Poor ovarian reserve **(Fig. 3)**:
AFC ≤5[8]

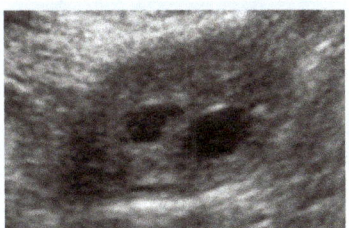

Fig 3: Poor ovarian reserve.

Ultrasonographic (US) features of polycystic ovaries:
- AFC >12–18
- Volume >10 cc
- Longest diameter >3.5 cm
- Predominant, hyperechogenic stroma
  – Intraovarian stromal PSV >10 cm/s (low resistance stromal flow) **(Fig. 4)**
- Stromal area: Ovarian area ratio >0.34
- High uterine artery PI

Note: All these features cannot be seen in all patients.

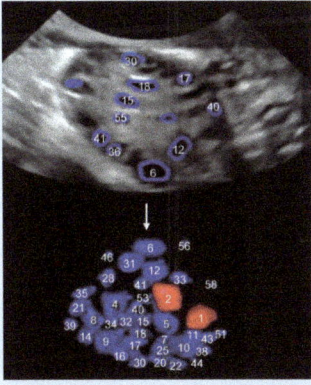

Fig. 4: Ultrasound features of polycystic ovaries.

(AFC: antral follicle count; PCOM: polycystic ovary morphology; PI: pulsatility index; PSV: peak systolic velocity)

> **BOX 1:** Features of mature follicle.
>
> - Rounded 16–18 mm sized
> - A sonolucent halo surrounding follicle (24 hours prior to ovulation)
> - Cumulus oophorus: A small projection from wall in follicular lumen is seen
> - Color Doppler-vascularity surrounding 3/4th of follicular circumference
> - On PD, the RI: 0.4–0.48, PSV >10 cm/s
> - Can wait till 24 mm for optimal flows
> - Perifollicular PSV rises >45 cm/s before an hour of rupture
> - Rising PSV with steady low RI: Close to rupture
> - Rising PSV with rising RI: Proceeding toward LUF[9]
>
> *Signs of rupture*[10,11]
>
> - Disappearance or sudden decrease in follicular size
> - Increased echogenicity inside follicle, indicating corpus luteum formation
> - Free fluid in pelvis (or pouch of Douglas)
> - Replacement of "triple-line appearance" of endometrium by homogenous, hyperechoic "luteinized" endometrium
>
> (LUF: luteinized unruptured follicle; PD: pouch of Douglas; PSV: peak systolic velocity; RI: resistance index)

Ovarian Cyst[12] *(Tables 2 and 3)*

TABLE 2: Nonseptate clear cysts—anechoic clear contents, no vascularity.[12,13]

Simple cyst paraovarian cyst **(Fig. 5)**

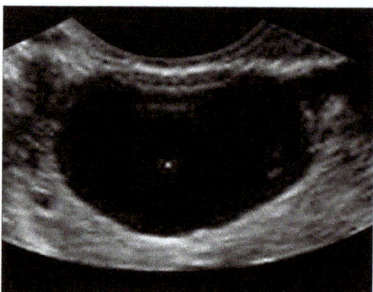

Fig. 5: Simple cyst paraovarian cyst.

Corpus luteum **(Fig. 6)**

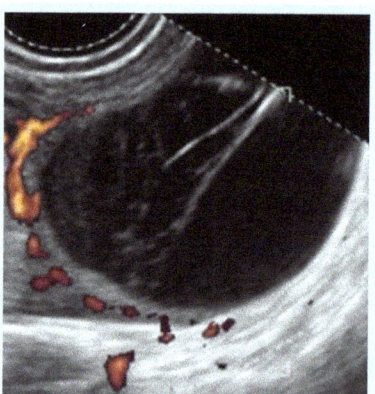

Fig. 6: Corpus luteum.

TABLE 3: Cysts with internal echoes—thick, echogenic wall, and internal echogenicity.[12,13]

Hemorrhagic cyst (Fig. 7):
- Fish net appearance
- Changes echogenicity over time due to fibrinolysis of a clot
- Scanty and high resistance blood flow

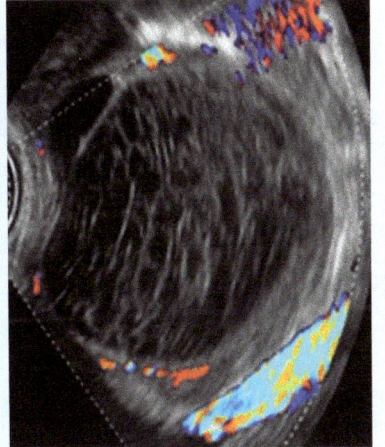

Fig. 7: Hemorrhagic cyst.

Endometrioma (Figs. 8A and B):
- 15% of infertile women
- Thick shaggy walls with or without internal septae
- Internal echogenicities, ground glass appearance, and fluid levels
- Mean gray value cut-off >15.56
- Avascular lesion indicates scarification—to be considered surgical therapy
- Pain on pressure with probe
- Bilateral in 1/3rd cases
- Streaming sign +

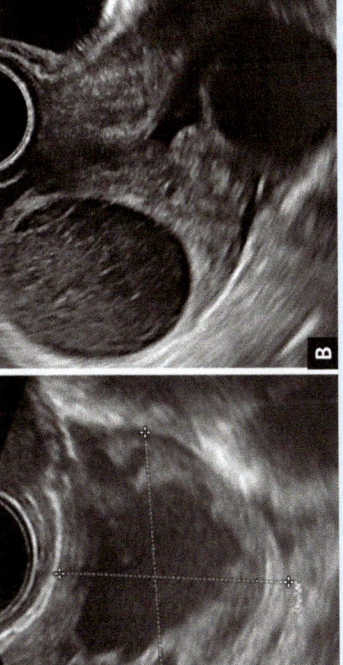

Figs. 8A and B: Endometrioma.

Ultrasound of Uterus (Box 2)

BOX 2: Ultrasound of uterus.[9,14,15]

*Baseline scan of uterus (**Fig. 9**):*
- Assess endocervical (EC) length: In longitudinal section of uterus measure EC length from fundal end of endometrium to external os
- Also known as functional/physiological uterocervical length
- Subendometrial flow on D2 indicates a low receptive endometrium
- Uterine artery RI >0.78 indicates that high doses of stimulation will be needed for endometrial maturation

(RI: resistance index)

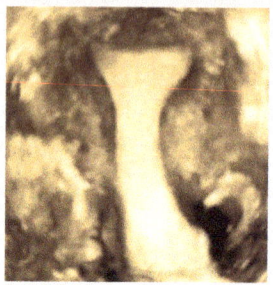

Fig. 9: Baseline scan of uterus.

Congenital Causes of Uterine Abnormalities[16] (Tables 4A and B)

- Incidence: 0.1–3.8%
- Infertile couples: 6.7%

TABLE 4A: Congenital causes of uterine abnormalities.

A. Failure of one or more Müllerian duct to develop or canalize	*Aplasia/hypoplasia of uterus (**Fig. 10**):* • Normal uterine body to cervix ratio 2:1 • Infantile type uterus 1:1 • Very small uterine cavity with long cervix

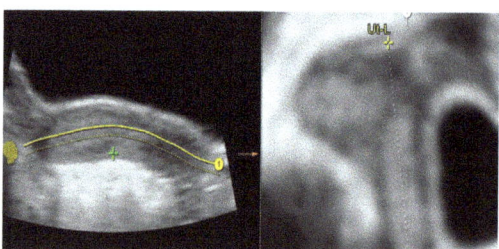

Fig. 10: Aplasia/hypoplasia of uterus.

*Unicornuate uterus (**Fig. 11**):*
- Uterus is not in midline
- Normal shape in long section
- One cornual projection
- Only one uterine artery
- 3D: Banana-shaped uterine cavity

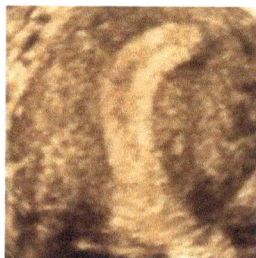

Fig. 11: Unicornuate uterus.

Contd...

Contd...

B. Failure to fuse or abnormal fusion	*Uterus didelphys (Fig. 12):*
	• Two separate uteri and cervix
	• Uteri are seen in midline or on lateral pelvic wall as two well-developed uterine structure
	• On transverse section, both uterine horns make a figure of eight
	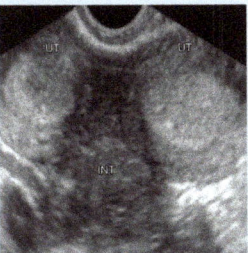
	Fig. 12: Uterus didelphys.
	
	Bicornuate uterus (Fig. 13):
	• Two separate uterine bodies and a single cervix
	• On transverse section widened fundus and division of endometrial cavity toward fundus
	  – Volume US:
	    - Fundus shows dimple
	    - Distance between the line joining the endometrial tips and the fundal dimple is <5 mm
	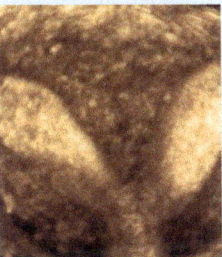
	Fig. 13: Bicornuate uterus.

C. Failure of resorption of midline septum	*Septate uterus (Fig. 14):* • Flat or convex external contour • Acute angle between endometrial cavities • Distance between line joining the tips of endocavity to the deepest point between the two cavities: >10 mm 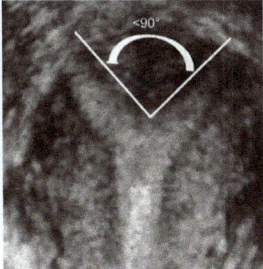 **Fig. 14:** Septate uterus.

Contd...

Contd...

Arcuate uterus **(Fig. 15)**:
- Convex external contour
- Obtuse angle between cavities
- Distance between line joining the tips of endocavity to the deepest point between the two cavities: <10 mm

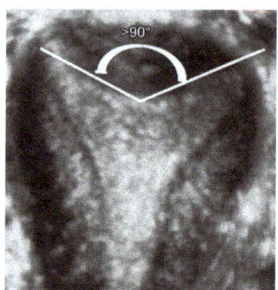

Fig. 15: Arcuate uterus.

TABLE 4B: Difference between septate and bicornuate uterus.

Septate uterus **(Fig. 16)**:
- Fundus: No dimple
- >5 mm uterine wall above the line joining tips of 2 uterine cavity
- Angle between 2 cavities <90°
- Medial margins of end cavity: Straight

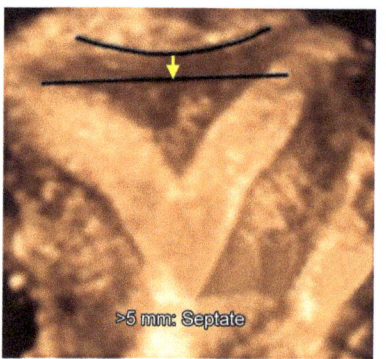

Fig. 16: Septate uterus.

Bicornuate uterus **(Fig. 17)**:
- Fundus-dimple
- <5 mm uterine wall above the line joining tips of 2 uterine cavity
- Angle between 2 cavities >90°
- Medial margins of endocavity: Convex

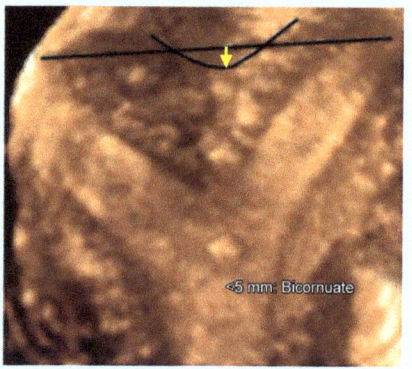

Fig. 17: Bicornuate uterus.

Acquired Causes of Uterine Abnormalities (Table 5)
Endometrial lesions

TABLE 5: Acquired causes of uterine abnormalities.

Endometritis **(Fig. 18):** Thick isoechoic endometrium with altered junctional zone, minimal fluid in endometrial cavity and altered vascularity	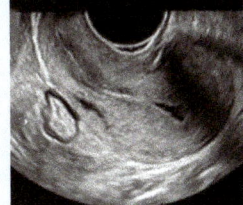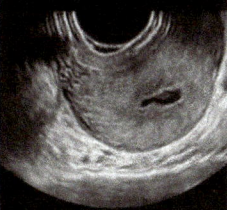 **Fig. 18:** Endometritis.
Endometrial hyperplasia **(Fig. 19):** • Localized overgrowth of endometrium—normal histology • Thick echogenic endometrium in part or entirely • ET >14 mm premenopausal and >5 mm in postmenopausal is hypertrophic. • ET is maintained and on Doppler shows regularly placed vessels	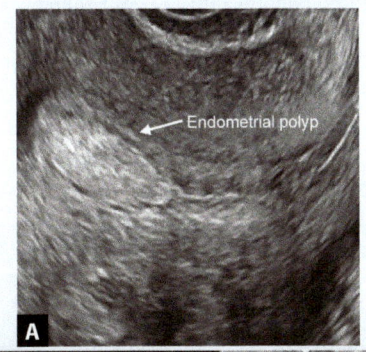 **Fig. 19:** Endometrial hyperplasia.
Polyp[17] **(Figs. 20A and B):** • May appear as just diffusely thickened endometrium, without visualization of discrete mass (mimics endometrial hyperplasia) • A feeding vessel may be seen extending to polyp on color Doppler imaging	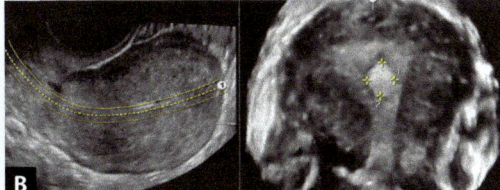 **Figs. 20A and B:** Polyp.

Contd...

Contd...

Synechiae[18] (Fig. 21):
- Hyperechoic bands traversing through the endometrial cavity due to infection/surgical results
- In thick synechiae, 3D US can be used for exact assessment of restriction of endometrial cavity. Sonohysterography 100% sensitive

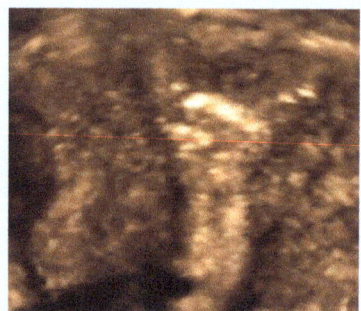

Fig. 21: Synechiae.

Submucous fibroid (Fig. 22):
- Grading (ESGE classification):
  - T0: Whole in endometrial cavity
  - T1: >50% in endometrial cavity
  - T2: <50% in endometrial cavity

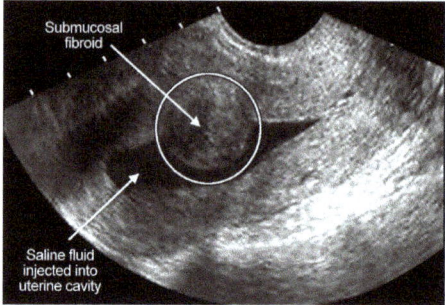

Fig. 22: Submucous fibroid.

Sonohysterography:
- 100% sensitive for differentiation of endometrial pathologies
- Lithotomy
- 6 Fr Foley's placed in cx
- Distended balloon with 1.5–2 mL fluid
- Slowly inject 5 mL of NS to distend uterine cavity
- Introduce TV probe in vagina with catheter in situ
- Endometrial lesions like synechiae, polyp will be easily seen

(ESGE: European Society of Gastrointestinal Endoscopy; ET: endometrial thickness)

Myometrial lesions (Table 6)

TABLE 6: Myometrial lesions.

Fibroid[19] (Fig. 23):
- Well-defined, hypoechoic, homogeneous, rounded lesions with peripheral hypoechoic rim
- Enlargement of the uterus and distortion of the contour
- Sometimes heterogeneity due to degeneration or calcification
- *Power Doppler: Peripheral vascularity*

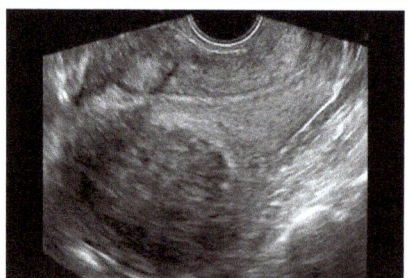

Fig. 23: Fibroid.

Contd...

Contd...

Adenomyoma/adenomyosis[20] (Fig. 24):
- Altered hyper- and hypoechoic zones—*Swiss cheese appearance*
- Generalized involving the whole uterus or localized to one portion (adenomyoma)
- *Power Doppler: Penetrating vascularity*

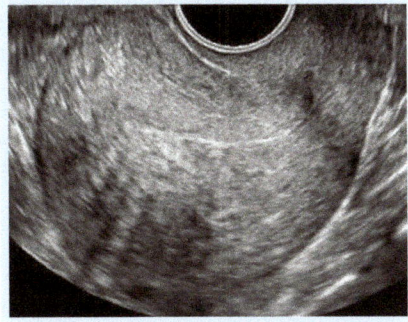

Fig. 24: Adenomyoma/adenomyosis.

Cervical lesions: Cervical malignancies.

Ultrasounds of Adnexal Diseases[21,22] (Table 7)

TABLE 7: Ultrasound of adnexal diseases.	
Ovarian lesions[21]	**Tubal lesions[22]**
Hydrosalpinx: • Fusiform cystic lesion • Cog wheel sign • Incomplete septae	Pelvic inflammatory disease (PID), cysts, and fibroids: • *Sonosalpingography:* To check for turbulence at the fimbrial end • String of pearl appearance • Waterfall sign

REFERENCES

1. Padubidri VG, Daftary SN. The pathology of conception. In: Padubidri VG, Daftary SN (Eds). Howkins and Bourne Shaw's Textbook of Gynaecology, 13th edition. New Delhi: Elsevier; 2004. pp. 194-216.
2. Adekunle RA. Gynaecological Anatomy. In: Arulkumaran S, Synmonds IM, Fowlie A (Eds). Oxford Handbook of Obstetrics and Gynaecology, 1st edition. New Delhi: Oxford University Press; 2004. pp. 453-8.
3. Rastogi R. Role of imaging in female infertility (Dr. K.M Rai Memorial Oration Award). Indian J Radiol Imaging. 2010;20(3):168-73.
4. Stimou S, Taheri H, Saadi H, Mimouni A. Place de l´échographieendovaginale dans l´exploration de l´infertilitéd´origineendométriale [The role of transvaginal ultrasound in the evaluation of endometrial infertility]. Pan Afr Med J. 2020;37:92.
5. The European Society of Human Reproduction and Embryology (ESHRE). (2019). Ultrasound: Oocyte Pick Up. Recommendations of the European Society of Human Reproduction and Embryology. [online] Available from https://www.google.com/url?sa= t&rct=j&q=&esrc=s&source=web&cd=&cad=rja&uact=8&ved= 2ahUKEwiC1q6f7pHwAhUgyDgGHYSbBiwQFjADegQIFBAD&url=https%3A%2F%2Fwww.eshre.eu%2F-%2Fmedia%2Fsitecore-files%2FGuidelines %2FUSS%2F Recommendations-for-good-practice-in-Ultrasound_062019.pdf%3Fla%3Den%26h ash%3D0D22FB08F742DDFC24C29AE1649FFD8720972621&usg=AOvVaw2W93wF y0gin2qwtU-VqCSN [Last accessed April, 2022].
6. Sihag P, Tandon A, Pal R, Jain BK, Bhatt S, Kaur S, et al. Sonography in male infertility: a look beyond the obvious. J Ultrasound. 2018;21(3):265-76.

7. European Society of Human Reproduction and Embryology. (2018). International Evidence-based Guideline for the Assessment and Management of Polycystic Ovary Syndrome (PCOS). [online] Available from https://www.eshre.eu/Guidelines-and-Legal/Guidelines/Polycystic-Ovary-Syndrome [Last accessed April, 2022].
8. Esteves SC, Alviggi C, Humaidan P, Fischer R, Andersen CY, Conforti A, et al. The POSEIDON Criteria and Its Measure of Success Through the Eyes of Clinicians and Embryologists. Front Endocrinol (Lausanne). 2019;10:814.
9. Bassil S, Magritte JP, Roth J, Nisolle M, Donnez J, Gordts S. Uterine vascularity during stimulation and its correlation with implantation in in-vitro fertilization. Hum Reprod. 1995;10(6):1497-501.
10. Matijevic R, Grgic O. Predictive values of ultrasound monitoring of the menstrual cycle. Curr Opin Obstet Gynecol. 2005;17(4):405-10.
11. Young JR, Jaffe RB. Strength-duration characteristics of estrogen effects on gonadotropin response to gonadotropin-releasing hormone in women. II. Effects of varying concentrations of estradiol. J Clin Endocrinol Metab. 1976;42(3):432-42.
12. Sayasneh A, Ekechi C, Ferrara L, Kaijser J, Stalder C, Sur S, et al. The characteristic ultrasound features of specific types of ovarian pathology (review). Int J Oncol. 2015;46(2):445-58.
13. Grabosch SM. (2018). Ovarian cysts workup. [online] Available from https://emedicine.medscape.com/article/255865-workup#c9 [Last accessed April, 2020].
14. Adibi A, Khadem M, Mardanian F, Hovsepian S. Uterine and arcuate arteries blood flow for predicting of ongoing pregnancy in in vitro fertilization. J Res Med Sci. 2015;20(9):879-84.
15. Silva Martins R, Helio Oliani A, Vaz Oliani D, Martinez de Oliveira J. Subendometrial resistance and pulsatility index assessment of endometrial receptivity in assisted reproductive technology cycles. Reprod Biol Endocrinol. 2019;17(1):62.
16. Caballero O, Bonilla F, Bonilla-Musoles F, Martin N, Esquembre MP, Castillo JC, et al. Uterine Malformations: Diagnosis with 3D-4D Ultrasound. Donald School J Ultrasound Obstet Gynecol. 2015;9(2):123-48.
17. Kamaya A, Yu PC, Lloyd CR, Chen BH, Desser TS, Maturen KE. Sonographic Evaluation for Endometrial Polyps: The Interrupted Mucosa Sign. J Ultrasound Med. 2016;35(11):2381-7.
18. Manchanda R, Rathore A. Intrauterine adhesions: Classification systems. In: Manchanda R, Rathore A (Eds). Intra Uterine Adhesions. Singapore: Springer Nature; 2021. pp. 21-32.
19. Wilde S, Scott-Barrett S. Radiological appearances of uterine fibroids. Indian J Radiol Imaging. 2009;19(3):222-31.
20. Cunningham RK, Horrow MM, Smith RJ, Springer J. Adenomyosis: A Sonographic Diagnosis. Radiographics. 2018;38(5):1576-89.
21. Benjaminov O, Atri M. Sonography of the Abnormal Fallopian Tube. AJR Am J Roentgenol. 2004;183(3):737-42.
22. Inki P, Palo P, Anttila L. Vaginal sonosalpingography in the evaluation of tubal patency. Acta Obstet Gynecol Scand. 1998;77(10):978-82.

6. Hysterolaparoscopy in Infertility

Parul Saoji, Chaitanya Shembekar

INTRODUCTION

To begin with laparoscopy was majorly done for the diagnosis of cause of infertility but in last one decade laparoscopy has been used to not only diagnose but also treat the various causes such as endometriosis, pelvic adhesions, and myomas. Laparoscopy helps in diagnosing the cause of infertility and hence in management of infertility.

In most of the cases of infertility, laparoscopy proves to be the final step in the line of investigation and management. It has been observed up to 50% infertile women have unsuspected pelvic pathology when they undergo laparoscopy.

According to many studies which have been published there is not one single noninvasive way of testing and predicting root cause and the existence of pelvic pathology and many factors are taken into consideration before suggesting and subjecting a patient for laparoscopy.

The indications for laparoscopy are any patient with probable risk factors, suspicious findings on pelvic examination or on hysterosalpingography (HSG) and unexplained infertility. The outcome of any infertility treatment is dependent on determinants such as age, duration of infertility so early diagnosis and timely intervention are mandatory for success.

As per the changing trends it is always hysterolaparoscopy, i.e., hysteroscopy followed by laparoscopy.

POLYCYSTIC OVARY SYNDROME

When to do laparoscopy in patients of polycystic ovary syndrome (PCOS)—is a question always?

Laparoscopy in PCOS patient having anovulation should be considered as first line of management for tubal patency in cases of suspected pelvic pathology such as tuberculosis (TB), pelvic inflammatory disease (PID) or in cases of endometriosis according to guidelines. Laparoscopic ovarian drilling (LOD) should be second line of management in cases of clomiphene citrate (cc)-resistant PCOS cases.

Laparoscopic ovarian drilling has certain advantages over gonadotropins usage being it results in monofollicular growth and risk for ovarian hyperstimulation syndrome (OHSS) is less. It is good for lean and thin PCOS with high luteinizing hormone (LH).

ECTOPIC PREGNANCY

The treatment modality is dependent on clinical condition of the patient, location of ectopic and also the desire for future pregnancies. Salpingectomy is the treatment of choice but other modalities such as salpingostomy, segmental resection and milking can be offered. Vermesh and coworkers demonstrated decreased hospitalization stay and cost in the laparoscopy group. In a prospective randomized trial comparing laparoscopy and laparotomy, Lundorff and coworkers in a randomized controlled trial (RCT) emphasized the importance of laparoscopy. In the laparoscopy group, the formation of peritubal adhesions was reduced with tubal patency rates comparable with those found in laparotomy.

Laparoscopy is definitely a wonderful choice though it requires surgical expertise and equipment.

ENDOMETRIOSIS

Endometriosis displays in many forms such as powder burn spots to large ovarian cysts, fulguration, excision can be done for patients with mild endometriosis. Depending on symptoms and location of endometriosis various surgeries can be done like adhesiolysis to ovarian cystectomy, resection and exploration of bowel, etc.

According to European Society of Human Reproduction and Embryology (ESHRE) guidelines, American Fertility Society (AFS) stage I/II should have operative laparoscopy rather than just diagnostic laparoscopy. According to ESHRE guidelines, there is no role of surgery prior to the in vitro fertilization (IVF) treatment for endometriomas >3 cm. The only reason why one should operate these endometriomas is to relieve the pain or to makes the ovaries and the follicles more accessible. Also the counseling is very important that after ovarian cystectomy the ovarian reserve also reduces. Drainage of cysts is responsible for 20% recurrence while it is 12% when cyst wall stripping is done.

For times immemorial laparotomy was offered to patients suffering from endometriosis but recent studies prove that laparoscopy can be offered to even in advanced stages.

According to 2022 ESHRE guidelines, laparoscopy is no longer the diagnostic gold standard and is only recommended in patients with negative imaging results and/or where empirical treatment was unsuccessful or inappropriate.

Endometriosis fertility index is one more step added in the treatment as it can support decision making for the most appropriate option to achieve pregnancy postsurgery.

As per the guidelines, the surgery is strongly recommended for patients having endometriosis associated pain. Cystectomy should be performed instead of drainage and coagulation. Also minimum ovarian damage should be kept in mind.

Center of expertise should be approached for deep infiltrating endometriosis and also surgeons should know where to have multidisciplinary approach.

PELVIC ADHESIONS

Preoperatively, diagnosis of pelvic adhesions is not difficult. Many times in HSG such pictures appear which may give an idea but are inconclusive and also at times there is a chance of not being able to anticipate the pelvic adhesions in view of negative history and physical examination findings.

Thus, laparoscopy is an important tool in detection of pelvic adhesions.

Pelvic adhesions usually impair fertility by disrupting the tubo-ovarian anatomy due to which ovum pick up, transport and fertilization is difficult.

To prove the importance of adhesioslysis in infertility cases, Tulandi and colleagues compared pregnancy outcome in women with periadnexal adhesions with and without laparotomy. After 2 years of follow-up, 45% of the treated group conceived compared with 16% in the untreated group. Many studies have been done to prove that adhesiolysis during surgeries is beneficial and helps in patients to conceive.

Based on results in animal many studies have been performed on animals and have shown less adhesion formation post laparoscopic surgeries. Although early studies in humans suggested superior results with laparoscopy, but latest work suggest equivalent pregnancy rates post laparoscopy or laparotomy ranging from 50 to 75%.

Postadhesiolysis adhesion reformation is the major concern and problem. A second look multicenter trial was performed in which 95% patients redeveloped adhesions and ovary being the most vulnerable sites being about 80%.

OVARIAN CYSTS

Ovarian cysts can be responsible for the infertility in women. One has to be very cautious when it comes to cystectomy. What is the role of cystectomy in patients with benign ovarian cysts and their outcome on pregnancy.

It has been noted that ovarian reserve reduces after the ovarian surgery and it has negative impact on infertility treatments and outcome.

Dermoid cysts: These do not have a negative impact on ovarian reserve up to 6 cm size. A Korean study also advocates that excision or no excision has no impact on anti-Müllerian hormone (AMH) levels.

Usually for the dermoids of size 4–6 cm the medium size ones need not to be removed and a careful follow-up is to be done as the growth of dermoid cysts is very slow, i.e., 1.7–1.8 mm/year.

If you have the opinion of removal of dermoid cysts then few things to keep in mind is that your approach should be laparoscopic cystectomy with minimum use of cautery that too it should be bipolar. There is no role of aspiration of dermoid cyst and the retrieval should be in bag. Even if we see no parenchyma after the cystectomy over a period of 6 months we will be able to notice that.

TUBAL BLOCK

Any insult to the distal oviduct results in complete or partial occlusion of tube which can be treated by microsurgical repair procedures resulting in 40% pregnancy rates. Due to lower fecundity rate these procedures are offered only to young patients.

Laparoscopic microsurgical techniques are better compared to laparotomy on the grounds of pregnancy rate, the expenditures, hospital stay, and recovery period postsurgery. Although not many studies have been published regarding the same so the most definitive treatment to treat distal tubal block remains an enigma.

Hydrosalpinges removal does improve the IVF success rates. As per the studies which are published improvement in pregnancy rates and implantation rates are seen.

FIBROIDS

Laparoscopic myomectomy is one of the finest surgeries which require a lot of acumen and surgical skill. It was started somewhere in 1980s. Myomectomy serves best for serosal or solitary intramural fibroid.

Laparoscopy myomectomy is associated with better outcome, short hospital stay and early resumption of activities.

Some studies and cases have been reported of uterine rupture after the laparoscopic myomectomy probably due to single layer closure. Adhesion formation is also observed following laparoscopy, but the degree of adhesions may be less compared to the abdominal myomectomies.

According to the guidelines, all submucous fibroids should be removed. No need to remove subserosal fibroids and for intramural fibroids >4 cm and affecting endomyometrial junction should be removed.

It is a boon for all the laparoscopic surgeons to do laparoscopic myomectomy especially when traditional way of dealing with them would not benefit the problem of infertility.

LOW OVARIAN RESERVE

In cases with low ovarian reserve, laparoscopic platelet-rich plasma (PRP) instillation can be done in both the ovaries and reassessment of the AMH levels can be done after 3 months.

HYSTEROSCOPY IN INFERTILITY

Infertility evaluation includes the following:
- Evaluation of cervical canal
- Endocervical canal
- Fallopian tubes
- Uterine cavity.

There are various methods to do the same such as HSG, endometrial biopsy but these techniques are associated with many drawbacks and thus necessitating the need for visualization of cervix, endocervical canal and uterine cavity.

Uterine pathologies such as submucous leiomyomas, intrauterine adhesions, tubal occlusions get benefitted from hysteroscopy.

The best time to do hysteroscopy is during the early follicular phase to avoid excess endometrium/debris, which hampers the proper visualization of the cavity.

Hysteroscopy offers to see and treat the pathology in contrary to HSG where the false positive rates are also very high.

Indications for hysteroscopy are:
- Abnormal HSG
- Abnormal uterine bleeding (AUB)
- Suspected intrauterine pathology
- Uterine anomalies
- Uterine infections (UI)
- Polyps
- Intrauterine adhesions
- Thin endometrium
- Misplaced or embedded foreign body
- Tubal cannulation.

The office hysteroscopy makes it possible for intruding the scope without any trauma or dilatation and also places such as endocervical canal and stenosis at internal os, cornual regions and uterotubal junction can be visualized.

Instruments can be guided visually and targeted to areas in the uterine cavity in need of treatment for uterine septa, intrauterine adhesions, polyps and submucous myomas, and tubal cornual occlusions.

Uterine Septa

It is responsible for 25% uterine anomalies. Earlier abdominal surgeries were performed for the same such as Jones and Tompkins metroplasty but due to advancement and introduction of hysteroscopy transcervically we can perform these surgeries.

Hysteroscopic scissors are used for the same and post procedure patient is given estrogen in doses of 1 tablet twice a day for 21 days.

Alternatively resectoscope can also be used where there is thick septum and bleeding is anticipated. Lasers with fiberoptic cables can also be used in cases of difficult dilatation and small size uterus.

Intrauterine Adhesions

Asherman's syndrome resulting in menstrual abnormalities and infertility can be treated hysteroscopically using a scissors and supplementing the further cycles with estrogen and progesterone. Many a times two-stage surgeries are required for extensive and dense adhesions.

Polyps and Submucous Leiomyoma

Submucous fibroids are known to symptomatic and cause excess bleeding. Hysteroscopic removal is warranted. Newer techniques of removing these fibroids laparoscopically are also being advocated due to advancement of 3D scans and USG machines, prior mapping. New guidelines advocate no change in pregnancy rates even if the cavity is opened so this new modality is picking up if the surgeons have the expertise and avoid all the hysteroscopic side effects.

TUBAL CORNUAL OCCLUSION

Many a times patients have a mucous plug, debris which occludes the tubal lumen or tubal spasms which give false results during HSG. Better catheters have come up which are soft, flexible, thin making tubal cannulation a safe and easy procedure. The wire guide is passed into the tubal lumen and the 3-French catheter then is guided over the guide wire, bypassing the intramural portion; the guide wire is removed and methylene is injected directly through the 3-French catheter.

Impacted and Misplaced Intrauterine Foreign Bodies

Hysteroscopy aids in the proper visualized of impacted foreign bodies or misplaced ones such as Cu-T which interfere with the fertility. Also the bony fragments of previous 1st or 2nd trimester abortion may also remain in the cavity and cause osseous metaplasia acting as a source. Blind removal is difficult. Hysteroscopy preceded by USG finding can be really useful in the correct visualized and depth of penetration if any in these patients.

Hysteroscopy as Pre-IVF Treatment

Many studies show that pre-IVF hysteroscopy is a must and increases the chances of conception.

Also if there is recurrent implantation failures/*thin endometrium* hysteroscopic instillation of PRP is done into the subendometrial zone resulting in better implantation rates and also better endometrium with good vascularity.

SUGGESTED READING

1. Adamson GD, Pasta DJ. Surgical treatment of endometriosis-associated infertility: meta-analysis compared with survival analysis. Am J Obstet Gynecol. 1994;171(6):1488-504.
2. Bateman BG, Kolp LA, Mills S. Endoscopic versus laparotomy management of endometriomas. Fertil Steril. 1994;62(4):690-5.
3. Blazar AS, Alexander K, Seifer DB. Absence of an effect of hydrosalpinx on pregnancy rate in vitro fertilization In: Blazar AS (Ed). 51st Annual Meeting of the American Fertility Society. Seattle, Washington: American Society for Reproductive Medicine; 1995.
4. Boyd IE, Holt EM. Tubal sterility: patency tests and results of operation. J Obstet Gynecol Br Commw. 1973;80:142-51.
5. Bronson RA, Wallach EE. Lysis of periadnexal adhesions for correction of infertility. Fertil Steril. 1977;28(6):613-9.
6. Brosens IA, Ballaer PV, Puttemans P, Deprest J. Reconstruction of the ovary containing large endometriomas by an extraovarian endosurgical technique. Fertil Steril. 1996;66(4):517-21.
7. Buttram VC Jr. Conservative surgery for endometriosis in the infertile female: a study of 206 patients with implications for both medical and surgical therapy. Fertil Steril. 1979;31(2):117-23.
8. Canis M, Mage G, Pouly JL, Manhes H, Wattiez A, Bruhat MA. Laparoscopic distal tuboplasty: report of 87 cases and a 4-year experience. Fertil Steril. 1991;56(4):616-21.
9. Canis M, Mages G, Manhes H. Laparoscopic treatment of endometriosis. Acta Obstet Gynecol Scand. 1989;150:15-20.
10. Centers for Disease Control and Prevention. Ectopic pregnancy. MMWR Morb Mortal Wkly Rep. 1995;44(3):46-8.
11. Chong AP, Keene ME, Thornton NL. Comparison of three modes of treatment for infertility patients with minimal pelvic endometriosis. Fertil Steril. 1990;53(3):407-10.
12. Crist T, Hulka JF, Williams P, Lee SH. Laparoscopic clip sterilization in a free-standing facility: an evaluation of cost and safety. NC Med J. 1983;44(9):546-9.
13. Crosignani PG, Vercellini P, Biffignandi F, Costantini W, Cortesi I, Imparato E. Laparoscopy versus laparotomy in conservative surgical treatment for severe endometriosis. Fertil Steril. 1996;66(5):706-11.
14. DeCherney A, Kase N. The conservative surgical management of unruptured ectopic pregnancy. Obstet Gynecol. 1979;54(4):451-5.
15. DeCherney AH, Diamond MP. Laparoscopic salpingostomy for ectopic pregnancy. Obstet Gynecol. 1987;70(6):948-50.
16. DeCherney AS, Boyers SP. Isthmic ectopic pregnancy: segmental resection as a treatment of choice. Fertil Steril. 1985;44(3):307-12.
17. Diamond E. Lysis of postoperative pelvic adhesions in infertility. Fertil Steril. 1979;31(3):287-95.
18. Donnez J, Nisolle M, Casanas-Roux F. CO_2 laser laparoscopy in infertile women with adnexal adhesions and women with tubal occlusion. J Gynecol Surg. 1989;5:47-53.

19. Dubuisson JB, Chavet X, Chapron C, Gregorakis SS, Morice P. Uterine rupture during pregnancy after laparoscopic myomectomy. Hum Reprod. 1995;10(6):1475-7.
20. Dubuisson JB, Joliniere JB, Aubriot FX, Daraï E, Foulot H, Mandelbrot L. Terminal tuboplasties by laparoscopy: 65 consecutive cases. Fertil Steril. 1990;54(3):401-3.
21. Fayez JA, Clark RR. Operative laparoscopy for the treatment of localized chronic pelvic-abdominal pain caused by postoperative adhesions. J Gynecol Surg. 1994;10(2):79-83.
22. Fayez JA, Collazo LM, Vernon C. Comparison of different modalities for treatment of minimal and mild endometriosis. Am J Obstet Gynecol. 1988;159(4):927-32.
23. Fayez JA, Collazo LM. Comparison between laparotomy and operative laparoscopy in the treatment of moderate and severe stages of endometriosis. Int J Fertil. 1990;35(5):272-9.
24. Gant NF. Infertility and endometriosis: comparison of pregnancy outcomes with laparotomy versus laparoscopic techniques. Am J Obstet Gynecol. 1992;166(4):1072-81.
25. Gomel V. Salpingostomy by laparoscopy. J Reprod Med. 1977;18(5):265-8.
26. Harris WJ. Uterine dehiscence following laparoscopic myomectomy. Obstet Gynecol. 1992;80(3 Pt 2):545-6.
27. Hulka JF, Fishburne JI, Mercer JP, Kumarasamy T, Omran KF, Phillips Jr JM, et al. Laparoscopic sterilization with a spring clip: a report of the first fifty cases. Am J Obstet Gynecol. 1973;116:715-20.
28. Jarvinen PA, Nummi S, Pietila K. Conservative operative treatment of tubal pregnancy with postoperative daily hydrotubation. Acta Obstet Gynecol Scand. 1972;51(2):169-70.
29. Lessey BA, Castelbaum AJ, Riben M. Effect of hydrosalpinges on markers of uterine receptivity and success in IVF. Presented at the 50th annual meeting of the American Fertility Society 1994. Seattle, Washington: American Fertility Society, program supplement; 1994:S45.
30. Levinson CJ. Endometriosis therapy: Rationale for expectant or minimal therapy in minimal/mild cases (AFSI). In: Levinson CJ (Ed). Proceedings of the Second World Congress on Gynecologic Endoscopy. France: Clermont-Ferrand; 1989.
31. Levy MJ, Murray D, Sagoskin A. The adverse effect of hydrosalpinges on IVF success rates are reversed equally well by salpingectomy, proximal tubal occlusion and neosalpingostomy. Presented at the meeting of the American Society for Reproductive Medicine 1996. Seattle, Washington: American Society for Reproductive Medicine, program supplement; 1996:S64.
32. Luciano AA, Maier DB, Koch EI, Nulsen JC, Whitman GF. A comparative study of postoperative adhesions following laser surgery by laparoscopy versus laparotomy in the rabbit model. Obstet Gynecol. 1989;74(2):220-4.
33. Lundorff P, Thorburn J, Hahlin M, Källfelt B, Lindblom B. Adhesion formation after laparoscopic surgery in tubal pregnancy: a randomized trial versus laparotomy. Fertil Steril. 1991;55(5):911-5.
34. Mage G, Pouly JL, Joliniere JB, Chabrand S, Riouallon A, Bruhat MA. A preoperative classification to predict the intrauterine and ectopic pregnancy rates after distal tubal microsurgery. Fertil Steril. 1986;46(5):807-10.
35. Marcoux S, Maheux R, Bérubé S. Laparoscopic surgery in infertile women with minimal or mild endometriosis. Canadian Collaborative Group on Endometriosis. N Engl J Med. 1997;337(4):217-22.
36. Martin DC, Hubert GD, Vander Zwaag R, el-Zeky FA. Laparoscopic appearances of peritoneal endometriosis. Fertil Steril. 1989;51(1):63-7.
37. McCausland A. Endosalpingosis ("endosalpingoblastosis") following laparoscopic tubal coagulation as an ectopic factor of ectopic pregnancy. Am J Obstet Gynecol. 1982;143(1):12-24.

38. Mettler L, Ironi S, Kapamadzija A, Semm K. Pelviscopic tubal surgery: the acceptable vogue. Hum Reprod. 1990;5(8):971-4.
39. Murphy AA, Schlaff WD, Hassiakos D, Durmusoglu F, Damewood MD, Rock JA. Laparoscopic cautery in the treatment of endometriosis related infertility. Fertil Steril. 1991;55(2):246-51.
40. Murray DL, Sagoskin AW, Widra EA, Levy MJ. The adverse effect of hydrosalpinges on in vitro fertilization pregnancy rates and the benefit of surgical correction. Fertil Steril. 1998;69(1):41-5.
41. Nezhat C, Crowgey S, Nezhat F. Videolaseroscopy for the treatment of endometriosis associated with infertility. Fertil Steril. 1989;51(2):237-40.
42. Olive DL, Lee KL. Analysis of sequential treatment protocols for endometriosis-associated infertility. Am J Obstet Gynecol. 1986;154(3):613-9.
43. Operative Laparoscopy Study Group: Postoperative adhesion development after operative laparoscopy: evaluation at early second-look procedures. Operative Laparoscopy Study Group. Fertil Steril. 1991;55(4):700-4.
44. Opsahl MS, Miller B, Klein TA. The predictive value of hysterosalpingography for tubal and peritoneal factors. Fertil Steril. 1993;60(3):444-8.
45. Paulson JD, Asmar P, Saffan DS. Mild and moderate endometriosis: comparison of treatment modalities for infertile couples. J Reprod Med. 1991;36(3):151-5.
46. Portuondo JA, Irala JP, Ibanez E, Echanojauregui AD. Clinical selection of infertile patients for laparoscopy. Int J Fertil. 1984;29(4):234-8.
47. Pouly JL, Mahnes H, Mage G, Canis M, Bruhat MA. Conservative laparoscopic treatment of 321 ectopic pregnancies. Fertil Steril. 1986;46(6):1093-7.
48. Reich H. Laparoscopic treatment of extensive pelvic adhesions, including hydrosalpinx. J Reprod Med. 1987;32(10):736-42.
49. Rock JA, Guzick DS, Sergos C, Schweditsch M, Sapp KC, Jones HW Jr. The conservative surgical treatment of endometriosis: evaluation of pregnancy success with respect to extent of disease as categorized using contemporary classification systems. Fertil Steril. 1981;35(2):131-7.
50. Saravelos HG, Li TC, Cooke ID. An analysis of the outcome of microsurgical and laparoscopic adhesiolysis for infertility. Hum Reprod. 1995;10(11):2887-94.
51. Seiler JC, Gidwani G, Ballard L. Laparoscopic cauterization of endometriosis for infertility: a controlled study. Fertil Steril. 1986;46(6):1098-100.
52. Semm K, Mettler L. Technical progress in pelvic surgery via operative laparoscopy. Am J Obstet Gynecol. 1980;138(2):121-7.
53. Shelton KE, Butler L, Toner JP, Oehninger S, Muasher SJ. Salpingectomy improves the pregnancy rate in in-vitro fertilization patients with hydrosalpinx. Hum Reprod. 1996;11(3):523-5.
54. Skulj V, Pavlic Z, Stoiljkovic C, Bacic G, Drazancicstoalkovic A. Conservative operative treatment of tubal pregnancy. Fertil Steril. 1967;15:634-9.
55. Stangel JJ, Gomel V. Techniques in conservative surgery for tubal gestation. Clin Obstet Gynecol. 1985;23:1221.
56. Stovall TG, Elder RF, Ling FW. Predictors of pelvic adhesions. J Reprod Med. 1989;34(5):345-8.
57. Sutton C, Hill D. Laser laparoscopy in the treatment of endometriosis: a 5-year study. Br J Obstet Gynecol. 1990;97(2):181-5.
58. Swart P, Mol BW, van der Veen F, van Beurden M, Redekop WK, Bossuyt PM. The accuracy of hysterosalpingography in the diagnosis of tubal pathology: a meta-analysis. Fertil Steril. 1995;64(3):486-91.
59. Taylor PJ, Leader A, George RE, Fick GH. Correlations between laparoscopic and hysteroscopic findings in 497 women with otherwise unexplained infertility. J Reprod Med. 1984;29(2):137-40.
60. Timonen S, Nieminen U. Tubal pregnancy: choice of operative method of treatment. Acta Obstet Gynecol Scand. 1967;46(3):327-39.

61. Trimbos-Kemper TC, Trimbos JB, van Hall EV. Adhesion formation after tubal surgery: results of the eight-day laparoscopy in 188 patients. Fertil Steril. 1985;43(3):395-400.
62. Tulandi T, Collins JA, Burrows E, Jarrell JF, McInnes RA, Wrixon W, et al. Treatment-dependent and treatment-independent pregnancy among women with periadnexal adhesions. Am J Obstet Gynecol. 1990;162(2):354-7.
63. Tulandi T, Murray C, Guralnick M. Adhesion formation and reproductive outcome after myomectomy and second-look laparoscopy. Obstet Gynecol. 1993;82(2):213-5.
64. Vercellini P, Vendola N, Bocciolone L, Colombo A, Rognoni MT, Bolis G. Laparoscopic aspiration of ovarian endometriomas. Effect with postoperative gonadotropin releasing hormone agonist treatment. J Reprod Med. 1992;37(7):577-80.
65. Vermesh M, Silva PD, Rosen GF, Stein AL, Fossum GT, Sauer MV. Management of unruptured ectopic gestation by linear salpingostomy: a prospective randomized clinical trial of laparoscopy versus laparotomy. Obstet Gynecol. 1989;73(3 Pt 1):400-4.
66. Wood C, Maher P, Hill D. Diagnosis and surgical management of endometriomas. Aust NZ J Obstet Gynecol. 1992;32(2):161-3.

CHAPTER 7: Evaluation and Management of Tubal Factors

Anjali Bhirud, Sarika Zunjare, Ashish Zarariya

INTRODUCTION

Tubal factor contributes to 25–30% of female factor infertility. Evaluation of fallopian tube patency is component of initial triad of investigation for infertile couples. It is third in line after evaluation of semen and ovulation. Advances in in vitro fertilization (IVF) technology have diminished the importance of tubal factor infertility but recent discoveries have shed a new light on (reproductive) tubal surgeries prior to IVF cycles.

CAUSES FOR TUBAL INFERTILITY

- *Congenital:* Developmental or inherent anomalies of fallopian tubes are rare.
- *Acquired:*
  - Pelvic inflammatory disease (PID) is the most frequent cause for tubal disease. Inflammatory damage to internal tubal mucosal architect cannot be detected easily but may nonetheless impair sperm or embryo transfer function.
  - Tubal affection could be due to obstruction or occlusion, endosalpingeal destruction, and periadnexal adhesions.
  - Eighty five percent of tubal infertility is due to distal tube disease. Distal tubal occlusive disease exhibits a spectrum ranging from mild (fimbrial agglutination), moderate (varying degree of fimbrial phimosis) to severe (complete obstruction).
  - Midtubal diseases are commonly due to PID, endometriosis, or prior surgeries.
  - Proximal tubal block may be pseudo-obstruction or true anatomical block. Pseudo blocks are mainly due to spasm or plugs of mucous secretions blocking the tube. Causes of true blocks are salpingitis isthmica nodosa (SIN), PID, cornual polyp or fibroids and intrauterine synechiae, and post abortion or intrauterine contraceptive device (IUCD). SIN is thought to arise from tubal inflammation of unspecified origin and affects proximal tube prominently.

HULL AND RUTHERFORD 2002 CLASSIFICATION OF TUBAL DAMAGE

Minor/Grade 1

- Tubal fibrosis absent even if tube occluded proximally.
- Tubal distention absent even if tube occluded distally.
- Mucosal appearances favorable.
- Flimsy adhesions.

Moderate/Grade 2

- Unilateral severe tubal damage.
- Contralateral minor disease present or absent.
- Limited dense adhesions of tubes/ovaries.

Severe/Grade 3

- Bilateral tubal damage.
- Extensive tubal fibrosis.
- Tubal distention >1.5 cm.
- Abnormal mucosal appearance.
- Bipolar occlusion.
- Extensive dense adhesions.

TUBAL ASSESSMENT TESTS

High index of suspicion for pelvic infection with history and clinical examination plays an invaluable role. Pelvic infection and active PID are absolute contraindications to performing tubal patency test **(Table 1 and Flowchart 1)**.

Hysterosalpingography

- Hysterosalpingography (HSG) is an inexpensive and widely available screening test.
- Conventional HSG is safe as radiation exposure is only 0.4–5.5 mGy, much below the safety threshold for teratogenicity.
- When HSG reveals obstruction there is still high probability (almost 60%) that tubes are open but when HSG demonstrates patency there is little chance that the tube is actually occluded (approximately 5%).

Sonohysterosalpingography

- Sonohysterosalpingography test is done by transcervical fluid instillation, the filling and flow of fluid is monitored by transvaginal ultrasonography.
- Two common methods used are Sion's test or saline infusion sonography (SIS) and hysterosalpingo-contrast sonography (HyCoSy). The uterine

Evaluation and Management of Tubal Factors

TABLE 1: Tubal assessment tests—summary.

Test	Sensitivity	Specificity	Limitations	Complications	Advantages
HSG	84%	74.5%	• Failure to catheterize/cannulate • Leak of dye around cervix • Tubal spasm or debris causing 15% false +ve report • Reporting errors	• Flare up of infection • Open fallopian tubes	Easily available
Sonosalpingography (saline infusion)					
HyCoSy	93.3%	89.7%	Expertise in transvaginal 3D sonography and Doppler study	PID	Better alternative to HSG
Laparoscopy	Unknown (No Comparator)	Unknown	• Invasive • General anesthesia • Skill requirement expensive	Bowel/urological/vascular injury 0.13%	Gold standard
Chlamydia antibody test	21–90%	29–100%	Immunological process may continue despite antibiotics (microbiological cure) so utility is limited.	None	• Cost effective • Helpful in subclinical salpingitis
USG	-	-	Very limited role as healthy tubes are not visualized	None	None

(HSG: hysterosalpingogram; HyCoSy: hysterosalpingo-contrast sonography; PID: pelvic inflammatory disease; USG: ultrasonography)

58 Evaluation and Management of Tubal Factors

Flowchart 1: Evaluation of tubal infertility.

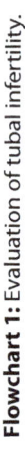

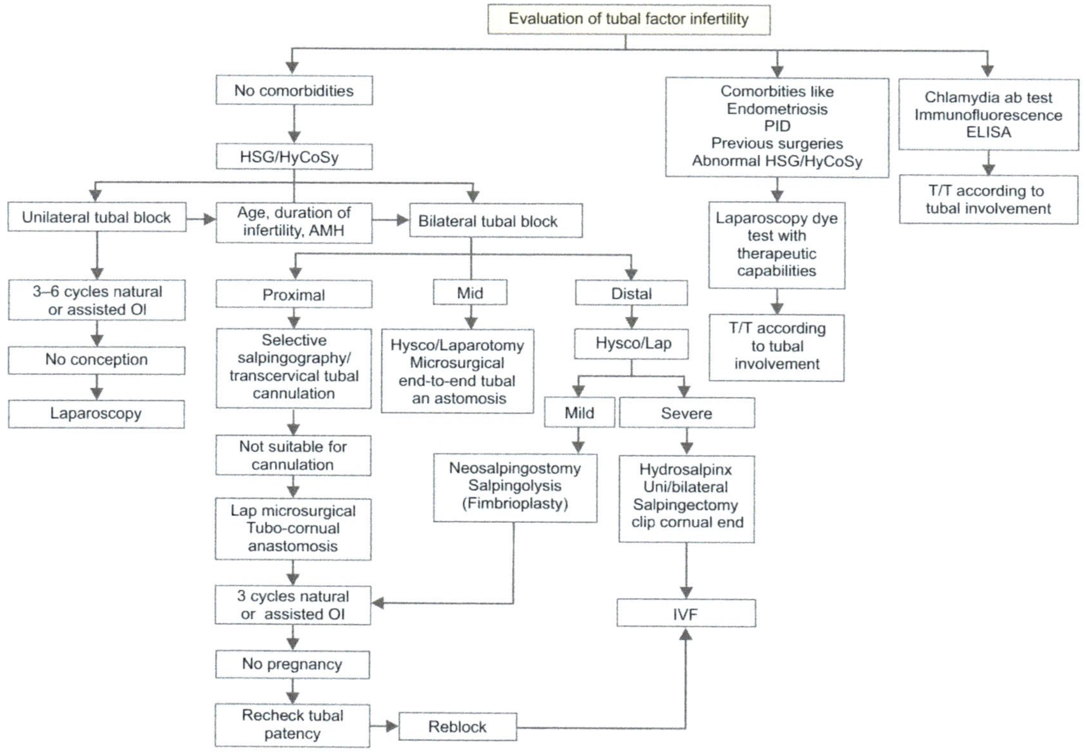

(AMH: anti-Müllerian hormone; ELISA: enzyme-linked immunosorbent assay; HSG: hysterosalpingogram; HyCoSy: hysterosalpingo-contrast sonography; IVF: in vitro fertilization; OI: ovulation induction; PID: pelvic inflammatory disease)

cavity is insufflated slowly with about 300 mL plain saline (Sion's test) or solution of galactose and 1% palmitic acid (HyCoSy).
- Standard two-dimensional (2D) image in sagittal and transverse plane is inadequate to visualize tubal anatomy. Three-dimensional (3D) coronal imaging and Doppler techniques improve visualization of fluid movement through fallopian tube.

Laparoscopy and Chromopertubation

- Laparoscopy is considered as gold standard and definitive test for evaluation of tubal patency.
- It is minimally invasive procedure which allows diagnosis, assessment and management of peritubal disease, adhesions, and endometriosis.
- Laparoscopy enables biopsy of suspicious region for further evaluation.

Chlamydia Antibody Test

- The role of Chlamydia antibody test in evaluation of infertile women has not been sufficiently defined.
- A positive test might alert one to the possibilities of tubal factors relating to previous Chlamydial infection not otherwise suspected.
- Due to pitfalls clinical utility of this test is limited.

Ultrasound Evaluation of Fallopian Tube

- The healthy fallopian tubes are not seen on routine two-dimension or three-dimension ultrasound imaging of pelvis unless filled or surrounded by fluid.
- Tubal wall is not sonologically discernible unless thickened or distended with fluid.
- Diseased distended fallopian tubes, on the other hand, can often be seen as adnexal masses.
- A "cogwheel" appearance and "beads on the string" appearance are noted on ultrasound with hydrosalpinges.

THE ROYAL COLLEGE OF OBSTETRICIANS AND GYNAECOLOGISTS GUIDELINES FOR TUBAL EVALUATION

- Hysterosalpingography is offered to the patients with no suspicion of comorbidity such as PID, previous ectopics, and endometriosis.
- Hysterosalpingo-contrast sonography screening for tubal patency should be considered as effective alternative to HSG for women without comorbidities.
- When comorbidity suspected laparoscopic chromopertubation should be offered.

TUBERCULOSIS AND TUBAL FACTOR INFERTILITY

- Female genital tuberculosis (FGTB) is usually secondary to lung TB or other organs.
- Fallopian tubes are affected in 90% women, infection reaching through hematogenous, lymphatic, or direct spread.
- Tubal involvement is bilateral in >90% cases.
- Endosalpingitis (swollen, edematous, and irregular), exosalpingitis (flimsy adhesion and miliary tubercles), beading, close tubes, hydrosalpinx, pyosalpinx, tubo-ovarian masses, and dense adhesions can occur in FGTB.
- Tubal conditions can be diagnosed and graded on HSG, HyCoSy, and laparoscopy as per type of adhesions, patency, morphology, and fimbrial stricture.
- Lymphocytosis, raised erythrocyte sedimentation rate (ESR), X-ray chest, Mantoux, and above-mentioned imaging methods help in diagnosing FGTB.
- Serological tests are not sensitive and specific so banned by the World Health Organization (WHO) and Government of India (GoI).
- All efforts should be made to achieve microbiological diagnosis by endometrial biopsy, curettage, aspiration (luteal phase), and multiple biopsy of suspect material in laparoscopy.
- Cartridge-based nucleic acid amplification test (CBNAAT)/Gene Xpert *Mycobacterium tuberculosis* (MTB)/resistance to rifampin (RIF) (WHO approved rapid diagnostic tests, polymerase chain reaction (PCR), liquid culture mycobacterial growth indicator tube (MGIT) with phenotypic drug sensitivity testing (DST) or genotypic DST by line probe assay can be done on biopsy sample along with microscopy.
- Directly observed treatment short-course (DOTS) is recommended by the WHO and GOI.
- Nondirectly observed treatment short course strategy of 2 HRZE (isoniazid + rifampicin + pyrazinamide + ethambutol) and 4 HRE (isoniazid + rifampicin + ethambutol) can also be given.
- Despite antitubercular treatment results for fertility is low conception rate is <20%.
- IVF is useful with blocked tubes and normal endometrium.

MANAGEMENT OF TUBAL FACTOR INFERTILITY

- For women with tubal factor infertility treatment options are reconstructive surgery and IVF **(Flowchart 1)**.
- IVF has become the treatment of choice for couples with other associated infertility factor and severe tubal diseases.

- However, reconstructive surgery remains appropriate options in young women with mild-to-moderate tubal disease and couple with ethical or religious objections for IVF.
- Reconstructive surgery should follow all principles of microsurgery like use of binocular microscope (20x), use of fine stitch materials (7-0 and 10-0) and with copious irrigation.
- Age, duration of infertility, ovarian reserve, presence/absence of other factors, and surgeons experience help in deciding management other than extent of tubal damage.
- Selective salpingography/proximal tubal canulation

Management of Proximal Tubal Disease

- Hysteroscopic proximal tubal cannulation or fluoroscopic selective salpingography is effective method to treat proximal tubal obstruction due to debris, sludge, and intraluminal adhesions.
- Proximal tubal cannulation is to be done only after confirmation of normalcy of distal tube using prior laparoscopic evaluation.
- Proximal tubal cannulation is preferred alternative to traditional microsurgical tubal repair as it is having less morbidity and lower cost.
- In case series regarding proximal tubal occlusion patency rate is between 60 and 80% and pregnancy rate is between 20 and 60% observed.

Management of Distal Tubal Disease

- Procedures like neosalpingostomy (opening up of blocked distal tube), fimbrioplasty (widening of stenosed distal tubal ostia), and salpingo-ovariolysis (to maintain tubo-ovarian relationship) are done routinely.
- Prognosis will inversely depend upon tubal mucosal damage and wall thickness of tube.
- Majority of pregnancies occur within first 2 years after surgical treatment of distal tube obstruction.

Management of Sterilization Reversal

- Success will depend on age, around 60% success is reported if age is <40 years.
- Ovarian reserve.
- Endoluminal status of tube.
- Isthmus to isthmus reanastomosis and longer final tube >4 cm has the best results.
- Laparoscopy is preferred method.

Tubal Delinking Followed by In Vitro Fertilization

- Reconstructive surgeries are not beneficial for women with severe and bipolar (proximal and distal) tubal disease.

- IVF outcome is poorer in women with extensive tubal disease with hydrosalpinges.
- 2010 systemic review including five randomized controlled trials (RCTs) of 646 women observed that odds of achieving an ongoing pregnancy were twice as great after laparoscopic salpingectomy and after laparoscopic tubal occlusion in case of hydrosalpinx. Effectiveness of ultrasound-guided aspiration of the hydrosalpinx at the time of oocyte retrieval has not been established.

SUGGESTED READING

1. Broeze KA, Opmeer BC, Coppus SF, Van Geloven N, Alves MF, Anestad G, et al. Chlamydia antibody testing and diagnosing tubal pathology in subfertile women: an individual patient data meta-analysis. Hum Reprod Update. 2011;17(3):301-10.
2. Cakmak H, Taylor HS. Implantation failure: molecular mechanisms and clinical treatment. Hum Reprod Update. 2011;17(2):242-53.
3. Déchaud H, Daurès JP, Arnal F, Humeau C, Hédon B. Does previous salpingectomy improve implantation and pregnancy rates in patients with severe tubal factor infertility who are undergoing in vitro fertilization? A pilot prospective randomized study. Fertil Steril. 1998;69(6):1020-5.
4. ESHRE Capri workshop group. Diagnosis and management of the infertile couple: missing information. Hum Reprod Update. 2004;10(4):295-307.
5. Honore GM, Holden AE, Schenken RS. Pathophysiology and management of proximal tubal blockage. Fertil Steril. 1997;71(5):785-95.
6. NICE Clinical Guideline. Fertility: assessment and treatment for people with fertility problems. London: RCOG; 2013. pp. 1-555.
7. Practice Committee of the American Society for Reproductive Medicine. Diagnostic evaluation of the infertile female: a committee opinion. Fertil Steril. 2015;103:e44-50.
8. Tripathy SN. Infertility and pregnancy outcome in female genital tuberculosis. Int J Gynecol Obs. 2002;76:159-63.
9. Watrelot A, Nisolle M, Chelli H, Hocke C, Rongières C, Racinet C; International Group for Fertiloscopy Evaluation. Is laparoscopy still the gold standard in infertility assessment? A comparison of fertiloscopy versus laparoscopy in infertility. Results of an international multicentre prospective trial: the 'FLY' (Fertiloscopy-LaparoscopY) study. Hum Reprod. 2003;4:834-9.

CHAPTER 8

Evaluation and Management of Uterine Factors in Infertility

Amrita Tandon, Sudha Tandon

INTRODUCTION

The uterus or *metra*, is the organ of procreation where the embryo implants and fetal nourishment takes place to achieve a successful pregnancy.

Any factor which leads to impairment in this uterine function leads to infertility.

Broadly uterine factors contribute to about 15-20% of all causes of infertility in a couple. Hence, evaluation and subsequent management of the uterine factor is crucial for any couple seeking fertility treatment.

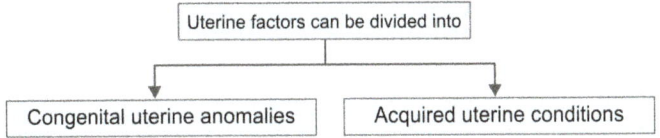

EVALUATION AND MANAGEMENT OF CONGENITAL UTERINE FACTORS

Congenital uterine anomalies result from developmental or fusion defects of the Müllerian duct during embryogenesis. The American Fertility Society has classified Müllerian anomalies in the following manner[1] as shown in **Figure 1**.

Investigations for Congenital Uterine Anomalies

- The female tract anatomy assessment in women of reproductive age is usually performed by gynecologic speculum examination and two-dimensional (2D) transvaginal ultrasound (TVUS). Two-dimensional TVUS is routinely used as it is easily available, with moderate cost involved and is noninvasive, but it has slight limitations. It is relatively not as sensitive as other methods, particularly for demonstration of the fundal contour.[2]
- Hysterosalpingography (HSG) is done as a routine investigation for uterine and tubal factor infertility, but it is not the ideal technique for detecting uterine malformation. The false-positive rate is 38%, and the

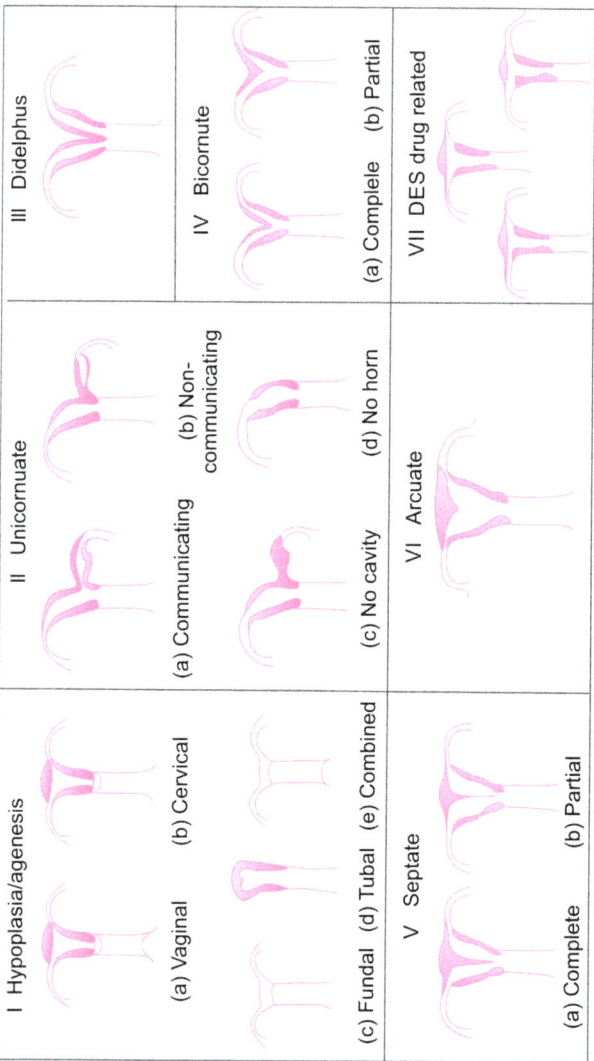

Fig. 1: Classification of Müllerian anomalies. (DES: diethylstilbestrol)

sensitivity is 44%. Particularly, the test cannot differentiate septate from bicornuate uterus.[3]
- Three-dimensional ultrasound has a noninvasive nature, and has the advantage of increased spatial awareness compared to 2D ultrasound, and thus, enables a detailed evaluation of uterine morphology. The additional coronal view of the uterus can be obtained in the three-dimensional ultrasound (3D-US) and this adds the value in differentiating between various congenital uterine anomalies.[2]
- Magnetic resonance imaging (MRI) of the pelvis is sensitive and specific for diagnosing uterine anomalies, particularly for endometrial defects and diagnosing uterine horns, for detecting aberrant gonadal location and renal anatomy. It is also less invasive than combined laparoscopy and hysteroscopy. Magnetic resonance imaging is useful for women with unconfirmed diagnosis on 3D ultrasound, and with suspected complex anomalies.[4]
- Recently, 3D-US along with 3D saline sonohysterography and sonovaginocervicography has been used to assess complex anatomical defects of the female genital tract, and this has led to reduced need for invasive methods such as hysteroscopy-laparoscopy for purely diagnostic purposes.[3]
- Renal and skeletal anomalies should be ruled out in all forms of Müllerian anomalies due to their high risk of association.

SEPTATE UTERUS

- The most common congenital structural uterine anomaly.
- It is a result of failure of complete resorption of the partition formed by the fused Müllerian ducts, leading to a partial or complete fibromuscular septum.
- It can lead to infertility, first and second trimester miscarriages and an adverse obstetric outcome **(Figs. 2 to 3)**.

Treatment

Hysteroscopic septal incision by resectoscope or scissors is the treatment of choice and minimally invasive surgery has now become a standard treatment of choice over the laparotomy and metroplasty surgeries. This may be performed under laparoscopic guidance or more recently under ultrasound guidance.

Whether to treat a uterine septum is a controversial subject. The American Society for Reproductive Medicine (ASRM) and European Society of Human Reproduction and Embryology (ESHRE)/European Society for Gynaecological Endoscopy (ESGE) classifications differ in the diagnosis of septate uterus. The ESHRE/ESGE classification system can at times overdiagnose septate uterus and lead to unnecessary treatment.

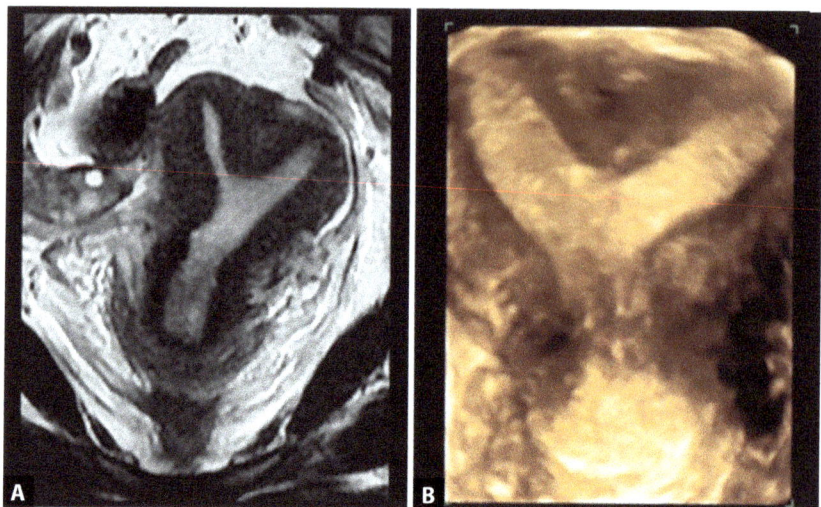

Figs. 2A and B: Subseptate uterus on—(A) Magnetic resonance imaging (MRI); and (B) Three-dimensional ultrasound sonography (3D-USG).
Source: radiopedia.org

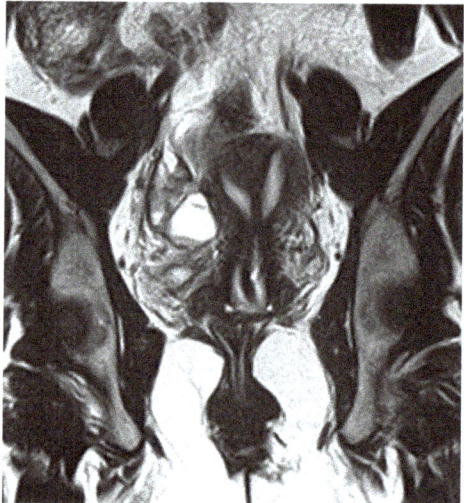

Fig. 3: Coronal, T2 magnetic resonance imaging (MRI) image of complete septate uterus.

There is not enough evidence to evaluate impact of septal resection for reproductive outcomes with the ESHRE/ESGE classification. Data suggests a septum of <1 cm is not associated with adverse clinical outcomes. Randomized trials are being performed to evaluate outcomes of uterine septum treatment versus expectant management.[5]

National Institute for Health and Care Excellence (NICE) guidelines 2013[6] suggest that further research is needed to prove benefit of surgical resection of septum on live birth rates in subfertile women.

UNICORNUATE UTERUS

- It results from failure of partial or complete development of Müllerian ducts. These can be of four types including—unicornuate uterus with a communicating rudimentary horn, with a noncommunicating rudimentary horn, with or without a cavity and an isolated unicornuate uterus.
- The unicornuate uterus is an uncommon anomaly, representing only 4.4% of uterine anomalies, and is associated with poor reproductive outcomes. Pregnancy occurring in the unicornuate uterus is associated with an increased risk of first-trimester miscarriage, second-trimester loss, cervical incompetence, and a number of obstetric complications such as intrauterine growth restriction (IUGR), preterm delivery, malpresentation, and intrauterine death.[7]
- The highest live birth rates are observed in women with a rudimentary horn, with or without a cavity.
- Treatment usually includes hysterolaparoscopy with laparoscopic removal of the rudimentary horn. Noncommunicating rudimentary horns with functional endometrium are generally removed.
- This can be done via laparotomy as well, but due to benefits of shorter hospital stay, lesser postoperative pain, laparoscopy is the preferred choice.
- Indications for removing rudimentary horns include dysmenorrhea, prevention of endometriosis, and avoiding a horn or tubal ectopic pregnancy.
- There is no consensus whether to remove communicating rudimentary horns or horns without functional endometrium.[1]
- The poor obstetric outcome in unicornuate uteri is associated with low uterine volume and a tubular uterine cavity, and the evidence suggesting that women with uncorrected unicornuate uteri have recurrent miscarriages at serially increasing gestational ages, the treatment should be directed toward metroplasty which increases the uterine volume and converts the tubular cavity into a triangular cavity.
- In smaller studies it has shown that hysteroscopic fundal and unilateral metroplasty, leads to increase in uterine cavity, and improves the reproductive outcomes in these women. Larger, randomized trials are needed before making this a universal recommendation.[8]

BICORNUATE UTERUS

- It results from failure of Müllerian ducts to fuse completely. It could be bicornuate unicollis or bicornuate bicollis.
- The bicornuate uterus is a common anomaly representing 26% of all anomalies. These women commonly encounter poor obstetric outcomes, and only a few may present with infertility.

- Bicornuate uterus rarely requires corrective surgery. Surgery is indicated in women who have experienced recurrent spontaneous abortion, mid-trimester loss, premature birth, and in whom no other cause has been identified.
- Strassmann's laparoscopic or transabdominal metroplasty for uterine unification, have shown to improve reproductive outcomes.[9]
- In 2005, Lolis et al. achieved 88% pregnancies and 100% take-home baby rate, concluding that reproductive capacity of women with bicornuate uterus was very good postsurgery and the procedure was reserved for selected women who had history of recurrent abortion or preterm birth.[10]

UTERINE DIDELPHYS

- It results from complete failure of fusion of the paired Müllerian ducts leading to duplication of the uterus and cervix and is usually associated with a longitudinal vaginal septum.
- It represents 11.1% of all uterine anomalies.
- Unification surgery is not routinely recommended for uterine didelphys as they are usually associated with good reproductive outcomes.[4]
- Resection of the longitudinal vaginal septum, if present, can be done, if associated with obstruction, dyspareunia, or infertility.[1]

MANAGEMENT OF OTHER COMPLEX MÜLLERIAN ANOMALIES

- Women with Müllerian agenesis can be offered either gestational surrogacy or uterine transplantation.[2]
- In a recent case series, patients of cervical agenesis or dysgenesis, treated with the use of uterovaginal anastomosis have demonstrated remarkable success, when combined with creation of a neovagina instead of hysterectomy which was performed traditionally. In one study of 18 cases, all of the women had successful reconstruction and only one woman experienced restenosis, which was treated successfully with the use of canalization. Pregnancy occurred without assistance in ten women, and four women had a successful delivery via cesarean section at 36–38 weeks.[2]
- Further larger randomized controlled trials (RCTs) are required to advocate reconstructive surgeries for improving reproductive outcomes in women with congenital uterine anomalies.

ACQUIRED UTERINE PATHOLOGIES

Uterine Fibroids

- The incidence of myomas in infertile women without any other cause of infertility is 1–2.4%.

- Submucosal fibroids negatively affect fertility, when compared to women without fibroids. Intramural fibroids above a certain size (>4 cm), even without cavity distortion, may also negatively influence fertility.
- The Society of Obstetricians and Gynaecologists of Canada (SOGC) guideline recommendations are as follows:[11]
  - Evaluation of fibroids:
    - In women with infertility, an effort should be made to adequately evaluate and classify fibroids, particularly those impinging on the endometrial cavity, using TVUS, hysteroscopy, hysterosonography, or MRI.
    - Preoperative assessment of submucosal fibroids should include, in addition to an assessment of fibroid size and location within the uterine cavity, evaluation of the degree of invasion of the cavity and thickness of residual myometrium to the serosa. A combination of hysteroscopy and TVUS or hysterosonography are the modalities of choice.
    - Magnetic resonance imaging has been well-studied in the evaluation of fibroid uteruses, especially for fibroid mapping and submucosal penetration. It was shown to be the most reliable method of evaluation when compared with vaginal ultrasound, hysterosonography, and hysteroscopy, with 100% sensitivity and 91% specificity.
  - Management:
    - Submucosal fibroids are managed hysteroscopically. The fibroid size should be <5 cm, although larger fibroids have been managed hysteroscopically, but repeat procedures are often necessary. There is fair evidence to recommend against myomectomy in women with intramural fibroids (hysteroscopically confirmed intact endometrium) and otherwise unexplained infertility, regardless of their size. (II-2D) If the patient has no other options, the benefits of myomectomy should be weighed against the risks, and management of intramural fibroids should be individualized. Subserosal fibroids do not appear to have an impact on fertility; the effect of intramural fibroids remains unclear. If intramural fibroids do have an impact on fertility, it appears to be small and to be even less significant when the endometrium is not involved. (II-3)

Adenomyosis

It is defined as the presence of endometrial glands and stroma distal to endomyometrial junction. Adenomyosis has been associated with other mild estrogen-dependent benign disorders such as endometriosis (70%), uterine fibroids (50%) and endometrial hyperplasia (35%).[12]

Adenomyosis has a negative effect on in vitro fertilization (IVF) pregnancy and the live birth rate, and an increased risk of miscarriage. Probable factors that cause infertility are abnormal uterotubal gamete and embryo transport, disruption of endometrial receptivity and function, and myometrial hyperactivity.[12]

Adenomyosis could be diffuse or focal. Diagnosis is usually by TVUS. Transvaginal ultrasound is a good imagine technique and can show ill-defined myometrial heterogeneity and myometrial cyst. Magnetic resonance imaging can be complementary to TVUS.

Limited evidence suggests gonadotropin-releasing hormone agonist (GnRH agonist) treatment, downregulates the pituitary leading to an antiproliferative effect on lesion, hence promoting apoptosis and size reduction. A few retrospective studies have shown treatment with a GnRH agonist before embryo transfer increases pregnancy rates.[13]

Laparoscopic conservative adenomyomectomy usually combined with GnRH agonist therapy has shown improved fertility outcomes. Most of these patients require some form of assisted reproductive technology (ART) treatment to achieve a successful pregnancy.[13]

Endometrial Polyps

- Endometrial polyps have been associated with infertility; the incidence of this disease in primary infertility is 3.8–38.5%, and 1.8–17% in secondary infertility. It has a combined infertility incidence of 1.9–24%[14]
- Transvaginal 2D ultrasound, especially done post menstrually is diagnostic of endometrial polyps. Saline infusion sonography (SIS) can also help diagnose polyps. Polyps can be distinguished from fibroids with the finding of a single pulsating feeding vessel seen at the base of the mass by color flow Doppler.[13]
- The overall prevalence of polyps in infertile women is apparently increased. In a large prospective trial of 1,000 women undergoing IVF, endometrial polyps were found in the prevalence of 32%.[13]
- There is an option for expectant management with no intervention. There is Class II evidence that polyps may spontaneously regress in approximately 25% of cases, with smaller polyps more likely to regress compared with polyps <10 mm in length.[15]
- Hysteroscopic polypectomy has been recommended to be the optimal treatment for the removal of endometrial polyps. There are a variety of methods practised to remove polyps at hysteroscopy; with use of resectoscope or scissors, however, there are no comparative studies for these methods with regard to efficacy or costs, and the method of choice is the one with which the clinician is trained in and most familiar.[15]
- While the efficacy and safety of hysteroscopic polypectomy in subfertile women is expectant management has been favorably reported in many

controlled studies, a sound evidence-based conclusion cannot be drawn due to the lack of data from any well conducted RCT.[16]
- According to the American Association of Gynecologic Laparoscopists (AAGL) practice guidelines published in 2012, for the infertile patient with a polyp, surgical removal is recommended to allow natural conception or ART a greater opportunity to be successful (level A evidence).[15]

Chronic Endometritis

- Its prevalence is about 30.3% in patients with repeated implantation failure at IVF. Women diagnosed with chronic endometritis (CE) have reduced implantation rates (11.5%) after IVF cycles. Common bacteria and mycoplasmas are the most frequently involved infectious agents.
- Due to its subtle pathology and often asymptomatic nature, it cannot be detected with ultrasound and HSG. Histological identification of plasma cells in the endometrial stroma is considered the gold standard for the diagnosis.
- Hysteroscopy is important for diagnosis of CE based on the demonstration of signs such as micropolyps, stromal edema and focal or diffuse hyperemia and endometrial biopsy taken simultaneously can be sent for microbiological examination.
- Treatment involves antibiotic therapy according to culture and sensitivity report. In case of gram negative bacteria, Ciprofloxacin 500 mg twice a day for 10 days can be given. For gram-positive bacteria, Amoxicillin + Clavulanate 1 g twice a day for 8 days can be given. In case of negative cultures, a treatment based on Ceftriaxone 250 mg IM in a single dose plus Doxycycline 100 mg orally twice a day for 14 days with Metronidazole 500 mg orally twice a day for 14 days, should be prescribed.
- Studies have shown that it is possible to evaluate the effectiveness of the antibiotic therapy in restoring a normal hysteroscopic picture of the endometrial cavity and histological examination by repeat hysteroscopy.
- Reproductive outcomes in terms of both implantation rates and live birth rates improved after antibiotic treatment of CE.[17]

Intrauterine Adhesions

- Asherman syndrome (AS) is scarring of the endometrial lining, usually secondary to postpartum hemorrhage or endometrial infection followed by aggressive curettage, due to retained products of conception. They can also develop after uterine surgery such as myomectomy or septal resection, endometrial tuberculosis, uterine artery embolization. The insult must be severe enough to remove or destroy the basal layer of the endometrium.[13,18]
- The prevalence of AS in women with impaired fertility ranges from 2.8 to 45.5% depending on the subpopulation.

- HSG shows filing defects, with low sensitivity and specificity.
- Saline infusion sonography or 3D-US can help diagnose intrauterine adhesions better than 2D TVS. Contrast sonohysterography has a high negative predictive value (98%), but a moderate positive predictive value (43%) when compared with hysteroscopy.[18]
- Confirmation is by visualization on hysteroscopic evaluation.
- For fertility, the initial goal of treatment is restoration of a normal calibrated uterine cavity covered with endometrial lining and free tubal ostia.
- Hysteroscopic adhesiolysis is the treatment of choice. Filmy adhesions can be lysed by using the tip of hysteroscope. Adhesiolysis performed with scissors biopsy forceps, sharp or blunt scissors and division of strings with energy such as monopolar diathermia, bipolar diathermia or laser.[18]
- The effect on fertility is influenced by several other factors, e.g., the age of the patient, and whether infertility is primary or secondary. The pregnancy rate ranges between 25 and 76% and the term delivery rate, in women who achieved pregnancy, between 25 and 79.7.[19] Success rate develops depending on severity of adhesions. Second-look hysteroscopy with division of newly formed filmy adherences has been studied in a retrospective setting of 151 patients, cumulative pregnancy rate (77% vs. 56%) and live birth rate (77% vs. 63%) seems to improve when early second-look is performed within two weeks to two months after primary adhesiolysis.[20]

REFERENCES

1. Taylor E, Gomel V. The uterus and fertility. Fertil Steril. 2008;89(1):1-16.
2. Ahmadi F, Zafarani F, Haghighi H, Niknejadi M, Dizaj AV. Application of 3D Ultrasonography in detection of uterine abnormalities. Int J Fertil Steril. 2011;4(4):144.
3. Alborzi S, Dehbashi S, Parsanezhad ME. Differential diagnosis of septate and bicornuate uterus by sonohysterography eliminates the need for laparoscopy. Fertil Steril. 2002;78(1):176-8.
4. Akhtar MA, Saravelos SH, Li TC, Jayaprakasan K, Royal College of Obstetricians and Gynaecologists. Reproductive implications and management of congenital uterine anomalies: Scientific Impact Paper No. 62 November 2019. BJOG. 2020;127(5):e1-3.
5. Ludwig A, Pfeifer SM. Reproductive surgery for Müllerian anomalies: a review of progress in the last decade. Fertil Steril. 2019;112(3):408-16.
6. Fertility problems: assessment and treatment: National Institute for Health and Care Excellence (NICE) Clinical guideline. London: NICE; 2013.
7. Xia EL, Li TC, Choi SN, Zhou QY. Reproductive outcome of transcervical uterine incision in unicornuate uterus. Chinese Med J. 2017;130(3):256.
8. Tandulwadkar S, Naralkar M. Unicornuate Uterus: Is There a Place for Hysteroscopic Management? In: Tinelli A, Alonso Pacheco L, Haimovich S (Eds). Hysteroscopy. Cham: Springer; 2018.
9. Karthik SD, Kriplani A, Mahey R, Kachhawa G. Successful reproductive outcome after laparoscopic Strassmann's metroplasty. J Hum Reprod Sci. 2017;10(3):231.
10. Lolis DE, Paschopoulos M, Makrydimas G, Zikopoulos K, Sotiriadis A, Paraskevaidis E. Reproductive outcome after Strassmann metroplasty in women with a bicornuate uterus. J Reprod Med. 2005;50:297-301.

11. Carranza-Mamane B, Havelock J, Hemmings R, Cheung A, Sierra S, Case A, et al. The management of uterine fibroids in women with otherwise unexplained infertility. J Obstet Gynaecol Can. 2015;37(3):277-85.
12. Szubert M, Koziróg E, Olszak O, Krygier-Kurz K, Kazmierczak J, Wilczynski J. Adenomyosis and Infertility—Review of Medical and Surgical Approaches. Int J Environ Res Pub Health. 2021;18(3):1235.
13. Hur C, Rehmer J, Flyckt R, Falcone T. Uterine factor infertility: a clinical review. Clin Obstet Gynecol. 2019;62(2):257-70.
14. Shokeir TA, Shalan HM, El-Shafei MM. Significance of endometrial polyps detected hysteroscopically in eumenorrheic infertile women. J Obstet Gynaecol Res. 2004;30(2):84-9.
15. American Association of Gynecologic Laparoscopists (AAGL) Advancing Minimally Invasive Gynecology Worldwide. AAGL practice report: practice guidelines for the diagnosis and management of endometrial polyps. Journal of Minimally Invasive Gynecology. 2012;19(1):3-10.
16. Jayaprakasan K, Sahu B, Thornton J, Raine-Fenning N. Surgical intervention versus expectant management for endometrial polyps in subfertile women (Protocol). Cochrane Database Syst Rev. 2014;2014(8):CD009592
17. Cicinelli E, Matteo M, Tinelli R, Lepera A, Alfonso R, Indraccolo U, et al. Prevalence of chronic endometritis in repeated unexplained implantation failure and the IVF success rate after antibiotic therapy. Hum Reprod. 2015;30(2):323-30.
18. Dreisler E, Kjer JJ. Asherman's syndrome: current perspectives on diagnosis and management. Int J Women Health. 2019;11:191.
19. Yamamoto N, Takeuchi R, Izuchi D, Yuge N, Miyazaki M, Yasunaga M, et al. Hysteroscopic adhesiolysis for patients with Asherman's syndrome: menstrual and fertility outcomes. Reprod Med Biol. 2013;12(4):159-66.
20. Xu W, Zhang Y, Yang Y, Zhang S, Lin X. Effect of early second-look hysteroscopy on reproductive outcomes after hysteroscopic adhesiolysis in patients with intrauterine adhesion, a retrospective study in China. Int J Surg. 2018;50:49-54.

CHAPTER 9

Evaluation of the Male Infertility Factors

Rishma Dhillon Pai, Balasaheb Khadbade

INTRODUCTION

- Male partner should be evaluated along with the female partner if they fail to achieve pregnancy within 1 year of unprotected intercourse. The initial evaluation should be general history along with the reproductive history and two properly performed semen analysis. Advanced evaluation of male partner should also be considered in couple with history of unexplained infertility or recurrent pregnancy loss **(Flowchart 1)**.
- Medical history:
  - A detailed medical and surgical history
  - Drug history
  - Lifestyle evaluation and exposures
  - History of past infections such as sexually transmitted diseases (STDs) and respiratory infection
- Physical examination:
  - American Urological Association (AUA) and American Society for Reproductive Medicine (ASRM) recommend one of the following factors in physical examinations—
    - Examine the penis, especially for the opening of the urethral meatus
    - Palpate the testes and measure their size (Normal 12-20 cc, if smaller testes indicates hypogonadism)
    - Existence and consistency of both the vasa and epididymides (absence indicates congenital bilateral of vas deferens, cause obstructive azoospermia)
    - Presence of a varicocele
    - Secondary sex characteristics including hair distribution body habitus and breast development
    - Rectal examination for seminal vesicles, prostatic adenoma and neoplasia
  - *Semen analysis:* Semen analysis is the mainstay for the assessment of the male partner and gives an overview of fertility potential of male. The sample is collected by masturbation or by intercourse using special semen collections condom that do not contain substances detrimental to sperm after a defined period of abstinence of 2-3 days.

Evaluation of the Male Infertility Factors

Flowchart 1: Assessment of male partner in an infertile couple.

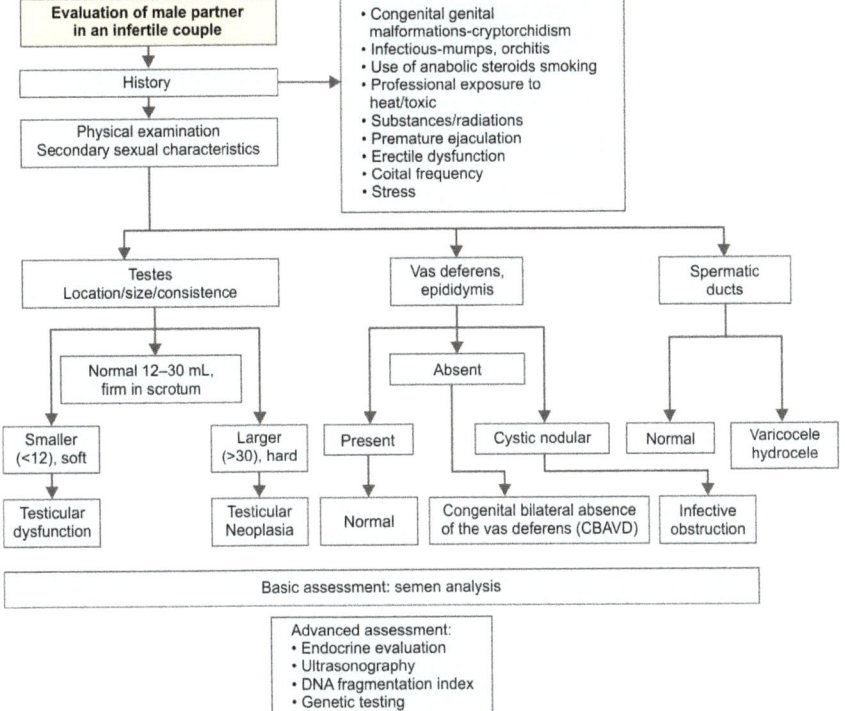

Although it is ideal to collect the sample at the laboratory, home collected sample may be accepted after mentioning the same in the report. When collected outside the laboratory, the specimen should be kept at room temperature during transport and examined within 1 hour of collection.

The semen analysis provides assessment of macroparameters such as semen volume as well as microparameters such as sperm concentration, motility and morphology. Levels that fall beyond the reference ranges (WHO) direct toward a male infertility that indicates need for additional clinical and laboratory evaluation. It must be stressed that the reference value for semen variable are not equivalent to the minimum value needed for conception, and that men with semen parameter outside the reference arrays may still be fertile. Patient with level within the reference range may still be fertile.

- *Endocrine evaluation:* Endocrine evaluation should include serum testosterone and follicle-stimulating hormone (FSH). It should be performed, if there is:
  - Low sperm count (<10 million/mL)
  - Impaired sexual function
  - Other finding suggestive of specific endocrinopathy

- *Ultrasound evaluation:* Ultrasound (USG) is not done as a part of routine investigation of male partner, but is performed only to confirm to rule out suspected abnormality either on examination or semen analysis. Scrotal USG, is done to evaluate the scrotal and testicular pathologies such as testicular masses, atrophic testis, varicocele, hydrocele, epididymal cyst, etc. Prostate can be evaluated using a transrectal USG (TRUS).

INTERPRETATION OF SEMEN ANALYSIS: MACROSCOPIC PARAMETERS

Semen analysis is the first step toward evaluation of the fertility potential of male. It measures the quantity and quality of the man's semen and sperm parameters. Values above the reference range are consider to have higher probability of pregnancy and values below this range are consider to have lower probability of pregnancy **(Table 1)**.

Macroscopic results sometimes are more relevant for clinical interpretation **(Flowchart 2)**.

- *Volume:* Normal value of semen sample is 1.5–4 mL. Pipetting is a better method of measuring volume. The variations in the volume help us to categorize various disorders, i.e., low volume associated with improper collection, partial retrograde ejaculation, congenital absence of vas deferens, obstruction of lower urinary tract whereas hyperspermia is associated with accessory gland infection or prolonged abstinence. In case of suspicious of infection, semen culture followed by antibiotic therapy.
- *pH:* Normal semen pH is 7.2–8.2 coagulated alkaline fluid coming from seminal vesicle the main component of semen and the prostatic acidic fluid is the second largest component. The alkaline pH of semen also gives protection to the sperm from the spermiolytic acidic condition of the vagina. Acidic semen of low volume indicates obstructive azoospermia.

TABLE 1: World Health Organization (WHO) reference value.

Semen characteristics	WHO, 2010
Volume (mL)	≥1.5
Count (10^6/mL)	≥15
Total count (10^6)	≥39
Motility (%)	≥40
Progressive (%)	≥32
Vitality (%)	≥58
Morphology (%)	≥4*
Leukocytes (10^6/mL)	1.0

*Strict (Tygerberg) criterion.

Evaluation of the Male Infertility Factors

Flowchart 2: Examination and processing of human semen.

WHO Semen Analysis

Macroscopic parameters of semen analysis and its clinical interpretation (WHO-5)

Volume
- Hyperspermia >6 mL
  - Increase day of abstinence
  - Urine contamination
  - Male accessory gland dysfunction
- Hypospermia
  - Spillage
  - Obstruction
  - Partial retrograde ejaculation
  - Absence of CBAVD

pH
- High
  - Duct obstruction
  - Absence of vas deference
  - Chronic infection
- Low
  - Acute prostatitis
  - Vasculitis

Appearance (grey opalescent)
- Yellow → Pus cell severe jaundice
- Red
  - UTI
  - Genital tract
  - Trauma
- Less opaque → Low concentration of sperm

Liquefaction time
- Absence of liquefaction → Prostate gland dysfunction
- Absence of coagulation
  - Ejaculatory duct obstruction
  - Congenital absence of seminal vesicle

Viscosity
- String test
  - Normal (<4 cm)
  - Equivocal (4–6 cm)
  - Hyperviscous
    - Zinc level
    - Antibody coated spermatozoa interfere with motility and concentration determination

(CBAVD: congenital bilateral absence of the vas deferens; UTI: urinary tract infection)

- *Appearance:* A normal semen sample is pearly white and opaque. Any variation is toward some clinical entity. Most common cause of reddish semen is genital tract trauma and tumor and needs to be evaluated by an andrologist. Yellow color semen denotes infection or severe jaundice which needs to culture therapy if is failing which there is high chance of endometritis during intrauterine insemination (IUI) or infection of culture media during in vitro fertilization (IVF).
- *Liquefaction time:* The semen is ejaculated in a coagulated state due to the presence of coagulation proteins secreted by seminal vesicle. This helps proper deposition of the sperm inside the vaginal cavity. The thinning eases the sperm mobility into the cervical canal. Normal time is 30–60 minutes. Failure of liquefaction is a sign of inadequate secretion of proteolytic enzymes of prostate whereas absence of coagulation pointed to toward ejaculatory duct obstruction or congenital vesicle. In case of high liquefaction, the sperm are exposed longer to the harsher vaginal environment reducing in the possibility to natural conception.
- *Viscosity:* Viscosity is defined as the resistant of seminal fluid to follow. Normal semen coagulates upon ejaculation and liquefies within 15–20 minutes. Viscosity is noted after liquefaction. Nonliquefaction should be differentiated from hyperviscosity. Highly viscos sample reduces sperm motility through the seminal fluid.

INTERPRETATION OF SEMEN ANALYSIS: MICROSCOPIC PARAMETERS

Introduction

The microscopic examination of semen is carried out after complete liquefaction of the sample using a small drop of it placed over a *Makler's chamber* and seen under a phase contrast microscope **(Flowchart 3)**.
- *Concentration and number:* It is very important prognostic factor for deciding time to pregnancy and conception. Concentration is number of sperm per mL of semen whereas total number is sperm concentration is multiplied by total volume. The lower reference number of sperm concentration is 15×10^6/mL and total sperm count is 39×10^6/mL ejaculate. There is different terminology, i.e.,
  - Polyzoospermia (>350 million sperm/mL)
  - Normozoospermia (>40 million sperm/mL)
  - Oligospermia (<20 million sperm/mL)
  - *Azoospermia (no sperm in ejaculate):* If there is azoospermia, centrifuge the sample at 3,000 rmp for 15 minutes and the pallet should be checked by two observers. A confirmation of azoospermia is given only after repeating the assessment a second time minimum 2 weeks apart. In case of abnormal result always repeat the test after 2 weeks.

Flowchart 3: Semen analysis: Microscopic parameters and its clinical interpretation.

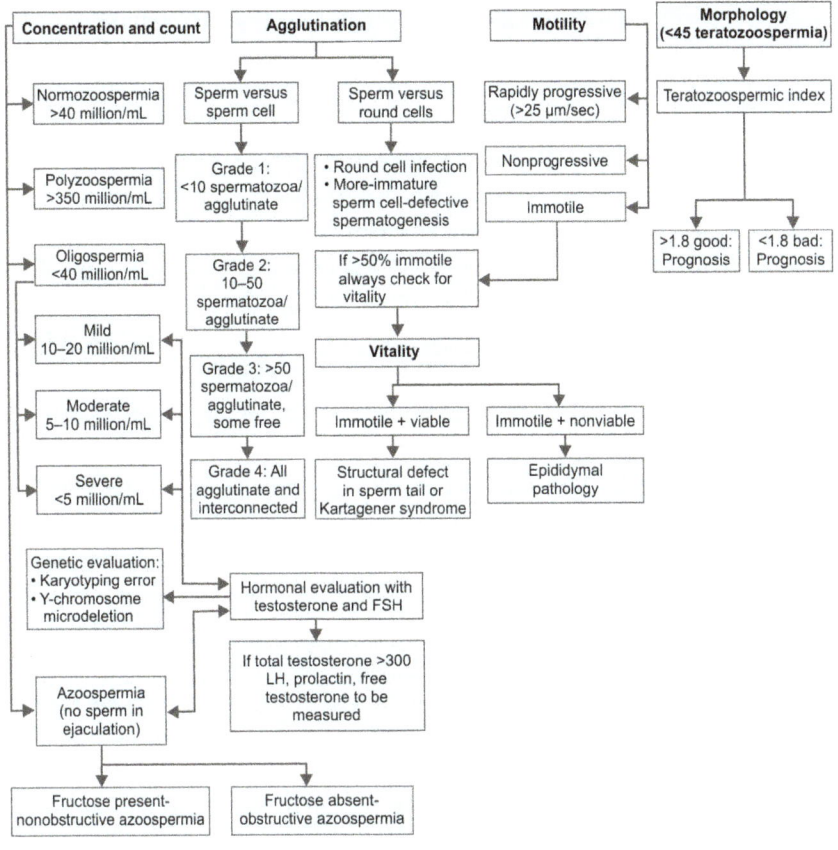

If the count is lower than 10 million sperm/mL then FSH total testosterone to be measured; low testosterone may be due to Leydig cell dysfunction or hypothalamic-pituitary-testicular axis dysfunction; if total testosterone <300 ng/dL then luteinizing hormone (LH), prolactin and free testosterone measured with the help of hormonal evaluation we get idea about clinical entity responsible for the abnormal result which help us to take treatment choices are assisted reproductive technology (ART) techniques. High FSH is found in testicular failure, and in testicular atrophy. Normal FSH is with normal testicular volume needs testicular sampling further to see for spermatogenesis. When spermatogenesis is normal, it is mostly due to obstruction to ejaculatory duct where vasovasostomy or vasoepididymostomy can be done or sperm retrieval by testicular sperm extraction/percutaneous epididymal sperm aspiration (TESE/PESA) followed by intracytoplasmic sperm injection (ICSI) to be done and if spermatogenesis is absent, it denotes destruction of tubular epithelium. Low and undetectable FSH is indicative of Kallmann syndrome. In case of azoospermia always check for fructose which decides whether it is of obstructive pathology. In severe oligospermia and azoospermia always do genetic evaluation to see karyotyping error or Y chromosome deletion.

- *Agglutination:* Agglutination of the sperms is seen in an unstained sample, it may be sperm versus sperm which can be—
  - Grade I (<10 spermatozoa per agglutinate)
  - Grade II (10–50 spermatozoa per agglutinate)
  - Grade III (>50 spermatozoa per agglutinate)
  - Grade IV (all spermatozoa agglutinated and agglutinates interconnected)

This agglutination may be between head-to-head, tail tip to tail tip, mixed and tangle. We plan the treatment accordingly, in case of case Grade I and Grade II, 2–3 cycle of IUI can be done whereas in Grade III and Grade IV better results are obtained by ICSI.

If it is with leukocytes and the leukocytes count is high then denotes infection, culture the semen sample and treat with antibiotics.

- *Motility:* The lower reference value for total motility is 40% and progressive motility is 32%. It can be broadly divided in three categories—rapidly progression (moving actively in linear speed), nonprogression (all pattern of motility without progressive), and immotile.
- *Vitality:* It differentiated dead sperm from live one. It can be done Eosin-Nigrosin (sperm with intact membrane are alive), hypo-osmotic swelling test swollen membrane when placed in a hypo-osmolar medium tests for the integrity of the sperm membrane. 1 µL of sperm are added to 250 µL of hypo-osmolar media available in the market and incubated for 60 minutes at room temperature and a minimum of 100 sperms per slide are observed for swollen tails demonstrating vitality. A vitality >58% is normal.
- *Morphology:* Morphology is scored by WHO classification by Kruger's strict criteria classification. The staining differentiates the quantitative normal and abnormal sperm morphological form in an ejaculate. It classifies abnormally shaped spermatozoa in different category on basis of head, tail, midpiece abnormality from the sperms recovered from postcoital cervical mucus or from surface of zona pellucida if sperms failed to meet, the strictly defined parameter of normal shape and they fall into abnormal category. The lower reference value is 4%. It can be head defect (double head, pyriform absence of acrosome, etc.), midpiece defect (bend neck and asymmetrical insertion into head), tail defect (short tail, hair pin, etc.). Teratozoospermic index is defined as the number of abnormality present per abnormal spermatozoa. If the value is >1.8, prognosis is poor and need ICSI and Intracytoplasmic morphologically selected sperm injection (IMSI).

MALE HYPOGONADISM

- The presence of symptoms or signs of testosterone deficiency with or without deficiency of spermatozoa production is defined as hypogonadism. In men with oligospermia hypogonadism should be suspected **(Flowchart 4)**. Hypogonadism may be due to primary disorder of the testes (primary hypogonadism) or be secondary toward defect in the hypothalamic pituitary axis (secondary hypogonadism). The diagnosis and cause of condition is made after assessing serum FSH and serum

Flowchart 4: Male hypogonadism.

Measure FSH, LH, and total serum testosterone

- FSH and LH elevated (>12 iU/mL) and testosterone low or low-normal → Primary (testicular) hypogonadism → Clinical suspicion for Klinefelter syndrome → Yes / No
- FSH and LH low or lower than expected for the level of testosterone and low testosterone (<300 g/dL) → Possible secondary gonadotropic hypogonadism → Measure serum prolactin and transferring saturation → Adolescent
  - No → Repeat hormone levels after 6 weeks
    - Normal levels → Temporary hypogonadism often due to temporary systemic illness
    - Persistently abnormal level → True hypogonadism → Measure serum prolactin and transferring saturation → Does the patient have any of the following?
      - Symptoms consistent with a pituitary tumor
      - Elevated prolactin level
      - Total testosterone level <200 ng/dL
      - Age <60 and no hemochromatosis or cushing disease
      - Yes → Obtain brain MRI or CT to rule out pituitary adenoma or other mass
      - No → Brain mass unlikely and neuroimaging unnecessary
  - Yes → Perform GnRH test
    - No increase in LH and FSH → True hypogonadism
    - Increase in FSH and LH → Delayed puberty
- FSH elevated or LH, FSH normal, and testosterone normal → Possible selective impairment of spermatogenesis

LH along with total (and when possible, free) serum testosterone levels measured concurrently. To evaluate serum testosterone, blood should be ideally drawn in morning (before 10 AM). The total testosterone normal range between 300 and 1,000 ng/dL.
- In primary hypogonadism, the testes fail to respond to FSH and LH secreted by pituitary. This results in reduced production of testosterone and failure of the negative feedback to pituitary inhibiting the production of FSH and LH, leading to elevated FSH and LH levels. Klinefelter syndrome is most common genetic cause of primary hypogonadism.
- In secondary hypogonadism, the hypothalamus fails to produce gonadotropin-releasing hormone (GnRH) or the pituitary gland fail to produce enough FSH and LH in respond to hypothalamic stimulation. In secondary hypogonadism, testosterone levels are low and levels of FSH and LH are low or borderline normal.
- If hypogonadism associated with testosterone deficiency manifest for first time in adulthood. The manifestation can be varied depending upon the degree and duration of the deficiency. Diminished libido, erectile dysfunction, cognitive skills, sleep disturbances and mood fluctuation are common. Features like gynecomastia, osteopenia, sparse body hair, decreased clean body mass, increased visceral parts, testicular atrophy etc. testosterone deficiency may increase risk of coronary artery disease and prostate cancer.
- *Diagnose:* Assessment of serum prolactin level (to screen the pituitary adenoma) and transferrin saturation (to screen for hemochromatosis) MRI and CT can be rule out pituitary macroadenoma or other mass in men following: (1) age <60 years with no other identified cause for hypogonadism; (2) very low total testosterone level <200 ng/dL; (3) elevated prolactin level; (4) symptoms consistent with a pituitary.
- *Treatment:* Testosterone replacement therapy (TRT)—
  - Primary hypogonadism with complete testicular failure, testosterone replacement therapy is mainly given for symptomatic treatment such as cognitive, sexual and physical symptoms. TRT should be avoided, especially when fertility is a concern, in secondary hypogonadism as exogenous testosterone supplementation impairs endogenous spermatogenesis (unless there is irreversible primary testicular failure). TRT can be considered for men who—(1) do not show any signs of puberty; (2) are near age 15; (3) after exclusion of secondary hypogonadism. They may be given long-acting testosterone enanthate 50 mg intramuscular (IM) once/month for 4-8 months. Testosterone cypionate is given at a dose that is increased gradually over 18-24 months from 50 mg to 100 mg to 200 mg IM every 1-2 weeks. Older adolescents on high doses of IM testosterone (100-200 mg every 2 weeks) are best transited to testosterone gel preparations at adult dosages.

- *Secondary hypogonadism:* Therapy begins with replacement of LH and FSH. LH replacement is initiated using human chorionic gonadotropin (hCG) AT doses of 1,500 IU subcutaneous (SC) three times/for a minimum of 12 weeks. FSH replacement, can be done using human menopausal gonadotropins (hMG) or human recombinant FSH, at doses of 150 IU three times/week. Doses may be adjusted based on the results of periodic testing with semen analysis and levels of serum FSH, LH, and testosterone. Therapy can be continued for a minimum of 6–12 months till sperm production is noticed. Most men who have secondary hypogonadism due to a hypothalamic defect (e.g., idiopathic hypogonadotropic hypogonadism, Kallmann syndrome) become fertile with treatment despite sperm counts that are low (e.g., <5 million/mL).

AZOOSPERMIA: EVALUATION (FLOWCHART 5)

Definition

It is complete absence of sperms in two semen samples even after centrifugation of semen sample **(Table 2)**. If sperms are seen after centrifugation, it is called cryptozoospermia and is different from azoospermia. Incidence of azoospermia in normal population is around 1 in 100. In infertile population, incidence is high as 1 in 10.

- Before making a diagnosis of azoospermia, it is essential to exclude any ejaculatory dysfunction. Meticulous and accurate history taking is the best tool to diagnose ejaculatory dysfunction such as anejaculation and retrograde ejaculation, the former is characterized by anorgasmia.
- Physically examination can give insight into the cause of azoospermia.
  Testis: Look for size and consistency, soft and small testis points toward testicular failure.
  In epididymis and vas deferens: Look for scarring or dilatation which suggests partial obstruction due to fibrosis and inflammation signs of post-testicular obstruction. Look for secondary sexual characters including body habitus, hair distribution and gynecomastia.
- Clinical varieties of azoospermia:
  - *Hypogonadotropic hypogonadism (pretesticular):* It mainly includes endocrinological abnormalities involving the hypothalamus pituitary or it can be receptor mutations **(Box 1)**.
  - *Hypergonadotropic hypogonadism (testicular):* It includes the defects that cause testicular failure leading to azoospermia **(Table 3)**.
  - *Normogonadotropic normogonadism (post-testicular obstructive):* 40% azoospermia men are normogonadotropic and obstruction of sperm delivery is the main cause.
- Endocrine tests are the major tools for the cause of azoospermia. Serum FSH is most important investigation to differentiate various types of

Flowchart 5: Evaluation and treatment of azoospermia.

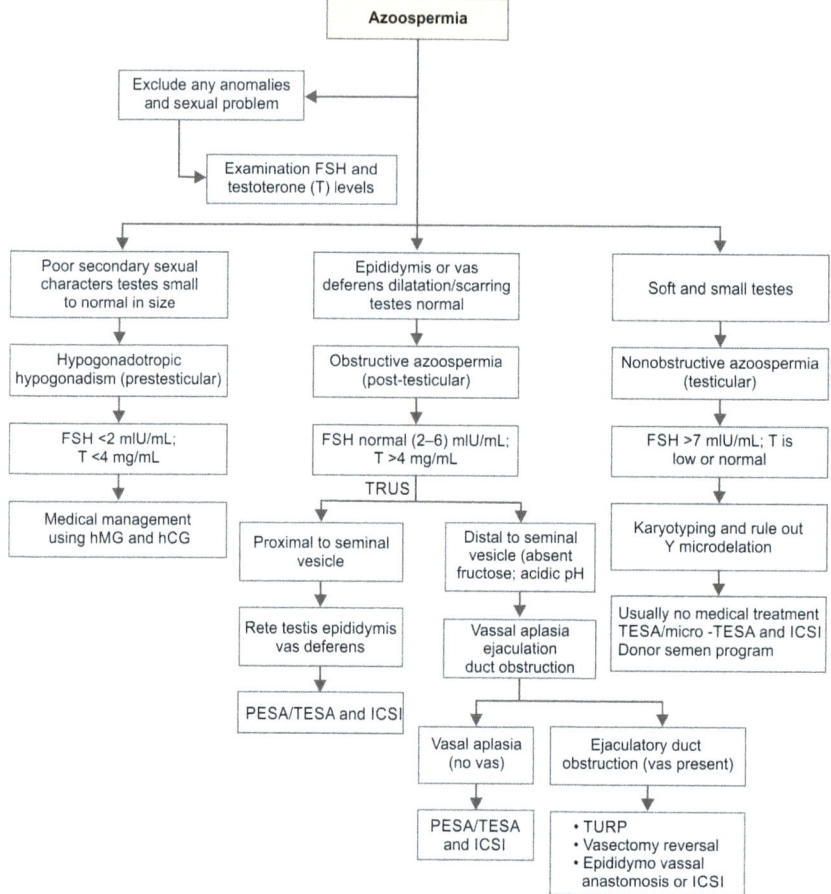

azoospermia. Elevated FSH >10 IU/L suggests testicular failure. It also has prognostic significance on sperm retrieval for ART higher the FSH less chance of sperm retrieval. FSH is markedly low in pretesticular cause such as hypogonadal-hypogonadism (secondary hypogonadism). FSH is unaffected in post-testicular cause such as in obstructive azoospermia.
- Ultrasound mostly TRUS has a role to play when an obstructive pathology is suspected. TRUS should look for presence or absence of vas deferens and seminal vesicle or ejaculatory duct distension.
- Genetic testing plays the role especially in nonobstructive cases. Karyotyping to detect chromosomal abnormalities resulting in impaired testicular function (e.g., Klinefelter syndrome), Y-chromosomal microdeletions leading to spermatogenic impairment. It helps as a tool to predict sperm retrieval in nonobstructive azoospermia. CFTR mutation testing in congenital bilateral absence of vas deferens, but incidence is low.

Evaluation of the Male Infertility Factors

TABLE 2: Azoospermia evaluation and treatment.

Testes	Epididymis	Vas deferens	FSH	Testosterone	Diagnosis	Treatment
Very small to normal size	Normal	Normal	Low (<2 mIU/mL)	<4 mg/mL	Hypogonadotropic hypogonadism	Gonadotropin therapy
Normal	Normal or distended	Absent/thickened/ beaded/discontinuous	Usually low normal around 5 mIU/mL	>4 mg/mL	Obstructive	PESA TESA Epididymo-vasal anastomosis
Soft atrophied to almost normal	Not delineated	Not delineated	High (>7 mIU/mL)	Low or normal	Nonobstructive	Micro-TESA

(PESA: percutaneous epididymal sperm aspiration; TESA: testicular sperm aspiration)

BOX 1: Causes of hypogonadotropic hypogonadism (pretesticular).

- Klinfelter syndrome
- Y chromosome deletions
- Cryptorchidism
- Infection (viral, TB)
- Drugs (alkylating agents, antiandrogen)
- Radiation
- Gonadotoxins

TABLE 3: Causes of nonobstructive azoospermia (testicular).

Congenital	Acquired
Kallmann syndrome	Trauma
Idiopathic isolated GnRH deficiency	Tumors, critical illness
Single gene mutation involving GnRH receptor, FSH/LH receptor	Infection (e.g., meningitis), infiltrative disorder like sarcoidosis

> **BOX 2:** Histopathological types of testicular biopsies.
> - Normal Spermatogenesis
> - Hypospermatogenesis
> - Maturation arrest
> - Sertoli only cell syndrome
> - Testicular atrophy

- Hypogonadotropic hypogonadism is probably the only group of azoospermic patients that responds well to medical management. The condition can be treated medically by gonadotropins (hMG), FSH or hCG for prolonged duration (1.5–2 years). Approximately 30% may respond well and have high chances if natural conception, and around 30% respond with minimal spermatogenesis and may need ART.
- The obstruction can be proximal to seminal vesicle (rete testis, epididymis, vas) to seminal vesicle (vasal aplasia or ejaculatory duct obstruction). Both distal varieties present with azoospermia acidic pH of semen, decreased semen value (<1 mL). Clinical examinations differentiate between vasal (vas absent) and ejaculatory duct obstruction (vas present). Treatment involves surgical sperm retrieval. Vasal recanalization is done in case postvasectomy. Ejaculatory duct obstruction may be treated with transurethral resection of the prostate (TURP).
- Most acceptable treatment of obstructive azoospermia is percutaneous epididymis sperm aspiration/testicular sperm aspiration (PESA/TESA) with ICSI, where there is an almost 100% sperm retrieval rate. The prognosis is good owing to retrieval of genetically normal sperm.
- No medical or surgical treatment is available or advisable for patients with testicular failure. Only chance to father the child is by attempting to retrieval sperm with the help of TESA/microtesticular sperm extraction (TESE). Micro-TESE has largely improved the sperm retrieval rate in this group of patients, wherein certain rate up to 60%. The treatment option where you do not retrieve sperm on any of this procedure or in couple who cannot afford to do an IVF treatment is to go for use of donor sperm.

Histopathological Types of Azoospermia

It is seen in a testicular biopsy specimen **(Box 2)**. However, testicular biopsy from particular site may not represent the total testicular function and is unreliable in predicting the prognosis.

ANEJACULATION

Anejaculation is defined as complete absence of ejaculation during sexual activity, despite normal erections or nocturnal emissions.
- Anejaculation should be differentiated from retrograde ejaculation by analyzing the postejaculation urine.

Anejaculation can be classified as:
- Orgasmic (organic) anejaculation
- Anorgasmic (psychogenic/idiopathic) anejaculation
- Situational anejaculation
- We can encounter different types of situational anejaculation:
  - Clinic anejaculation (can collect semen at home, but has anejaculation in clinic)
  - Periovulatory anejaculation (unable to ejaculate at ovulation, but can ejaculate on other days)
  - Unexpected anejaculation (first time failure of ejaculation on day of ovulation)
  - Masturbatory anejaculation (ejaculates during intercourse, but not by masturbation)
  - Intercourse anejaculation (ejaculates by masturbation, but not during intercourse).
- Situational anejaculation mostly means existence of ejaculation by masturbation, but not during sexual intercourse and it can be because of performance anxiety or hostility toward the partner or psychosexual development, and unconscious desire to avoid pregnancy.

Management of Anejaculation on the Day of Ovum Pickup

- Anxiety most likely plays a major role in these reported cases. Acute ejaculation failure can occur in patients who previously had no problems with semen production on demand in the clinic.
- Sildenafil citrate (Viagra) has been recommended after failed trails of more than 1 hour to produce semen.
- A prior proper history and counseling is important to diagnose such problems. Each clinic should discuss the possible difficulties associated with sperm procurement with the couple on initial medical consultations and also during the in vitro fertilization (IVF) counseling session with andrologist. If a problem is detected, the possibility of cryopreserving sperm for backup use should always be offered.
- Anejaculation, or lack of ejaculation, can occur in men with pelvic nerve damage from diabetes mellitus, retroperitoneal surgery, multiple sclerosis, spinal cord injury, or psychological causes. The use of penile vibratory stimulation (PVS) or rectal probe electroejaculation (EEJ) can help to procure a semen sample containing sperm for use with assisted reproductive technique (ART). In particular, PVS, which often does not require general anesthesia, works best in men with complete spinal cord injuries above T10, with up to 86% of patients able to achieve ejaculation with PVS. On the other hand, only 0–15% of men with spinal cord injuries below T10 were able to achieve ejaculation with PVS. In men

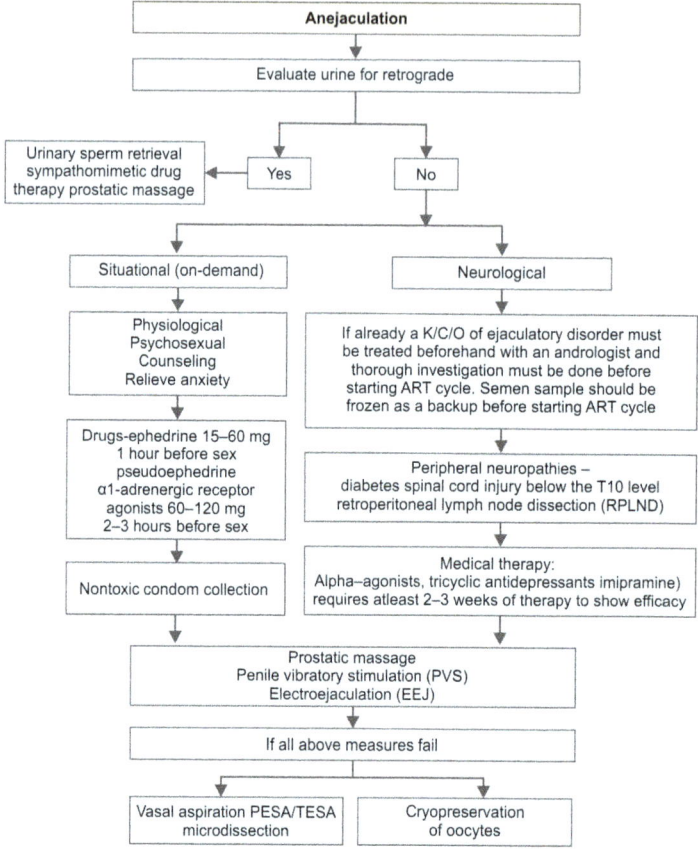

Flowchart 6: Evaluation and treatment of anejaculation.

with anejaculation from other etiologies or after failure with PVS, EEJ is preferred and can produce ejaculation in 92% of men with anejaculation from spinal cord injury. Of note, since both PVS and EEJ can cause autonomic dysreflexia in men with spinal cord injuries at or above T6, blood pressure monitoring and premedication with nifedipine should be considered.

- If noninvasive methods to obtain a sperm sample fail, invasive techniques should be used with caution and cryopreservation of oocytes can be also offered as last resort. If invasive method is required for sperm collection, testicular sperm aspiration should be preferred means of extraction. Performing a percutaneous epididymal sperm aspiration from a normal epididymis might not only be difficult but also has lower probability of obtaining sperms and higher chances of damaging the epididymis **(Flowchart 6)**.

CONCLUSION

Evaluation of male infertility is an important aspect of evaluation in infertile couple. Detailed history, physical examination and hormonal evaluation provide important insights for treatment to the clinician.

SUGGESTED READING

1. Fritz MA, Speroff L. Clinical Gynecologic Endocrinology and Infertility, 8th edition. Philadelphia: Lippincott Williams & Wilkins; 2010.
2. Gardner DK, Weissman A, Howles CM, Shoham Z. Textbook of Assisted Reproductive Technique, Clinical Perspectives, 5th edition. Florida: CRC Press; 2018.
3. Male infertility best practice policy committee of the American Urological Association, practice committee of the American Society for Reproductive Medicine. Report on optimal evaluation of the infertile male. Fertil Steril. 2006;86(5 Suppl 1):S202-9.
4. World Health Organization. WHO laboratory manual for the examination and processing of human semen. Geneva: WHO; 2010.

CHAPTER 10

Evaluation and Management of Azoospermia

Sheetal Sawankar, Satish Patki

INTRODUCTION

The prevalence of azoospermia is approximately 1% among all men and ranges between 10 and 15% among infertile men. Thus, this group of patients represents a significant population in the field of male infertility.

DEFINITION

Azoospermia is defined as complete absence of sperm in the ejaculate sample. If no sperms are seen in the wet preparation of the semen sample, The World Health Organization (WHO) recommends centrifugation of the semen sample at 3,000 × g or greater for 15 minutes at room temperature followed by a high-powered microscopic examination of the pellet formed. If still no sperms are seen, a second semen analysis with similar centrifugation is repeated at least 2 weeks apart. If no sperms are seen in two successive samples, the man can be labeled as azoospermic. If even a few sperms are seen in the pellet, the condition is described as cryptozoospermia **(Flowchart 1)**.

Flowchart 1: Classification of azoospermia.

```
         Etiology and classification of azoospermia
                          │
         ┌────────────────┴────────────────┐
         ▼                                 ▼
    Nonobstructive              Obstructive azoospermia
     azoospermia                     Less common:
                                  15–20% of all cases
         │                                 │
    ┌────┴────┐                            │
    ▼         ▼                            ▼
```

Pretesticular causes:	Testicular causes:	Post-testicular causes:
• Congenital: Kallmann's syndrome • *Acquired*: Hypothalamic or pituitary disorders • *Secondary*: Adverse effect from medication	• Congenital: Anorchia • Cryptorchidism • Y-chromosome deletions • *Sertoli cell*: Only tumors • *Acquired*: Trauma, torsion, infection (mumps orchitis)	• Ejaculatory disorders and obstruction • Congenital bilateral absence of the vas deferens (CBAVD) • Acquired due to infection or surgery

EVALUATION OF AN AZOOSPERMIC MALE

A good history taking and thorough physical examination are of paramount importance in evaluation of azoospermic males **(Tables 1, 2 and Flowchart 2)**.

Semen Examination

A good semen examination can give us insight into the cause of azoospermia.

- *Semen volume:* A low semen volume <1.5 mL is usually found in the following conditions—
  - Ejaculatory duct dysfunction
  - Ejaculatory duct obstruction

TABLE 1: History taking.

General information	Examples and areas of focus
Infertility history	• Duration of infertility • Whether the infertility is primary or secondary • Any treatments to date • Libido • Sexual function • Sexual activity
The general health of the man	• Diabetes • Respiratory issues • Recent illnesses
Any proven or suspected genitourinary infections, testicular infections or inflammation	• Sexually transmitted infections • Epididymo-orchitis • Mumps orchitis
Any surgery of the reproductive tract	• Testis cancer • Undescended testis • Hydrocelectomies • Spermatocelectomies

TABLE 2: Physical examination.

Type of examination	Examples and areas of focus
State of virilization	
Scrotal examination	• Size and consistency of the testis • Presence and grade of varicoceles • Palpable vas deferens
Abdominal examination	Presence of scars in the inguinal area indicative of previous inguinal surgery or treatment of undescended testis

92 Evaluation and Management of Azoospermia

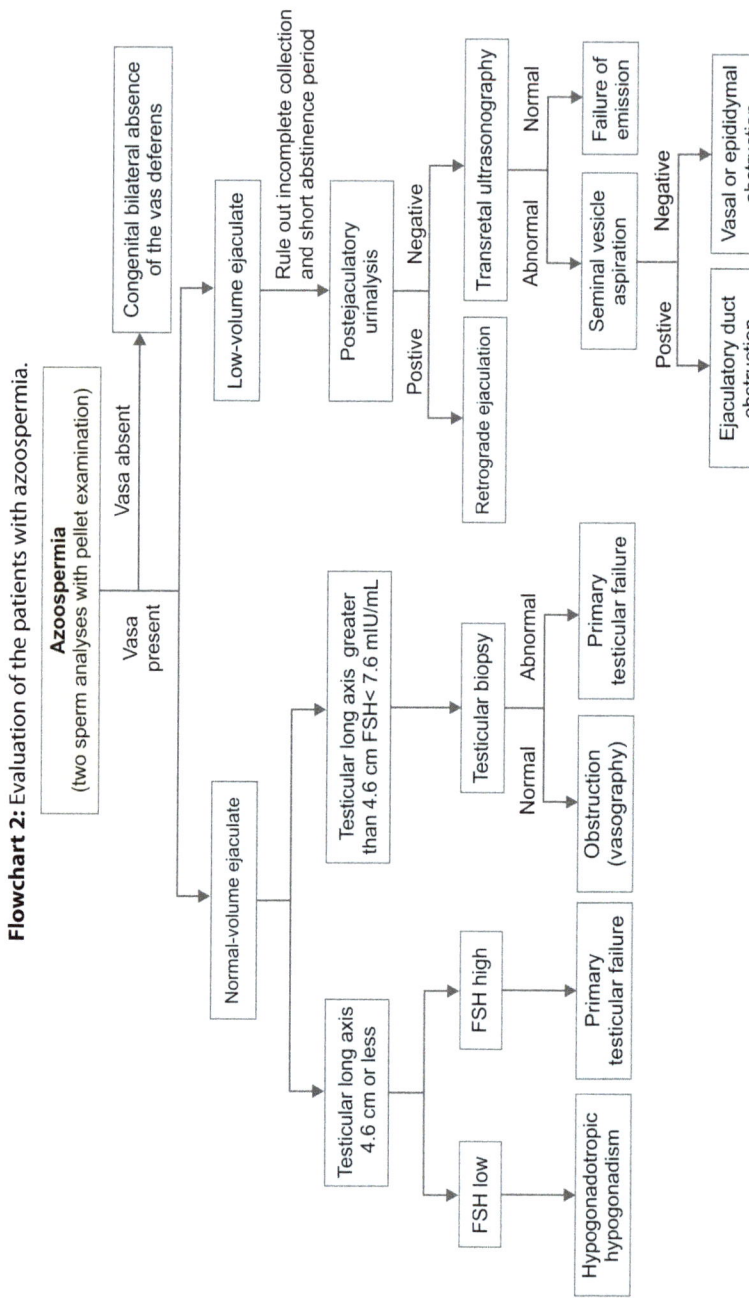

Flowchart 2: Evaluation of the patients with azoospermia.

(FSH: follicle-stimulating hormone)

- Cases of retrograde ejaculation in which sperms can be isolated from the post coital urine sample on centrifugation
- *Semen pH:* A low semen pH goes in favor of obstruction at the level of the ejaculatory ducts
- *Fructose in semen:* Absence or low levels of fructose in semen again suggest obstruction at the level of the ejaculatory ducts.

Radiological Evaluation

Scrotal ultrasonography (USG) to rule out varicocele, transrectal ultrasonography (TRUS), TRUS-guided seminal vesiculography, endorectal magnetic resonance imaging, abdominal USG, and cranial imaging are the various methods which can be used to evaluate males with azoospermia.

Endocrinological Examination

The endocrinological examination primarily involves measurement of serum follicle-stimulating hormone (FSH), luteinizing hormone (LH), testosterone, prolactin and a thyroid profile.
- Elevated prolactin levels can suppress gonadotropin releasing hormone (GnRH) pulsatile release from the hypothalamus, occasionally causing azoospermia
- Elevated FSH and LH levels with decreased testosterone levels suggests primary testicular failure
- A low FSH, LH and testosterone levels suggests hypogonadotropic hypogonadism
- A normal FSH, LH and testosterone level in an azoospermic patient suggests an obstructive cause of azoospermia.

Testicular Biopsy

A testicular biopsy [testicular sperm extraction (TESE) or micro-TESE] can be performed as a confirmation tool in cases of azoospermia. In cases where the cause of azoospermia is obstruction at any level in the ejaculatory system, TESE or micro-TESE should be able to yield adequate number of sperms to perform intracytoplasmic sperm injection (ICSI) for the couple.

In conditions where the FSH levels are normal, a testicular biopsy may help differentiate between a normally functioning testis and disorders of spermatogenesis such as maturation arrest, Sertoli cell only syndrome, etc.

Genetic Examination

A genetic examination and karyotyping should be performed in men with testicular causes of azoospermia cytogenetic tests such as Y-chromosome microdeletion (YCMD) test and cystic fibrosis transmembrane conductance regulator (CFTR) gene mutation should be looked for.

MANAGEMENT OF CASES OF AZOOSPERMIA (FLOWCHART 3)

Obstructive Azoospermia

- *Reversal of obstruction:*
  - *Vasovasostomy:* Most commonly done procedure and is the gold standard for vassal reconstructive procedures. 86% patency rates and 52% pregnancy outcomes.

  Natural conception is shown in **Figure 1**.

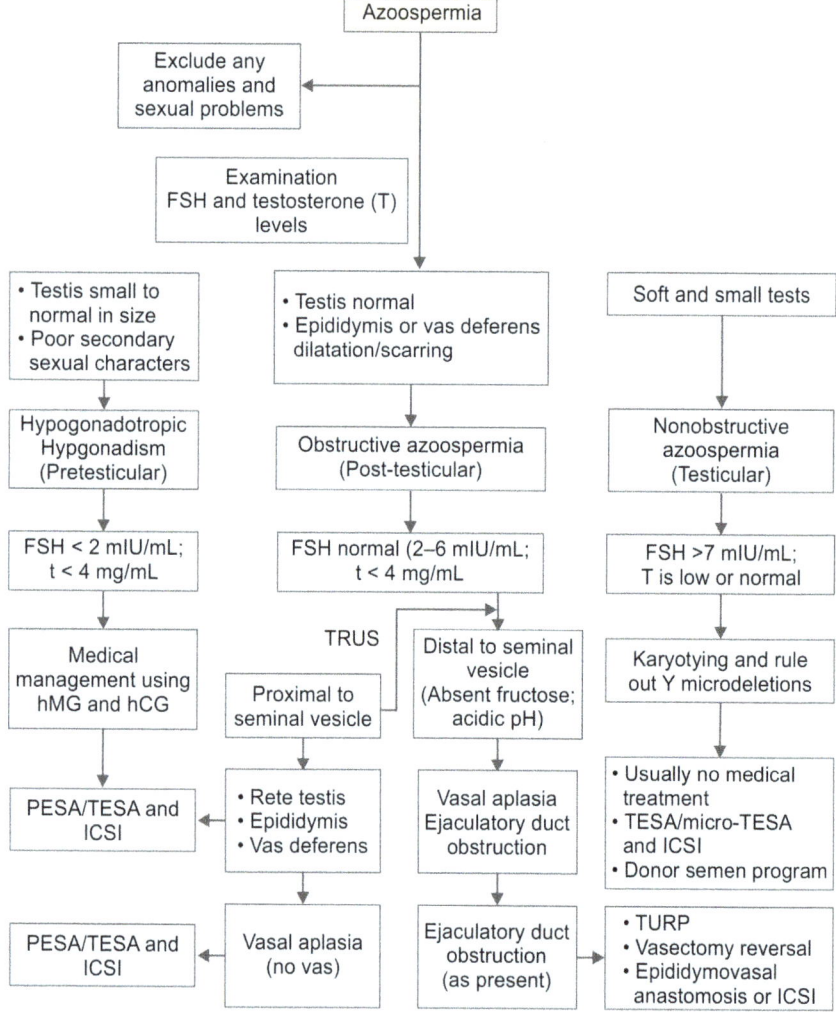

Flowchart 3: Differential diagnosis and management of azoospermia.

(FSH: follicle-stimulating hormone; ICSI: intracytoplasmic sperm injection; PESA: percutaneous epididymal sperm aspiration; TESA: testicular sperm aspiration; TURP: transurethral resection of the prostate; TURS: transrectal ultrasonography)

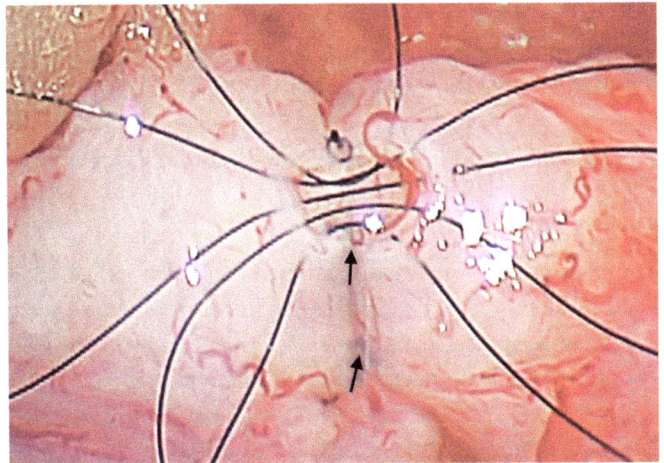

Fig. 1: Vasovasostomy.

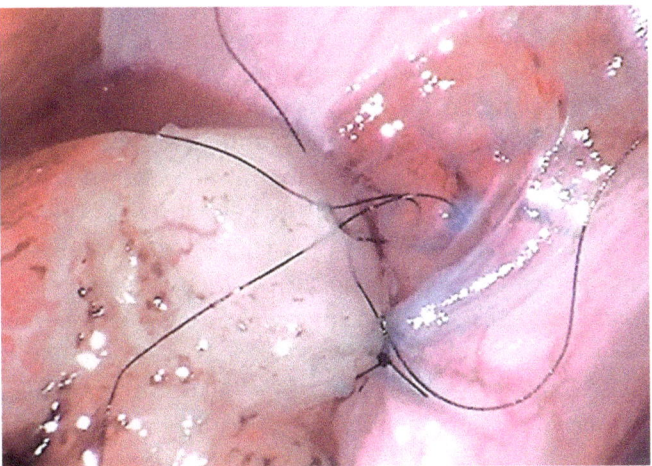

Fig. 2: Vasoepididymostomy.

- *Vasoepididymostomy:* It is done in cases of proximal vas blockage. 20-40% couples achieve pregnancy through timed intercourse **(Fig. 2)**.
- *Transurethral resection of ejaculatory ducts (TURED):* Treatment of choice in cases of ejaculatory duct obstruction.
  After TURED sperms return to the ejaculate in approximately 50-75% men and almost 20% men achieve pregnancy.
  Complications can include hematuria, hematospermia, UTI, and a watery ejaculate due to reflux of urine.
- *Sperm retrieved from the reproductive tract* (close to 100% chance of finding sperm) to be used in an ICSI program. The method of sperm

retrieval used may be a percutaneous or an open microscopic aspiration of sperm from the epididymis or a percutaneous or open biopsy of the testis. Microdissectional TESE is known to have the highest sperm retrieval rate as compared to c-TESE or testicular sperm aspiration (TESA)/percutaneous epididymal sperm aspiration (PESA).

Nonobstructive Azoospermia

This could be due to either a testicular failure or a failure of the hypothalamo-hypophyseal pituitary axis to secrete adequate hormones to stimulate the testis to perform proper spermatogenesis. Intrinsic testicular impairment rarely responds to medication. Options of management include:

- *Human chorionic gonadotropin (hCG) supplementation:* Biweekly or thrice a week administration of hCG 2,500 units subcutaneously for 3-6 months can induce spermatogenesis. This is especially useful in cases of hypogonadotropic hypogonadism.
- *FSH and gonadotropin administration:* FSH when administered in doses of 37.5-150 IU thrice a week for 3-6 months especially in conjunction with HCG administration can significantly improve spermatogenesis. FSH is known to help in the completion of spermiogenesis.
- *Antioxidant administration:* The role of antioxidants in the management of cases of spermatogenesis arrest is highly debatable with a number of papers both supporting and opposing the outcomes. The proponents suggest that increased oxidative stress can cause spermatogenesis arrest and this can be reversed by prolonged use of antioxidants.
- *Aromatase inhibitors:* In men with non-obstructive azoospermia having low testosterone levels and high estradiol levels, administration of aromatase inhibitors such as letrozole or anastrozole can help correct this imbalance by preventing the peripheral conversion of testosterone to estradiol. This correction is known to facilitate spermatogenesis by increasing intratesticular levels of testosterone.
- *Management of varicocele associated nonobstructive azoospermia:* In rare cases grade 3 and 4 varicocele may be associated with nonobstructive azoospermia with raised FSH levels. Surgical correction of the varicocele is known to restore sperm in the ejaculate in up to 44% patients according to a recent review. As the restoration of sperm to the ejaculate is often transient it is often advisable to freeze the semen sample containing the sperm for future use.
- *Genetic evaluation of patients with nonobstructive azoospermia:* This may reveal a variety of conditions such as Klinefelter's syndrome, Y chromosomal microdeletions, etc. This diagnosis requires concurrent management with a genetic counselor who can advise on the impact of the genetic condition on the health of the patients as well as the possibility of

successful surgical sperm retrieval through microdissection techniques. In these conditions such as Y chromosome microdeletions where the patient harbors complete AZF-a or AZF-b deletion the patient should be advise to opt for donor sperm IUI or ICSI.
- In patients having AZF chromosome microdeletion, they should be forewarned that any male child that they may conceive will also likely suffer from nonobstructive azoospermia.
- *Pulsatile administration of GnRH:* GnRH can be administered subcutaneously/intravenously/intranasally. It is used as a second-line treatment when treatment with gonadotropins fails. It will only be effective if the man has an intact pituitary gland. The dose administered is 5–20 μg subcutaneously every 2 hours for 12–24 months. Spermatogenesis results in 77% of azoospermic men. However, it is an expensive treatment and the frequency of doses makes compliance an issue. It is again useful in cases of hypogonadotropic hypogonadism.

The use of androgens is contraindicated in men with azoospermia (Level of Evidence 1, Grade of Recommendation A).

Men with nonobstructive azoospermia with serum FSH levels >7.6 mIU/mL and low testosterone levels are likely to have a lower chance of sperm retrieval with either TESA, PESA conventional or microdissection TESE. They will benefit from donor sperm treatment or adoption.

CONCLUSION

- Majority of etiologies of azoospermia are treatable/manageable
- Establish nonobstructive azoospermia versus obstructive azoospermia with at minimum H and P, testosterone + FSH level
- Patients with testicular nonobstructive azoospermia always need a karyotype + YCMD
- Purely diagnostic testicular biopsy is no longer indicated
- With advances in ART, most azoospermic men are best treated in the setting of a fertility clinic where sperm can be banked or utilized on-site
- Even men with severe forms of azoospermia can still have a family.

SUGGESTED READING

1. Cocuzza M, Alvarenga C, Pagani R. Epidemiology and etiology of azoospermia. Clinics (Sao Paulo). 2013;68(Suppl 1):15-26.
2. Coward M. Novel approaches to the evaluation and management of azoospermia. Fertil Steril. 2018;109(5):777-82.
3. Esteves SC, Miyaoka R, Roque M, Agarwal A. Outcome of varicocele repair in men with non-obstructive azoospermia: systematic review and meta-analysis. Asian J Androl. 2016;18(2):246-53.
4. Gopinathan KK, Gopinath P. Azoospermia: Evaluation. In: Reddy AP, Agarwal R (Eds). Decision Making in Infertility, Ist edition. New Delhi: Jaypee Brothers Medical Publishers (P) Ltd.; 2020.

5. Gudeloglu A, Parekattil S. Update in the evaluation of the azoospermic male. Clinics (Sao Paulo). 2013;68(Suppl 1):27-34.
6. Jarvi K, Lo K, Grober E, Mak V, Fischer A, Grantmyre J, et al. The workup and management of azoospermic males. Can Urol Assoc J. 2015;9(7-8): 222-35.
7. Practice Committee of the American Society for Reproductive Medicine. Management of non-obstructive azoospermia: a committee opinion. Fertil Steril. 2018;110(7):1239-45.
8. Shiraishi K, Ohmi C, Shimabukuro T, Matsuyama H. Human chorionic gonadotrophin treatment prior to microdissection testicular sperm extraction in non-obstructive azoospermia. Hum Reprod. 2012;27:331-9.

CHAPTER 11

Step by Step Management of Infertility in Polycystic Ovary Syndrome

Girish Godbole, Manjiri Valsangkar

INTRODUCTION

Polycystic ovary syndrome (PCOS) is most common endocrine disorder affecting 3–28% of Indian women.[1] It has a multifactorial etiology and is the most common cause of infertility in Indian women. PCOS is defined universally by the Rotterdam criteria given in **Flowcharts 1 and 2**.

Clinically diagnosing PCOS is a challenge as it has a varied presentation commonly as infertility, acne, hirsutism, uncontrolled weight gain, central alopecia, and acanthosis nigricans are common clinical features.[2]

Polycystic ovary syndrome may coexist with comorbidities such as hypertension, dyslipidemia, insulin resistance, hyperandrogenemia, and congenital heart disease (CHD), hypothyroidism, hyperprolactinemia, endometriosis, etc. Diagnosis of PCOS is confirmed using hormonal

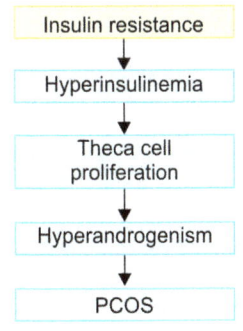

Flowchart 1: Pathogenesis of polycystic ovary syndrome (PCOS).

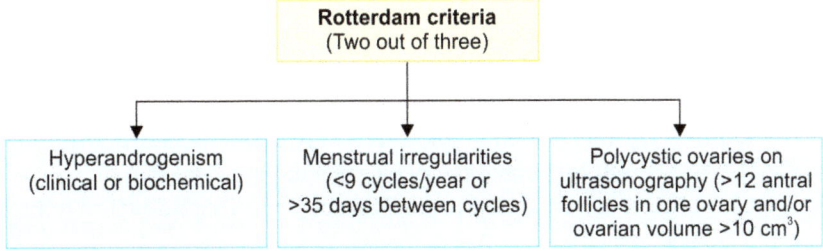

Flowchart 2: Rotterdam criteria.

TABLE 1: Sonomorphology of PCOS.	
Volume	**>10 CC**
AFC	>12
Stromal RI	<0.5
Stromal PSV	10
Stromal/total volume	>3/4
Stromal FI	>15

(AFC: antral follicle count; FI: flow index; PCOS: polycystic ovary syndrome; PSV: peak systolic blood flow velocity; RI: resistance index)

investigations such as anti-Müllerian hormone (AMH), HbA1c, serum-free testosterone along with sonography for antral follicle count (AFC) and volume studies which helps in diagnosing PCOS **(Table 1)**.

MANAGEMENT OF PCOS—OI IN PCOS-FERTIL-STERIL 2008

The primary goal of ovulation induction is to stimulate monofollicular development resulting in a successful singleton pregnancy **(Flowcharts 3 and 4)**.[3]

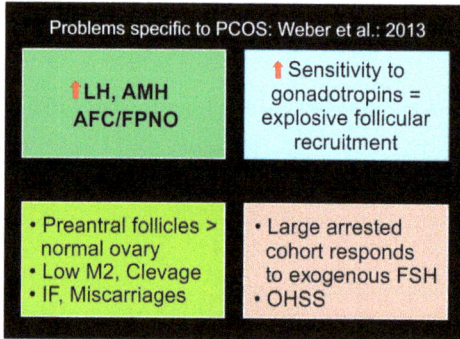

(AFC: antral follicle count; AMH: anti-Müllerian hormone; FNPO: follicle number per ovary; FSH: follicle-stimulating hormone; LH: luteinizing hormone; OHSS: ovarian hyperstimulation syndrome; PCOS: polycystic ovary syndrome)

- Gonadotropins in intrauterine insemination (IUI) for PCOS
    - Second line of ovulation induction (OI) in PCOS
    - Anovulatory PCOS not responding to oral agents for more than three cycles/CCR
    - Unexplained infertility, endometriosis
    - Counseling the patients for ovarian hyperstimulation syndrome (OHSS), multiple pregnancy, cycle cancellations, and cost
    - Chronic low-dose step up protocol is ideal than step down to reduce OHSS.

- Recommended starting doses in PCOS are 37.5 or 75 IU rFSH/hMG/day

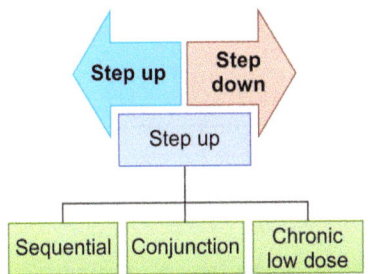

If no follicle, cancellation of cycle
If more than four follicles convert to IVF

Flowchart 3: Ovulation induction for IUI in PCOS.

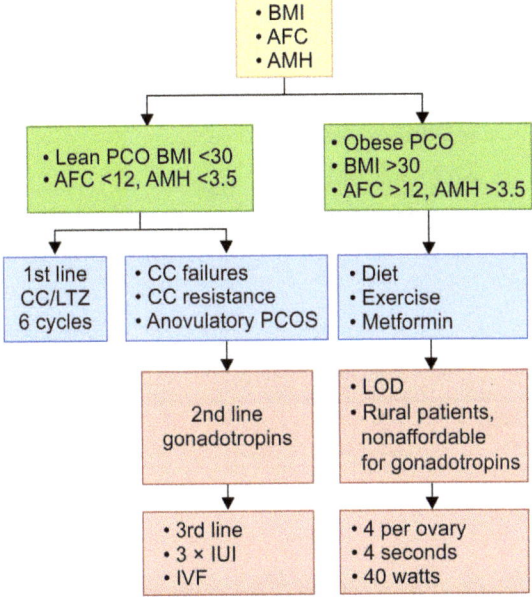

(AFC: antral follicle count; AMH: anti-Müllerian hormone; BMI: body mass index; CC: clomiphene citrate; IUI: intrauterine insemination; IVF: in vitro fertilization; LOD: limit of detection; LTZ: letrozole; PCOS: polycystic ovary syndrome)

Flowchart 4: Oral ovulogens.

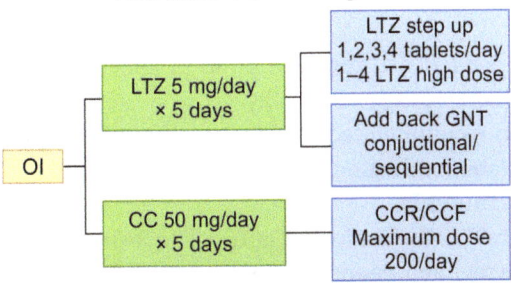

(OI: ovulation induction)

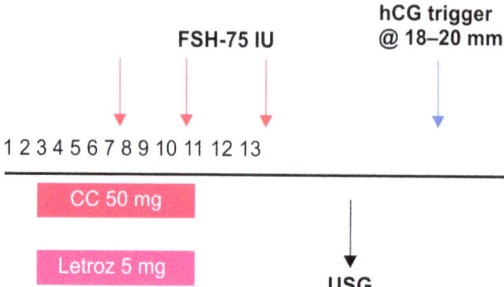

Fig. 1: Conjunction regimen step-up protocol.

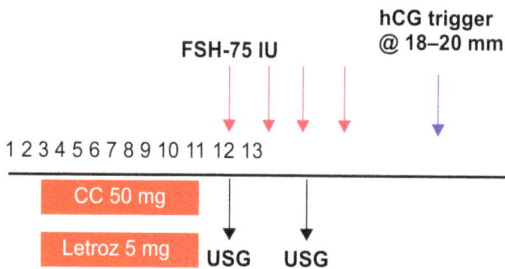

Fig. 2: Sequential regimen step-up protocol.

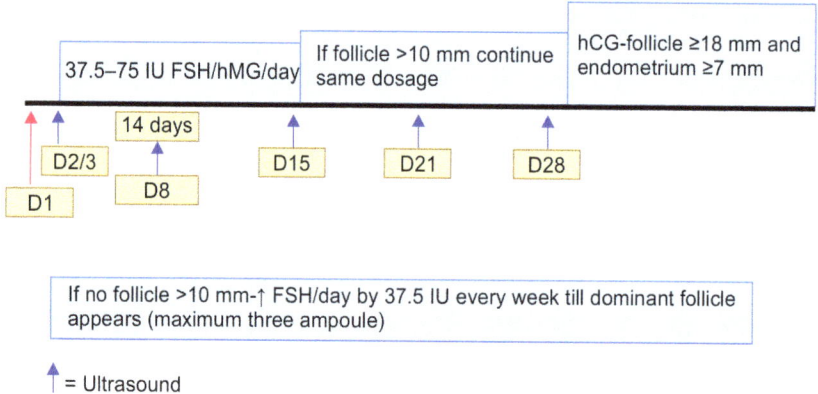

Fig. 3: Chronic low dose step-up protocol.

- *Indications for IUI*: IUI must be done in anovulatory subfertile PCOS women with male factor subfertility
- IUI must be recommended to three unsuccessful conception attempts despite ovulation induction
- Unexplained infertility
- Mild-moderate endometriosis. **Figures 1 to 3** show step-up protocol for conjunction regimen, sequential regimen and chronic low dose.
- In vitro fertilization (IVF) for PCOS is recommended who fail to conceive after OI six attempt or male subfertility.

Step by Step Management of Infertility in Polycystic Ovary Syndrome

- Gonadotropin-releasing hormone (GnRH) antagonist protocol **(Fig. 4)** must be preferred over agonist protocol due to reduced OHSS and safety, efficacy.
- Recommended starting dose: 75–150 IU
- Trigger with agonist whenever required with elective cryopreservation/split cycles **(Figs. 5 and 6)**.

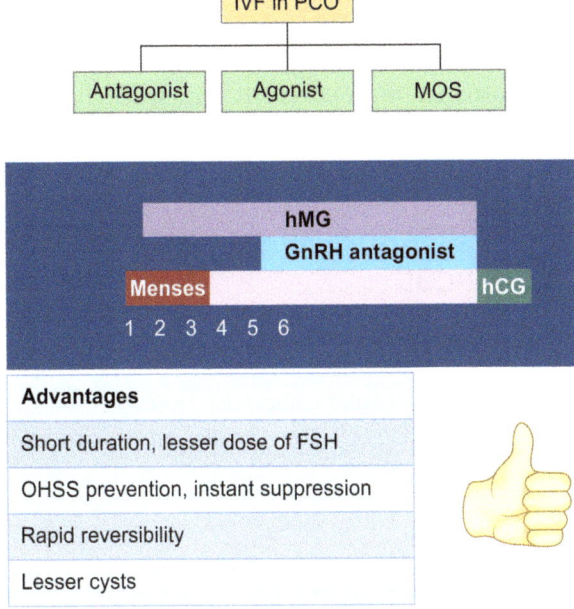

Fig. 4: Antagonist protocol.

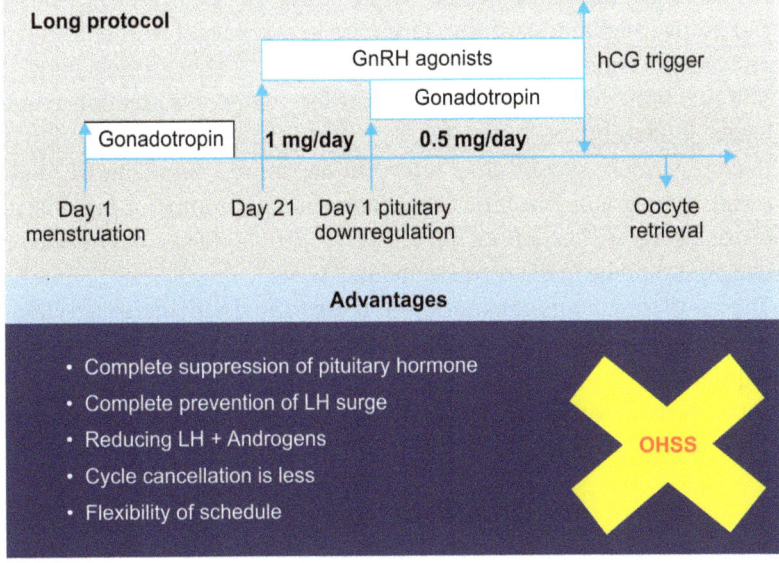

Fig. 5: Agonist protocol.

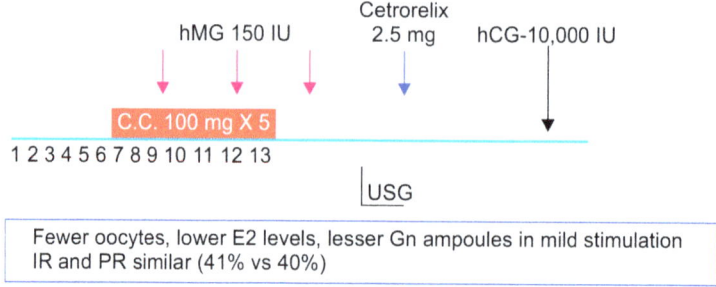

Fig. 6: Minimal ovarian stimulation protocol.
Source: Hwang JL, Huang LW, Hsieh BC, Tsai YL, Huang SC, Chen CY, et al. Ovarian stimulation by clomiphene citrate and hMG in combination with cetrorelix acetate for ICSI cycles. Hum Reprod. 2003;18(1):45-92003;18(1):45-9

STRATEGIES TO IMPROVE PREGNANCY RATES IN IVF IN PCOS

- Minimal ovarian stimulation protocol
- Early antagonist protocol
- Fixed antagonist versus flexible antagonist protocol
- Synchronization of follicles by downregulation with medroxyprogesterone, luteal phase estradiol.

CONCLUSION[4]

- Evaluation of women with presumed PCOS desiring pregnancy should exclude any other health issues in the woman or infertility problems in the couple. Before any intervention is initiated, preconceptional counseling should be provided emphasizing the importance of lifestyle, especially weight reduction and exercise in overweight women, smoking, and alcohol consumption.
- The recommended first-line treatment for ovulation induction remains letrozole/clomiphene citrate (CC)
- Recommended second-line intervention should letrozole/CC fail to result in pregnancy is either exogenous gonadotropins or laparoscopic ovarian surgery (LOS). Both have distinct advantages and drawbacks. The choice should be made on an individual basis.
- The use of exogenous gonadotropins is associated with increased chances for multiple pregnancy, so intense monitoring of ovarian response is required.
- Laparoscopic ovarian surgery is usually effective in <50% of women, and additional ovulation induction is required under those circumstances.

- Overall, ovulation induction (representing the CC–gonadotropin paradigm) is reported to be highly effective, with a cumulative singleton live-birth rate of 72%.
- Recommended third-line treatment is IVF because this treatment is effective in women with PCOS.

REFERENCES

1. Malik S, Jain K, Talwar P, Prasad S, Dhorepatil B, Devi G, et al. Management of polycystic ovary syndrome in India. Fertil Sci Res. 2014;1:23-43.
2. Wang, et al. Rotterdam criteria for PCO. Hum Reprod; 2007.
3. Weber, et al. OI in PCOS Fertility Sterility; 2008.
4. ESHRE ASRM Joint consensus PCOS; 2008.

CHAPTER 12 | Thyroid Disorders and Hyperprolactinemia in Infertility

Milind R Shah, Jhelam Deshmukh

INTRODUCTION

Different endocrine and immune factors play an important role in the process of fertility. There are great advances in the field of infertility. Many scientists have tried to identify risk factors that contribute to infertility. Thyroid autoimmunity (TAI) and thyroid dysfunction are important risk factors among them. Therefore, in the initial work-up of infertility, screening for thyroid-stimulating hormone (TSH) and anti-thyroperoxidase antibodies (TPO-Abs) should be done.

THYROID DISORDERS AND FEMALE INFERTILITY

The incidence of hypothyroidism ranges between 2 and 4%.[1] Compared to clinical thyroid dysfunction, subclinical thyroid anomalies, subclinical hypothyroidism, hypothyroxinemia and/or isolated TAI are much more frequent. In women with TPO-Abs, the risk of female infertility is increased in patients with TPO-Abs.[1] Patients with recurrent miscarriages also have a higher incidence of Tg- and/or TPO-Abs (25%).[2] **Figure 1** depicts the effect of thyroid abnormalities on female reproductive organs.

Pathophysiology

The ovarian surface epithelium and oocytes of primordial, primary, and secondary follicles have presence of TSH receptor and thyroid hormone receptors (TR-a1 and TR-b1)[4] **(Fig. 1)**. Thyroid hormones synergize with follicle-stimulating hormone (FSH) action on these oocytes. Thyroid hormone also cause direct stimulatory effects on granulosa cell functions, such as morphologic differentiation, luteinizing hormone (LH)/human chorionic gonadotropin (hCG) receptor formation, and induction of 3-beta-hydroxysteroid dehydrogenase and aromatase.[5] Thyroid hormones also can alter gonadotropin releasing hormone (GnRH) and prolactin secretion, sex hormone-binding globulin (SHBG) levels and coagulation factors.

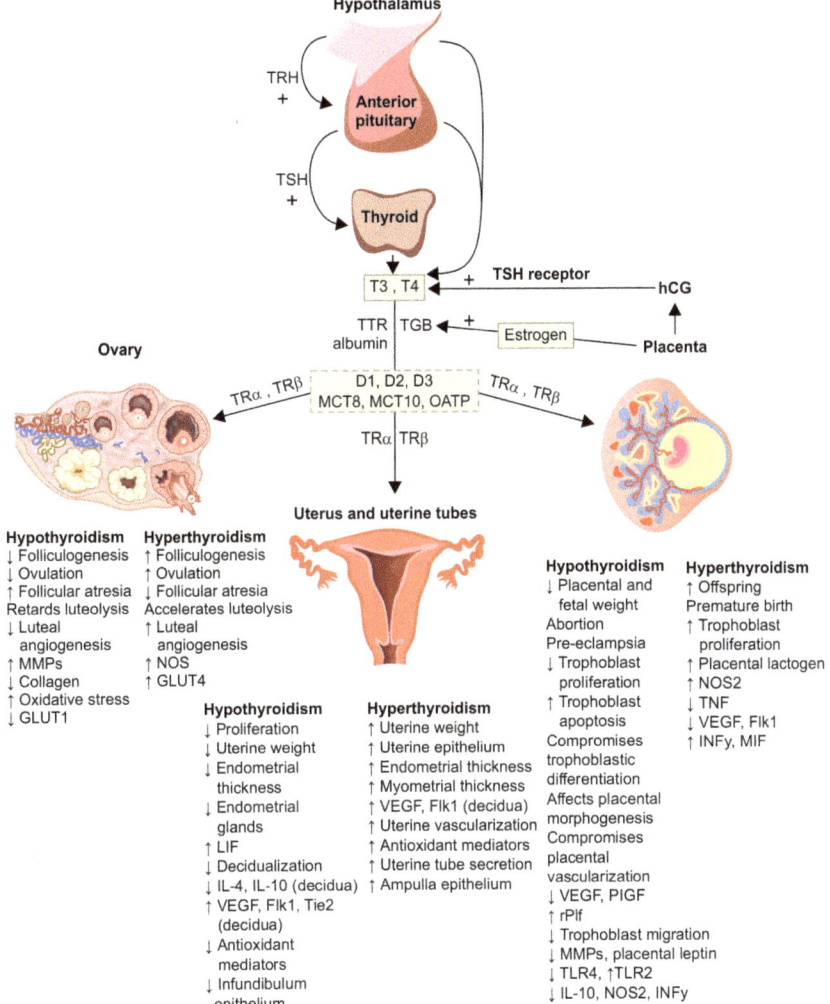

Fig. 1: Hypothalamic-pituitary-thyroid axis and effects of hypo- and hyperthyroidism on the morphophysiology of the ovary, uterine tube, uterus, and placenta.[3]

Thyroid Dysfunction and Female Infertility

Effect of hyperthyroidism on female infertility is shown in **Figure 2**. Subclinical and overt hypothyroidism and female infertility are shown in **Figure 3**.

Prolactin can cause ovulatory dysfunction by impairing pulsatile secretion of GnRH. It also causes insufficiency of the corpus luteum leading to low progesterone secretion in the luteal phase of the cycle.[6] Oligomenorrhea is the main menstrual problem with prolactinemia.[6] Even though in literature, the association of infertility and subclinical hypothyroidism (SCH) is not consistent, patients with fertility issues often showed higher mean TSH compared to fertile women.[1]

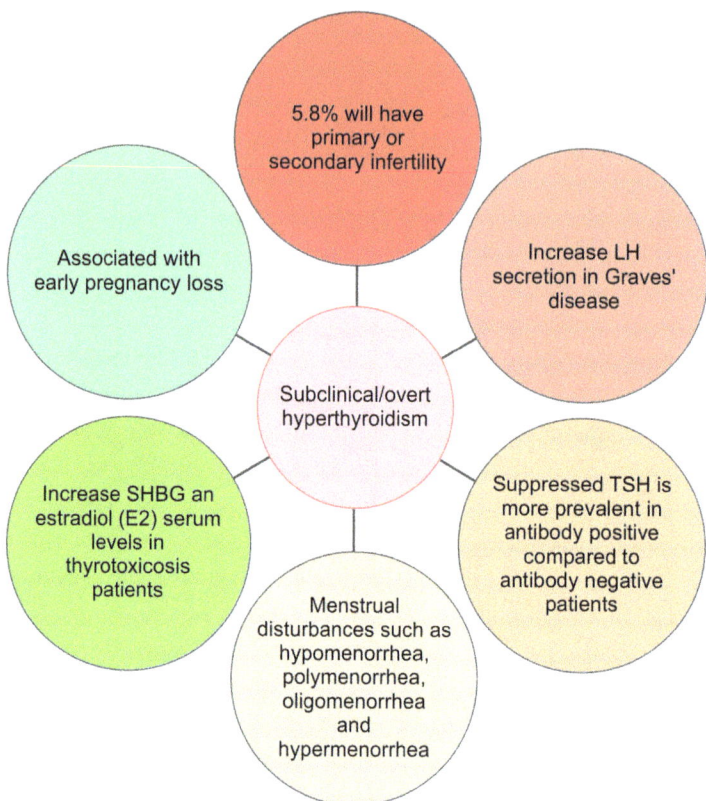

Fig. 2: Subclinical and overt hyperthyroidism and female infertility.[1,6-8]

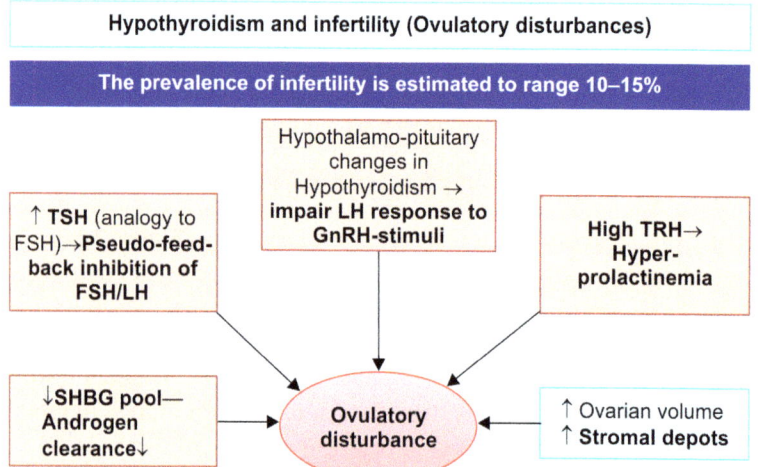

Fig. 3: Ovulatory disturbance in hypothyroidism.[9]

Thyroid Autoimmunity and Female Infertility

The prevalence of TAI is estimated at around 10%.[10] In unexplained subfertility, the thyroid antibodies are frequently associated in euthyroid patients.[11]

The prevalence of TAI is increased in patients with polycystic ovary syndrome (PCOS). There is polymorphism of the PCOS-related gene for fibrillin-3, which influences the activity of TGF-beta, which is a major immune regulator. Thus, the factors that contribute to autoimmunity are lower TGF-β, low vitamin D levels and the high estrogen-to-progesterone ratio.[12] Some of the evidence suggests endometriosis is associated with a variety of immunological changes which includes antibodies to endometrial antigens.

Thyroid Autoimmunity and Assisted Reproductive Technology

Thyroid autoimmunity is important peripheral marker of a general immune imbalance, which can lead to failure of fertilization, implantation failure and sustained pregnancy **(Flowchart 1)**.

Thyroid Cancer Treatment and Radioactive Iodine Treatment

In women undergoing radioactive iodine (RAI), anti-Müllerian hormone (AMH) levels can drop more than 70% till 3 months and then partially recover at 12 months (~30% lower than normal).[16] In men undergoing RAI treatment, the sperm count fell at 3 months and fully recovered at 13 months. However, these patients have frequent chromosomal abnormalities mainly aneuploidies.[17]

Flowchart 1: The mechanism of thyroid autoimmunity (TAI) affecting fertilization.[13-15]

Quantitative and qualitative changes in the profile of endometrial T cells with reduced secretion of IL-4 and IL-10 along with hypersecretion of interferon-γ

↓

TAI alters the immune and hormonal response of the uterus in patients with TAI due to hyperactivity and increased migration of cytotoxic natural killer cells

↓

In TAI, Polyclonal B cell activation is common. It is also associated with increased titers of non-organ specific autoantibodies

↓

The thyroid antibodies cross the "follicle-blood" barrier during maturation of a secondary follicle. They cause cytotoxicity and damage the maturing oocyte. This leads to reduced oocyte quality (grade A) and decrease in fertilization potential

Levothyroxine Treatment and Assisted Reproductive Technology

Overt Hypothyroidism

The latest American Thyroid Association (ATA) guidelines recommend that, in patients treated for clinical hypothyroidism, the TSH concentration should be targeted below 2.5 mIU/L.[18]

Subclinical Hypothyroidism

The effect of levothyroxine treatment in SCH is studied in four main randomized controlled trials (RCTs). They have evaluated different aspect of spontaneous pregnancy outcomes in SCH. Negro et al. showed that improvement in adverse pregnancy outcome in TPO-Abs positive women, with TSH levels exceeding 2.5 mIU/L can be achieved with treatment with levothyroxine.[19] Nazapour et al. also showed a decrease in preterm delivery in TPO-Abs positive patients with TSH levels exceeding 4.0 mIU/L after treatment with levothyroxine.[20] They also suggested, in TPO-Abs negative women with TSH levels above 4 mIU/L there is beneficial effect of LT4 therapy in reducing preterm delivery. The study conducted by Zhang et al. indicated that the risk of miscarriage is increased significantly in patients without intervention than those who underwent effective drug treatments.[21] In the case of ART, TAI positive euthyroid women do not benefit from levothyroxine treatment. Recently, a multicentric, double blinded RCT, the TABLET trial evaluated the results of levothyroxine 50 mg daily in TPO-Abs positive euthyroid women before conception. Women with a medical history of (recurrent) miscarriage or receiving treatment for infertility were included. There results showed that levothyroxine treatment did not result in a higher live birth or pregnancy rate compared with placebo.[22] Despite the low evidence, recommendations from both ATA and American Society for Reproductive Medicine (ASRM) guidelines suggest that treatment may be initiated for any TSH elevation >2.5 mIU/L before ART, considering its potential benefits in comparison to its minimal risk.[18,23]

Summary

- The assessment of SCH in women who plan to become pregnant by ART, the nonpregnant reference range can be used.
- Association with adverse fertility outcomes is more common with TSH levels above 4.0 mIU/L.
- There is no strong evidence to advise levothyroxine treatment for TSH levels between 2.5 and 4.0 mIU/L.
- According to various scientific papers, the cut-off value of 4 mIU/L for TSH is a reasonable intervention level for treatment of SCH in women with and without TAI in ART **(Flowchart 2)**.

Thyroid Disorders and Hyperprolactinemia in Infertility

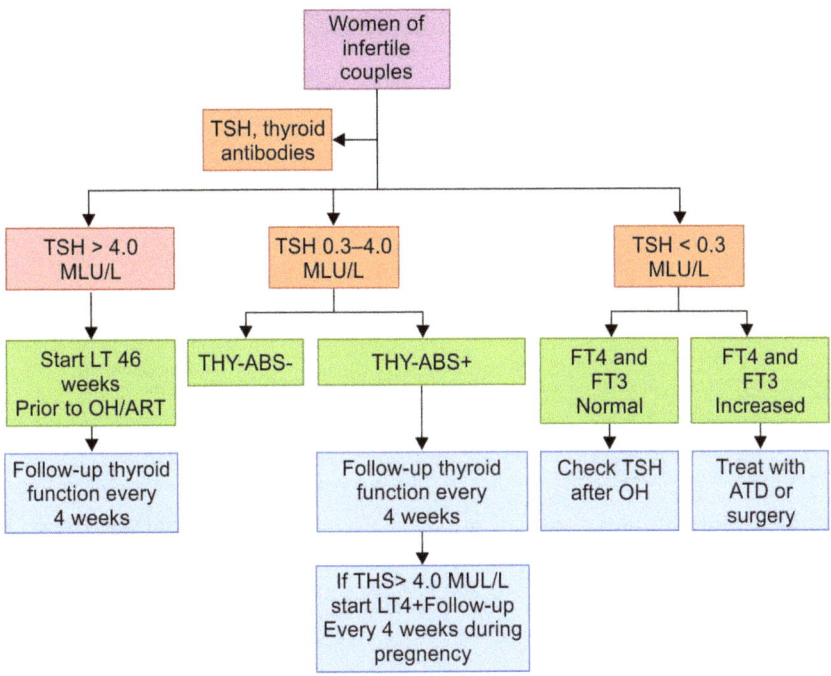

Flowchart 2: Algorithm for clinical approach of thyroid disorders in infertile women considering ART.[24]

HYPERPROLACTINEMIA

Prolactin is a pituitary-derived hormone that plays a pivotal role in the reproduction process. Causes of hyperprolactinemia are shown in **Figure 4**.

Clinical Presentations of Hyperprolactinemia

Premenopausal women:
- Marked prolactin excess (>100 µg/L) is commonly associated with hypogonadism, galactorrhea and amenorrhea
- Moderate prolactin excess (51–75 µg/L) is associated with oligomenorrhea
- Mild prolactin excess (31–50 µg/L) is associated with short luteal phase, decreased libido and infertility.

Men:
- Hyperprolactinemia presents with decreased libido, impotence, decreased sperm production, infertility, gynecomastia and rarely, galactorrhea
- Impotence due to hyperprolactinemia is unresponsive to testosterone treatment and is associated with decreased muscle mass, body hair and osteoporosis

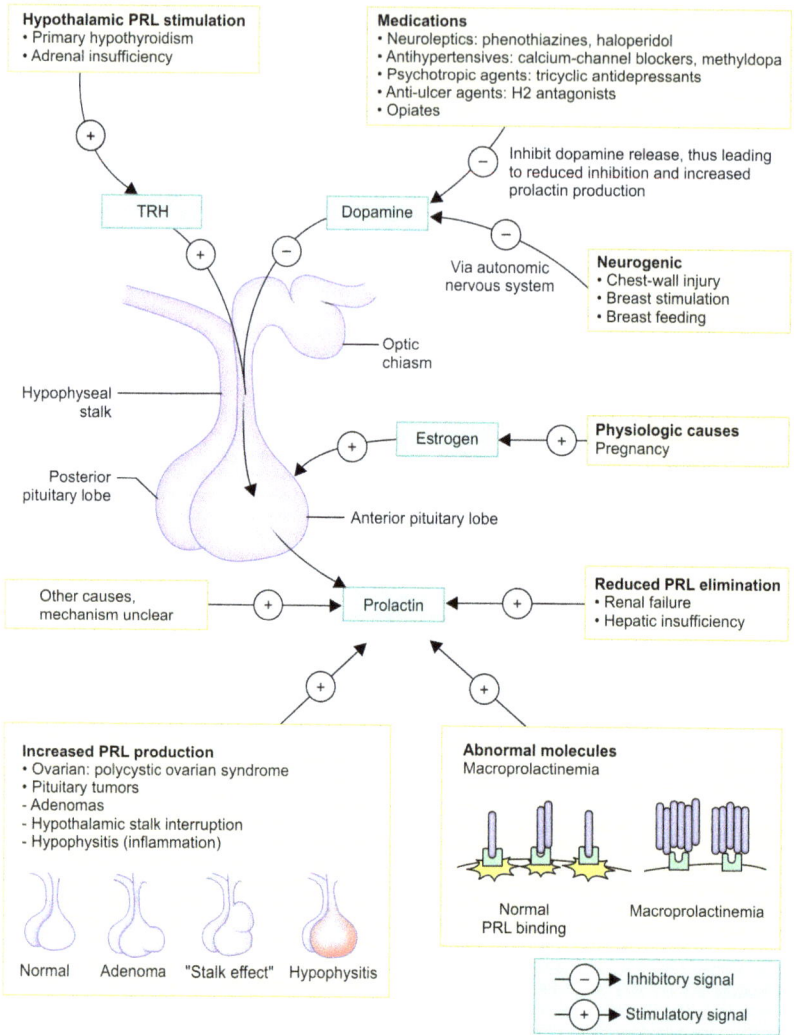

Fig. 4: Causes of hyperprolactinemia.[25]

Approach to a Case of Hyperprolactinemia[25] (Flowchart 3)

- Repeat measurement
- Rule out secondary causes such as hypothyroidism and antidopaminergic drugs
- MRI of pituitary in case of pathological hyperprolactinemia.

Monitoring and Follow-up

Dopamine agonist are first line of therapy for hyperprolactinemia, different dopamine agonist are discussed in **Table 1**. Biochemical and clinical

Thyroid Disorders and Hyperprolactinemia in Infertility

Flowchart 3: Approach to a case of hyperprolactinemia.[25]

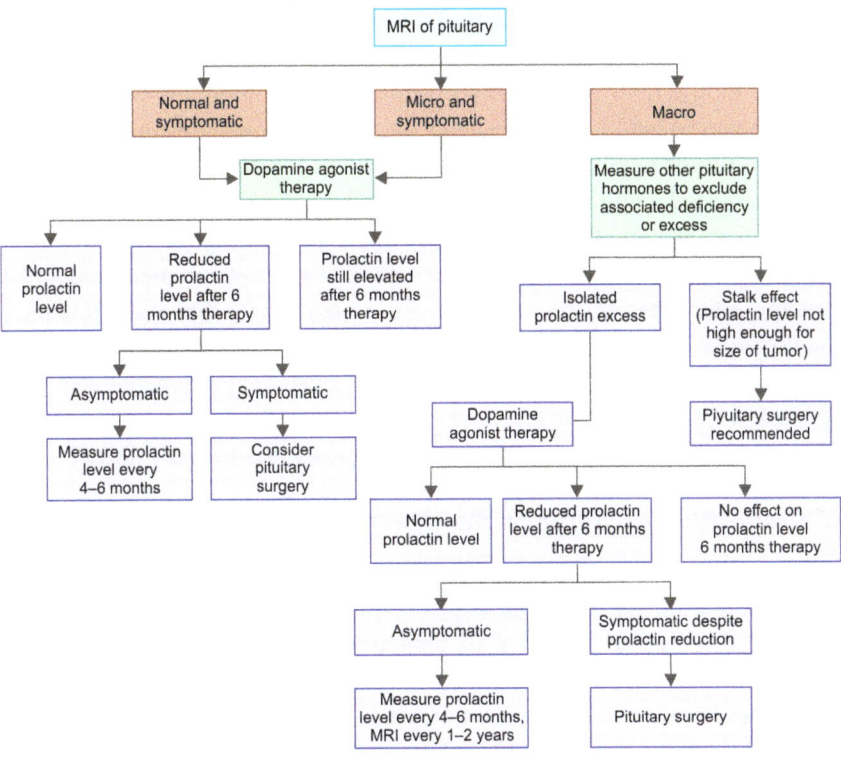

TABLE 1: Advantages, disadvantages and cost of different dopamine agonist agent.[25]			
Drug	*Advantages*	*Disadvantages*	**Dose**
Bromocriptine	Oldest track record	High frequency of gastrointestinal upset and sedation	2.5 mg/day
Cabergoline	Highly efficacious; low frequency of adverse effects; indicated in cases of bromocriptine resistance or intolerance	Experience during pregnancy relatively limited	0.5 mg/week
Quinagolide	Pituitary selectivity; indicated in cases of bromocriptine resistance or intolerance	Limited access, daily use	0.075 mg/day
Pergolide	Beneficial in resistant cases occasionally	High frequency of adverse events	0.25 mg/day

improvements in response to dopamine agonist therapy are apparent in most patients. Tumor shrinkage can be expected in about 80% of macroadenomas.[26] A major drawback of medical therapy is the potential need for long-term treatment. Discontinuation of bromocriptine therapy has been shown to lead to recurrence of hyperprolactinemia in many patients and also tumor regrowth if treatment duration has been <2 years.[27] Passos et al.[27] reported maintenance of normal prolactin levels and absence of adenoma re-expansion after withdrawal of dopamine agonist therapy in about 6.6–37.5% of patients. There is no indication to continue dopamine agonist therapy after attaining menopause.[27] It is suggested that the dopamine agonist dose can be decreased after 2 or 3 years of normal prolactin levels and therapy can be stopped if the prolactin levels remain unchanged after 1 year at the reduced dose. The dose can be reduced by half over the course of 3 months while prolactin levels are advised to be measured monthly.[25]

Management of Hyperprolactinemia in Pregnancy[28]

- There is no clear evidence of increased teratogenicity associated with bromocriptine or cabergoline use during pregnancy.
- Also, there is no evidence of increased risk of abortion or multiple pregnancies with dopamine agonist use.
- Dopamine agonist therapy is stopped during pregnancy when the tumor size before pregnancy is <10 mm, because the risk of tumor expansion is low.
- Bromocriptine use is advised during pregnancy, if the tumor size before pregnancy is ≥10 mm. This is to avoid significant tumor expansion.
- All patients must be evaluated every 2 months during pregnancy.

Summary

Mild hyperprolactinyemia is often seen in patient undergoing treatment for infertility. Correction of hypothyroidism is crucial for correction of hyperprolactinemia.

Medical management with cabergolin and bromocriptine is very effective. Only few patients require surgical management.

CONCLUSION

Several aspects of reproduction get affected by thyroid dysfunction and same is applicable to pregnancy. As all these hormones are secreted by pituitary gland, even hyperprolactinemia also adversely affects the fertility potential by affecting pulsatile secretion of GnRH and hence interfering with ovulation. Understanding all this synchrony and harmony is of utmost importance while dealing with a case of infertility.

REFERENCES

1. Poppe K, Glinoer D, Steirteghem AV, Tournaye H, Devroey P, Schiettecatte J, et al. Thyroid dysfunction and autoimmunity in infertile women. Thyroid. 2002;12(11):997-1001.
2. Kutteh WH, Schoolcraft WB, Scott RT Jr. Antithyroid antibodies do not affect pregnancy outcome in women undergoing assisted reproduction. Hum Reprod. 1999;14(11):2886-90.
3. Silva JF, Ocarino NM, Serakides R. Thyroid hormones and female reproduction[†]. Biology of Reproduction. 2018;99(5):907-21.
4. Aghajanova L, Lindeberg M, Carlsson IB, Stavreus-Evers A, Zhang P, Scott JE, et al. Receptors for thyroid-stimulating hormone and thyroid hormones in human ovarian tissue. Reprod Biomed Online. 2009;18(3):337-47.
5. Anasti JN, Flack MR, Froehlich J, Nelson LM, Nisula BC. A potential novel mechanism for precocious puberty in juvenile hypothyroidism. J Clin Endocrinol Metab. 1995;80(1):276-9.
6. Joshi JV, Bhandarkar SD, Chadha M, Balaiah D, Shah R. Menstrual irregularities and lactation failure may precede thyroid dysfunction or goitre. J Postgrad Med. 1993;39(3):137-41.
7. Krassas GE, Poppe K, Glinoer D. Thyroid function and human reproductive health. Endocr Rev. 2010;31(5):702-55.
8. Millar LK, Wing DA, Leung AS, Koonings PP, Montoro MN, Mestman JH. Low birth weight and preeclampsia in pregnancies complicated by hyperthyroidism. Obstet Gynecol. 1994;84(6):946-9.
9. Poppe K, Velkeniers B, Glinoer D. Thyroid disease and female reproduction. Clin Endocrinol (Oxf). 2007;66(3):309-21.
10. Hollowell JG, Staehling NW, Flanders WD, Hannon WH, Gunter EW, Spencer CA, et al. Serum TSH, T4, and thyroid antibodies in the United States population (1988 to 1994): National Health and Nutrition Examination Survey (NHANES III). J Clin Endocrinol Metab. 2002;87(2):489-99.
11. van den Boogaard E, Vissenberg R, Land JA, van Wely M, van der Post JAM, Goddijn M, et al. Significance of (sub)clinical thyroid dysfunction and thyroid autoimmunity before conception and in early pregnancy: a systematic review. Hum Reprod Update. 2011;17(5):605-19.
12. Gaberšček S, Zaletel K, Schwetz V, Pieber T, Obermayer-Pietsch B, Lerchbaum E. Mechanisms in endocrinology: thyroid and polycystic ovary syndrome. Eur J Endocrinol. 2015;172(1):R9-21.
13. Twig G, Shina A, Amital H, Shoenfeld Y. Pathogenesis of infertility and recurrent pregnancy loss in thyroid autoimmunity. J Autoimmun. 2012;38(2-3):J275-81.
14. Roberts J, Jenkins C, Wilson R, Pearson C, Franklin IA, MacLean MA, et al. Recurrent miscarriage is associated with increased numbers of CD5/20 positive lymphocytes and an increased incidence of thyroid antibodies. Eur J Endocrinol. 1996;134(1):84-6.
15. Monteleone P, Parrini D, Faviana P, Carletti E, Casarosa E, Uccelli A, et al. Female infertility related to thyroid autoimmunity: the ovarian follicle hypothesis. Am J Reprod Immunol. 2011;66(2):108-14.
16. Dosiou C. Thyroid and fertility: recent advances. Thyroid. 2020;30(4):479-86.
17. Bourcigaux N, Rubino C, Berthaud I, Toubert ME, Donadille B, Leenhardt L, et al. Impact on testicular function of a single ablative activity of 3.7 GBq radioactive iodine for differentiated thyroid carcinoma. Hum Reprod. 2018;33(8):1408-16.
18. Alexander EK, Pearce EN, Brent GA, Brown RS, Chen H, Dosiou C, et al. 2017 Guidelines of the American Thyroid Association for the diagnosis and management of thyroid disease during pregnancy and the postpartum. Thyroid. 2017;27(3):315-89.

19. Negro R, Mangieri T, Coppola L, Presicce G, Casavola EC, Gismondi R, et al. Levothyroxine treatment in thyroid peroxidase antibody-positive women undergoing assisted reproduction technologies: a prospective study. Hum Reprod. 2005;20(6):1529-33.
20. Nazarpour S, Ramezani Tehrani F, Simbar M, Tohidi M, Minooee S, Rahmati M, et al. Effects of levothyroxine on pregnant women with subclinical hypothyroidism, negative for thyroid peroxidase antibodies. J Clin Endocrinol Metab. 2018;103(3):926-35.
21. Zhang Y, Wang H, Pan X, Teng W, Shan Z. Patients with subclinical hypothyroidism before 20 weeks of pregnancy have a higher risk of miscarriage: a systematic review and meta-analysis. PLoS One. 2017;12(4):e0175708.
22. Dhillon-Smith RK, Middleton LJ, Sunner KK, Cheed V, Baker K, Farrell-Carver S, et al. Levothyroxine in women with thyroid peroxidase antibodies before conception. N Engl J Med. 2019;380:1316-25.
23. Practice Committee of the American Society for Reproductive Medicine. Subclinical hypothyroidism in the infertile female population: a guideline. Fertil Steril. 2015;104(3):545-53.
24. Unuane D, Velkeniers B. Impact of thyroid disease on fertility and assisted conception. Best Pract Res Clin Endocrinol Metab. 2020;34(4):101378.
25. Serri O, Chik CL, Ur E, Ezzat S. Diagnosis and management of hyperprolactinemia. CMAJ. 2003;169(6):575-81.
26. Webster J, Piscitelli G, Polli A, Ferrari CI, Ismail I, Scanlon MF. A Comparison of cabergoline and bromocriptine in the treatment of hyperprolactinemic amenorrhea. Cabergoline Comparative Study Group. N Engl J Med. 1994;331(14):904-9.
27. Passos VQ, Souza JJS, Musolino NRC, Bronstein MD. Long-term follow-up of prolactinomas: normoprolactinemia after bromocriptine withdrawal. J Clin Endocrinol Metab. 2002;87(8):3578-82.
28. Melmed S, Casanueva FF, Hoffman AR, Kleinberg DL, Montori VM, Schlechte JA, et al. Diagnosis and treatment of hyperprolactinemia: an Endocrine Society Clinical Practice Guideline. J Clin Endocrinol Metab. 2011;96(2):273-88.

CHAPTER 13: Endometriosis and Infertility

Ashish Kale, Ashwini Yelikar Kale

INTRODUCTION

Endometriosis is a common, challenging, chronic inflammatory estrogen-dependent disease in women of reproductive age, defined as the presence of endometrial-like tissue outside the uterus, which induces a chronic, inflammatory reaction. It is estimated that endometriosis affect up to 10–15% of women of reproductive age and 50% of infertile women.[1,2] In normal couples in the reproductive age the estimated fecundity rates are 15–20%, while in untreated endometriosis women, the estimated fecundity rate ranges from 2 to 20%.[3,4] The spontaneous conception rates are reduced in women with endometriosis depending upon the extent of the disease, approximately 50% of them with minimal/mild disease and 25% of women with moderate disease conceive without any treatment. However, only few women with severe endometriosis conceive spontaneously.[5] The etiopathogenesis of endometriosis is not well understood. Retrograde menstruation, celomic metaplasia, dysfunctional immune response, and genetics are discussed in current literature to explain the pathogenesis of endometriosis. The mechanism by which endometriosis affects fertility are still not well explained.[6,7]

PROPOSED BIOLOGICAL MECHANISMS TO EXPLAIN INFERTILITY IN ENDOMETRIOSIS

Many evidences demonstrate an association between endometriosis and infertility. Several mechanisms have been discussed in the literature to explain the association of endometriosis and infertility. However, a causal relationship between the proposed mechanisms and endometriosis has not been established.[3,8] The American Society for Reproductive Medicine Classification System for Endometriosis (ASRM 1996) is the commonly used staging system for endometriosis.

Pelvic Anatomy Distortion

Pelvic anatomical disruption in severe endometriosis causes infertility. Pelvic and peritubal adhesions resulting from endometriosis disrupt tubo-ovarian anatomy which can lead to impaired release of ovum or transport of ovum in the fallopian tube, altered sperm transport, altered myometrial contractions, and adversely affect fertilization and embryo transport. Extensive pelvic adhesions may result in occlusion of the tubal ostium, which disturb sperm transport, leading to infertility.[9,10] Anatomical disruptions in endometriosis may result in development of hydrosalpinx, which leads to reduced in vitro fertilization (IVF) success rate.

In women with minimal and mild endometriosis there is little anatomical distortion. However, these women also have less chance of spontaneous pregnancy. Following mechanisms are proposed by which minimal and mild disease impacts fertility.

Changed Peritoneal Functions

Several studies have shown that in women with endometriosis the volume of peritoneal fluid, and peritoneal fluid concentrations of prostaglandins, proteases, and inflammatory cytokines such as interleukin-1 (IL-1), IL-6, tumor necrosis factor-alpha (TNF alpha), and angiogenic cytokines, such as IL-8 and vascular endothelial growth factor (VEGF) produced by macrophages are increased. The numbers of leukocytes and macrophages are increased in the peritoneal fluid and in endometrial implants. Moreover, it is also observed that serum levels of inflammatory cytokines are increased in women with endometriosis. These changes could have unfavorable effect on egg, sperm, embryo, or fallopian tube.[3,11,12] The increased IL-6 levels in peritoneal fluid in women with endometriosis may reduce sperm motility and contribute to pathogenesis of endometriosis associated infertility. Inflammatory mediators of the peritoneal fluid may also contribute to sperm DNA damage. High levels of inflammatory cytokines impede tubal motility, impair gamete transport, fertilization and embryo transport. In addition, there is increased oxidative stress in endometriosis which is also implicated as one of the factors responsible for impaired embryo development, implantation.[9,10]

IMPAIRED ENDOCRINE FUNCTION, FOLLICULOGENESIS AND OVULATORY FUNCTIONS IN ENDOMETRIOSIS

It has been observed that in women with endometriosis the ovarian folliculogenesis is impaired. The number of preovulatory follicles, follicular growth, size of the dominant follicle, and levels of estradiol in the follicle are reduced.[13] In these women, mechanisms of normal ovulation are disturbed. Increased apoptosis of cumulus cells surrounding the oocyte is observed in women with endometriosis. Ovarian cells apoptosis is an indicator of poor oocyte quality. Premature as well as multiple luteinizing hormone (LH) surges and reduced follicular LH receptors are observed, which affect ovulation. The prevalence of luteinized unruptured follicle syndrome (LUFS), is higher in women with endometriosis. It has been proposed that women with endometriosis may have luteal phase dysfunction. Evidence shows there may be a longer follicular phase with reduced luteal phase progesterone secretion.[3,10,13,14]

Effect on Oocyte, Sperm and Embryo Quality in Endometriosis

Endometriosis associated infertility may be related to poor quality of oocyte and subsequent embryo development. Altered progesterone and cytokine concentrations found in follicular fluid from women with endometriosis support this concept. It has also been suggested that changes in peritoneal fluid impair sperm quality (e.g., increased sperm DNA fragmentation), sperm function and increase sperm phagocytosis by activated macrophages. Endometriomas produce substances which are harmful to maturing oocytes. The increased number of inflammatory cells in the peritoneal fluid have toxic effect on the embryo. Moreover, it has also been shown that there is an increase in free radicals in endometrium causing adverse effect on embryo and results in decreased embryo quality. Women with endometriosis undergoing assisted reproductive technology (ART) have reduced rate of fertilization. Further it affects cleavage following fertilization. When compared to embryos produced from women with tubal illness, endometriosis-derived embryos tend to mature more slowly.[9,13,15-18]

Impact on Endometrium and Implantation

Studies have reported that women with endometriosis experience higher implantation failure compared to controls.[13] There is raised aromatase enzyme in eutopic as well as in ectopic endometrium in endometriosis. This leads to raised estrogen production in endometrium which may affect the endometrial receptivity. The increased endometrial estrogen may lead to resistance to progesterone. The progesterone resistance and dysregulation in isoforms of the progesterone receptor in eutopic endometrium results in an unopposed estrogen state—a condition which is not appropriate for implantation of embryo. Raised endometrial estrogen possibly impairs peristaltic activity of the myometrium. The levels of enzyme involved in the synthesis of the endometrial ligand for L-selectin are reduced in infertile women with endometriosis. It has been observed that some women with endometriosis have reduced expression of $\alpha v \beta 3$-integrin (an adhesion molecule) at the time of implantation.[3,9,19,20] In normal women, during the mid-luteal phase, endometrial expression of genes for *HOXA10* increases, which is necessary for endometrial receptivity. However, in women with endometriosis there is no increase in *HOXA10* gene during mid-luteal phase.[9] The endometrium is less sensitive to progesterone in women with endometriosis. Matrix metalloproteinases (MMPs), enzymes that break down extracellular matrices, are normally inhibited by progesterone during the secretory phase. In women with endometriosis due to progesterone resistance the MMPs are not inhibited and remain elevated during period of implantation, which lead to degradation of the extracellular matrix and makes the endometrium hostile for implantation.[9,21] There may be increased lymphocytes in the endometrium of women with endometriosis. Endometrial antibodies are increased in some women with endometriosis. These autoantibodies bind to endometrial antigens and may alter endometrial receptivity and affect implantation.[3,22,23]

Effects of Endometriosis on Ovarian Reserve

Endometriosis damages ovarian tissue disrupts ovarian follicular development and adversely affects ovarian reserve. The results of studies have reported that ovarian endometriosis reduces ovarian reserve. The reduction in ovarian reserve is mainly observed in severe cases. Enlargement of endometriomas destroys ovarian tissue and leads to reduction in ovarian reserve. Kasapoglu et al. showed that there is a faster reduction in serum anti-Müllerian hormone (AMH) levels in endometriosis women, compared to the healthy controls. These evidences indicate that women with endometriosis may reach menopause earlier than those women without endometriosis history.[18,24,25]

Effects of Endometriosis on Early Pregnancy Loss

Although the association between the miscarriage rates and endometriosis is not proven, women with endometriosis may have an increased risk of miscarriage **(Table 1)**. The possible causes suggested for the observed increased risk of spontaneous miscarriage in women with endometriosis are defective embryogenesis, autoantibodies, or inadequate endometrial support.[13]

Treatment Options in Infertile Women with Endometriosis

Current treatment of endometriosis-associated infertility includes various treatment options including expectant management, surgical treatment, and ART. The treatment of infertility in women with endometriosis should be individualized taking account the various parameters such as age, stage and extent of the disease. The drugs most commonly used for medical treatments of endometriosis include oral contraceptives, progestins, and gonadotropin-releasing hormone (GnRH) agonists. These drugs inhibit ovulation resulting in contraception. Therefore, current medical treatments of endometriosis cannot be used for the treatment of infertility associated with endometriosis.[26]

TABLE 1: Probable theories in pathogenesis of endometriosis-associated infertility.

S. No.	Theory	Mechanism
1.	Distortion of pelvic anatomy	• Pelvic adhesions disrupt the tubo ovarian anatomy, impair release of ovum or transport in the fallopian tube, alter sperm transport, tubal ostium occlusion • Impaired fertilization and embryo transport
2.	Changed peritoneal functions	• Increased peritoneal fluid concentrations of prostaglandins, proteases, and inflammatory cytokines • Increased macrophages • Impaired tubal motility, gamete transport, fertilization and embryo transport
3.	Impaired endocrine function, folliculogenesis and ovulatory functions	• Altered ovarian folliculogenesis • Increased apoptosis of cumulus cells, poor oocyte quality • Impaired ovulation, luteinized unruptured follicle syndrome (LUFS) • Luteal phase dysfunction
4.	Effect on oocyte, sperm and embryo quality in endometriosis	• Poor oocyte quality • Impaired sperm quality, sperm function and increased sperm phagocytosis • Impaired embryo development and quality • Toxic effect on the embryo • Reduced rate of fertilization and impaired cleavage in assisted reproductive technology (ART)
5.	Impact on endometrium and implantation	• Raised aromatase enzyme—raised endometrial estrogen production, progesterone resistance, an unopposed estrogen state • Reduced levels of enzyme involved in the synthesis of endometrial ligand for L-selectin • Reduced expression of endometrial $\alpha v \beta 3$-integrin (an adhesion molecule) at the time of implantation • Altered *HOXA10* gene expression • Elevated endometrial matrix metalloproteinases (MMPs) • Increased endometrial antibodies • Impaired peristaltic activity of the myometrium • Reduced endometrial receptivity and affect implantation
6.	Effects of endometriosis on ovarian reserve	• Damages ovarian tissue, disrupts ovarian follicular development and adversely affects ovarian reserve
7.	Effects of endometriosis on early pregnancy loss	• Defective embryogenesis • Autoantibodies, inadequate endometrial support • Altered endometrial receptivity

Surgery as a Treatment Option for Infertile Women with Endometriosis

When considering surgery for treatment of infertility associated with endometriosis, clinician should take into account the stage of the disease and results of surgical treatment compared with other treatments. In women with endometriosis, the disease itself as well as surgery for endometriosis can reduce ovarian reserve.[27] The women should be counseled regarding the impact of endometriosis and surgery on ovarian reserve. A Cochrane review reported that operative laparoscopy (excision or ablation of the endometriosis lesions including adhesiolysis) may improve pregnancy rates in women with minimal and mild endometriosis.[1,9] In such women operative laparoscopy should be preferred as compared to diagnostic laparoscopy only.[1] As per ASRM committee opinion, "the benefit of laparoscopic treatment of minimal or mild endometriosis is insufficient to recommend laparoscopy solely to increase the likelihood of pregnancy. When laparoscopy is performed for other indications, the surgeon may consider safely ablating or excising visible lesions of endometriosis."[3]

There are no randomized controlled trials comparing conservative surgical treatment in women with moderate/severe endometriosis-associated infertility and expectant treatment. Cohort studies have reported higher spontaneous pregnancy rate following laparoscopic surgery as compared to expectant treatment in women with moderate to severe endometriosis.[1] Operative laparoscopy can be considered in infertile women with American Fertility Society (AFS)/ASRM stage III/IV endometriosis, instead of no treatment, to improve spontaneous pregnancy rates.[1] Surgical treatment of endometrioma by excision of endometrioma capsule results in better spontaneous postoperative pregnancy rate as compared to drainage and electrocoagulation of the endometrioma wall.[1] However, surgical treatment of endometriomas has been controversial as there is a risk of reduction in ovarian reserve following surgery. The patient should be counseled regarding the risks of reduced ovarian reserve after surgery and the possible loss of the ovary.[1]

Assisted Reproduction

Assisted reproductive technology methods such as intrauterine insemination (IUI) and IVF are being widely used for the management of endometriosis associated infertility. In vitro fertilization is currently the most effective treatment of endometriosis-associated infertility.[9]

Intrauterine Insemination

Intrauterine insemination with controlled ovarian stimulation results in higher live birth rate compared to expectant management and also as compared to IUI alone in infertile women with AFS/ASRM stage I/II endometriosis.[1] As per ASRM committee opinion, "in younger women

(<35 years) with stage I/II endometriosis-associated infertility, expectant management or superovulation and intrauterine insemination (SO/IUI) can be considered as first-line therapy. In women 35 years of age or older, more aggressive treatment, such as SO/IUI or IVF may be considered".[3] In infertile women with AFS/ASRM stage I/II endometriosis achieve lower success rates with stimulation and IUI compared with women with unexplained infertility. However, in these women IUI with controlled ovarian stimulation within 6 months after surgical treatment results in pregnancy rates similar to those achieved in unexplained infertility.[1]

In Vitro Fertilization and Embryo Transfer

According to the best available evidence, in all stages of endometriosis, IVF seems to be the most successful treatment option for endometriosis associated infertilty.[9] In vitro fertilization is recommended in endometriosis associated infertility if there is associated compromised tubal function, male factor infertility and if other treatments have failed in moderate-to-severe endometriosis.[1] Ovarian responsiveness to hyperstimulation is an important factor determining the success of IVF.[28] Studies have reported fewer oocytes retrieved, lower implantation rate, and lower birth rate in IVF in women with moderate/severe endometriosis.[29-31] Recent meta-analyses reported that IVF in women with minimal/mild endometriosis and IVF in women with other indications resulted in similar live birth rate. However, the same meta-analyses reported that IVF in women with moderate/severe endometriosis, resulted in fewer oocytes retrieved, lower implantation rate, and lower birth rate as compared to IVF in women with other indications for IVF. The reported IVF success rates in women with endometriosis stage III and IV is less compared to women with tubal factor infertility.[30,31] However, the Society for Assisted Reproductive Technology (SART) database shows that endometriosis does not adversely affect pregnancy rates.[1] For women with stage III/IV endometriosis who fail to conceive following conservative surgery or because of advancing reproductive age, IVF-ET is an effective alternative.[3]

It has been reported that downregulation for 3-6 months with a GnRH agonist in women with endometriosis increases clinical pregnancy rate. As per the recent European Society of Human Reproduction and Embryology (ESHRE) guidelines on management of women with endometriosis, "Clinicians can prescribe GnRH agonists for a period of 3-6 months prior to treatment with ART to improve clinical pregnancy rates in infertile women with endometriosis".[1]

Surgery before ART in Women with Endometriosis-associated Infertility

Whether surgery for endometriosis improve pregnancy rate in women with endometriosis associated infertility is controversial. In infertile women

> **BOX 1:** Risks associated with surgical treatment of endometrioma prior to assisted reproductive technology (ART).[18]
> - *Surgical risks:* Bleeding, infection, pain, injury to viscera
> - Impact to ovarian reserve
> - Premature ovarian failure
> - Incomplete surgery and recurrence of disease
> - Learning curve and competency of the surgeon
> - Probable delay of ART

with AFS/ASRM stage I/II endometriosis undergoing laparoscopy prior to treatment with ART, clinicians may consider the complete surgical removal of endometriosis to improve live birth rate, although the benefit is not well established. The evidence indicates that surgical treatment in women with moderate to severe endometriosis can reduce ovarian reserve and reduce the subsequent IVF outcomes. As per the recent ESHRE guidelines on management of women with endometriosis, surgical excision is not routinely recommended before performing ART.[1] There is an increased risk of reduced ovarian reserve/functions following surgical treatment of endometrioma. Women with endometrioma should be counseled regarding this risk **(Box 1)**.[1,18]

There is no evidence that cystectomy of endometrioma >3 cm before ART improves pregnancy rates. Cystectomy of endometrioma >3 cm before ART should be considered only to improve endometriosis-associated pain or the accessibility of follicles.[1] The effectiveness of surgical excision of deep-infiltrating endometriosis before performing ART in women with endometriosis is not conclusive with regard to reproductive outcome.[1]

ENDOMETRIOSIS FERTILITY INDEX

Recently endometriosis fertility index (EFI) a score ranging from 0 to 10 points is being used to predict probability of pregnancy with non-IVF treatment in women with endometriosis associated infertility. This classification system is based on the surgical least function score, historical factors, and the AFS score. A systemic review and meta-analysis by S Vesali et al. reported that EFI score performed well in predicting the non-ART pregnancy rate.[32]

CONCLUSION

Endometriosis is a common, complex, estrogen dependent disease affecting women of reproductive age. It is one of the major causes of infertility. The causes of infertility associated with endometriosis are multifactorial. The proposed mechanisms of infertility associated with mild endometriosis include peritoneal inflammation, altered endocrine and ovulatory functions. These changes lead to impaired gamete quality and transport, impaired embryo development and quality, reduced endometrial receptivity, disordered uterine peristalsis and impaired implantation. In addition to above mentioned factors, distorted pelvic anatomy in severe endometriosis leads to impairment in oocyte release, oocyte pick-up, alteration in sperm motility, disordered myometrial contractions, impaired fertilization, and embryo transport.

Medical treatment of endometriosis is not effective in improving fertility. Surgery or ARTs are the treatment options for endometriosis associated infertility. Laparoscopic surgery improves spontaneous pregnancy rate in minimal-mild endometriosis. However, surgical removal of endometriomas has been controversial as there is a risk of reduction in ovarian reserve following surgery. In infertile women with AFS/ASRM stage I/II endometriosis, superovulation with IUI after surgical treatment increases chances of pregnancy. The most effective treatment for endometriosis associated infertility is IVF. The results of IVF in women with minimal/mild endometriosis are comparable to the results of IVF performed for other indications. In women with sever endometriosis the success rates of IVF are lower.

REFERENCES

1. Dunselman GAJ, Vermeulen N, Becker C, Calhaz-Jorge C, D'Hooghe T, De Bie B, et al. ESHRE guideline: management of women with endometriosis. Hum Reprod. 2014;29:400-12.
2. Olive DL, Pritts EA. Treatment of endometriosis. N Engl J Med. 2001;345(4):266-75.
3. Practice Committee of the American Society for Reproductive Medicine. Endometriosis and infertility: A committee opinion. Fertil Steril. 2012;98(3):591-8.
4. Hughes EG, Fedorkow DM, Collins JA. A quantitative overview of controlled trials in endometriosis-associated infertility. Fertil Steril. 1993;59(5):963-70.
5. Olive DL, Stohs GF, Metzger DA, Franklin RR. Expectant management and hydrotubations in the treatment of endometriosis-associated infertility. Fertil Steril. 1985;44(1):35-41.
6. Rocha ALL, Reis FM, Petraglia F. New trends for the medical treatment of endometriosis. Expert Opin Investig Drugs. 2012;21(7):905-19.
7. Giudice LC, Kao LC. Endometriosis. Lancet. 2004;364 (9447):1789-99.
8. Schenken RS. Treatment of human infertility: the special case of endometriosis. In: Adashi EY, Rock JA, Rosenwaks Z (Eds). Reproductive endocrinology, surgery and technology. Philadelphia: Lippincott-Raven; 1996:2122-39.
9. Macer ML, Taylor HS. Endometriosis and infertility: A review of the pathogenesis and treatment of endometriosis-associated infertility. Obstet Gynecol Clin North Am. 2012;39(4):535-49.
10. Tanbo T, Fedorcsak P. Endometriosis-associated infertility: aspects of pathophysiological mechanisms and treatment options. Acta Obstet Gynecol Scand. 2017;96(6):659-67.
11. Bedaiwy MA, Falcone T, Sharma RK, Goldberg JM, Attaran M, Nelson DR, et al. Prediction of endometriosis with serum and peritoneal fluid markers: a prospective controlled trial. Hum Reprod. 2002;17(2):426-31.
12. Pizzo A, Salmeri FM, Ardita FV, Sofo V, Tripepi M, Marsico S. Behaviour of cytokine levels in serum and peritoneal fluid of women with endometriosis. Gynecol Obstet Invest. 2002;54(2):82-7.
13. Stilley JAW, Birt JA, Sharpe-Timms KL. Cellular and molecular basis for endometriosis-associated infertility. Cell Tissue Res. 2012;349(3):849-62.

14. Cunha-Filho JS, Gross JL, Bastos de Souza CA, Lemos NA, Giugliani C, Freitas F, et al. Physiopathological aspects of corpus luteum defect in infertile women with mild/minimal endometriosis. J Assist Reprod Genet. 2003;20(3):117-21.
15. Garrido N, Navarro J, Remohi J, Simon C, Pellicer A. Follicular hormonal environment and embryo quality in women with endometriosis. Hum Reprod Update. 2000;6(1):67-74.
16. Pellicer A, Oliveira N, Ruiz A, Remohi J, Simon C. Exploring the mechanism(s) of endometriosis-related infertility: an analysis of embryo development and implantation in assisted reproduction. Hum Reprod. 1995;10(Suppl 2):91-7.
17. Gupta S, Goldberg JM, Aziz N, Goldberg E, Krajcir N, Agarwal A. Pathogenic mechanisms in endometriosis-associated infertility. Fertil Steril. 2008;90(2):247-57.
18. Hamdan M, Dunselman G, Li TC, Cheong Y. The impact of endometrioma on IVF/ICSI outcomes: a systematic review and meta-analysis. Hum Reprod Update. 2015;21(6):809-25.
19. Burney RO, Talbi S, Hamilton AE, Vo KC, Nyegaard M, Nezhat CR, et al. Gene expression analysis of endometrium reveals progesterone resistance and candidate susceptibility genes in women with endometriosis. Endocrinology. 2007;148(8): 3814-26.
20. Mendelson CR. Minireview: fetal-maternal hormonal signaling in pregnancy and labor. Mol Endocrinol. 2009;23(7):947-54.
21. Osteen KG, Keller NR, Feltus FA, Melner MH. Paracrine regulation of matrix metalloproteinase expression in the normal human endometrium. Gynecol Obstet Invest. 1999;48(Suppl 1):2-13.
22. Lebovic DI, Mueller MD, Taylor RN. Immunobiology of endometriosis. Fertil Steril. 2001;75:1-10.
23. de Ziegler D, Borghese B, Chapron C. Endometriosis and infertility: pathophysiology and management. Lancet. 2010;376(9742):730-8.
24. Kasapoglu I, Ata B, Uyaniklar O, Seyhan A, Orhan A, Yildiz Oguz S, et al. Endometrioma-related reduction in ovarian reserve (ERROR): a prospective longitudinal study. Fertil Steril. 2018;110(1):122-7
25. Lee D, Kim SK, Lee JR, Jee BC. Management of endometriosis-related infertility: Considerations and treatment options. Clin Exp Reprod Med. 2020;47(1):1-11.
26. Hughes E, Brown J, Collins JJ, Farquhar C, Fedorkow DM, Vandekerckhove P. Ovulation suppression for endometriosis. Cochrane Database Syst Rev. 2007; 2007(3):CD000155.
27. Yap C, Furness S, Farquhar C. Pre- and postoperative medical therapy for endometriosis surgery. Cochrane Database Syst Rev. 2004;2004(3):CD003678.
28. Garcia-Velasco JA, Somigliana E. Management of endometriomasn in women requiring IVF: to touch or not to touch. Hum Reprod. 2009;24(3):496-501.
29. Benaglia L, Bermejo A, Somigliana E, Faulisi S, Ragni G, Fedele L, et al. In vitro fertilization outcome in women with unoperated bilateral endometriomas. Fertil Steril. 2013;99(6):1714-9.
30. Hamdan M, Omar SZ, Dunselman G, Cheong Y. Influence of endometriosis on assisted reproductive technology outcomes: a systematic review and meta-analysis. Obstet Gynecol. 2015;125(1):79-88.
31. Harb HM, Gallos ID, Chu J, Harb M, Coomarasamy A. The effect of endometriosis on in vitro fertilisation outcome: a systematic review and meta-analysis. BJOG. 2013;120(11):1308-20.
32. Vesali S, Razavi M, Rezaeinejad M, Hajiagha AM, Maroufizadeh S, Sepidarkish M, et al. Endometriosis fertility index for predicting non-assisted reproductive technology pregnancy after endometriosis surgery: a systematic review and meta-analysis. BJOG. 2020;127(7):800-9.

CHAPTER 14 | Fibroids and Fertility

Chaitanya Shembekar, Parul Saoji

INTRODUCTION

Do fibroids affect fertility? Which fibroids affect fertility? How do fibroids have an impact on fertility? To treat or not to treat?

In this chapter, we will try to evaluate the precise impact of fibroids on fertility. We all know the widely accepted fact that submucosal fibroids need treatment and have a direct impact on fertility. It would be more interesting to study the fibroids in other locations. Apart from a traditional myomectomy, various other modalities will be discussed in detail.

Leiomyomas are benign tumors of the uterus. Bleeding, pain, and infertility are the three major presentations of fibroid.[1] Fibroids affect approximately 35-77% of women of reproductive age group.[2-4]

Fibroids are seen in 5-10% of infertile patients and alone are the cause of infertility in 1-2.4% of patients.[5,6] A randomized and prospective study evaluating spontaneous conception in infertile women with or without fibroids was conducted by Bulletti et al.[7] in 1999. Authors noted that there was a significant discrepancy in pregnancy rate of 11% versus 25% in infertile women with or without fibroids. Removing fibroids increased the pregnancy rate supporting the fact that fibroids have an impact on fertility. The effect of fibroids on ART has been elucidated through numerous studies on ART patients.[8-11] We all know that mechanical impact and blockage of fallopian tubes affect fertility in fibroids. Fibroids also compromise fertility by altering endometrial receptivity negatively. This affects embryo implantation and chances of pregnancy.[12,13]

FIBROIDS—EVALUATION AND CLASSIFICATION

Imaging is a necessary tool in the preoperative evaluation of myomas. It has a great role to play, especially for uterus-sparing procedures.

Ultrasound has been shown to be a rapid, safe, and cost-effective means. It helps in evaluating the size, number, and location of fibroids. Fibroids of up to 4-5 mm in diameter are identified by transvaginal ultrasound. The ultrasound may be suboptimal for multiple fibroids, because of acoustic shadowing, and for the proper evaluation of endometrial impingement.

Magnetic resonance imaging (MRI) has a major role in the evaluation of fibroid uteruses, especially for fibroid mapping and submucosal penetration. When compared with vaginal ultrasound, hysterosonography, and hysteroscopy, it is the most reliable method of evaluation with 100% sensitivity and 91% specificity (pathological examination was the gold standard). The main drawbacks of MRI evaluation are high cost and lack of accessibility, especially in rural areas of India.

Hysterosalpingography is routinely performed to assess tubal patency in women with infertility and to exclude intrauterine pathology. The sensitivity and positive predictive value of this test for the identification of intrauterine lesions can be as low as 50% and 28.6%, respectively. Thus, hysterosalpingography cannot be considered reliable to exclude endometrial distortion due to submucosal myomas.

Hysterosonography has been advocated as superior to transvaginal ultrasound alone and equal to hysteroscopy in the evaluation of endometrial impingement.

Hysteroscopy is the gold standard in the diagnosis and evaluation of submucosal fibroids. It not only helps in the diagnosis but also can be used as a tool for the removal of submucosal fibroids.

RECOMMENDATIONS

1. In women with infertility, an effort should be made to adequately evaluate and classify fibroids, particularly those impinging on the endometrial cavity, using transvaginal ultrasound, hysteroscopy, hysterosonography, or MRI. (III-A)
2. Preoperative assessment of submucosal fibroids should include, in addition to an assessment of fibroid size and location within the uterine cavity, an evaluation of the degree of invasion of the cavity and thickness of residual myometrium to the serosa. A combination of hysteroscopy and transvaginal ultrasound or hysterosonography are the modalities of choice. (III-B)
3. Submucosal fibroids are managed hysteroscopically. The fibroid size should be <5 cm, although larger fibroids have been managed hysteroscopically, but repeat procedures are often necessary. (III-B)
4. A hysterosalpingogram is not an appropriate exam to evaluate and classify fibroids. (III-D)

CLASSIFICATION OF ESGE/FIGO PALM-COEIN

The classifications of European Society of Gastrointestinal Endoscopy (ESGE)/The International Federation of Gynecology and Obstetrics (FIGO) PALM-COEIN are shown in **Tables 1 and 2**.

TABLE 1: ESGE/FIGO PALM-COEIN classification.

Polyp

Adenomyosis

Leiomyoma
- Submucosal
- Other

Malignancy and hyperplasia

Coagulopathy

Ovulatory dysfunction

Endometrial

Iatrogenic

Not yet classified

Leiomyoma subclassification system

Submucosal	0	Pedunculated intracavitary
	1	<50% intramural
	2	≥50% intramural
Other	3	Contacts endometrium; 100% intramural
	4	Intramural
	5	Subserosal >50% intramural
	6	Subserosal <50% intramural
	7	Subserosal pedunculated
	8	Other (specify, e.g., cervical, parasitic)
Hybrid leiomyomas (impact both endometrium and serosa)	\multicolumn{2}{l}{Two numbers are listed separated by a hyphen. By convention, the first refers to the relationship with the endometrium, while the second refers to the relationship with the serosa. One example below:}
	2-5	Submucosal and subserosal, each with less than half the diameters in the endometrial and peritoneal cavities, respectively

(ESGE: European Society of Gastrointestinal Endoscopy; FIGO: The International Federation of Gynecology and Obstetrics; PALM-COEIN: polyp; adenomyosis; leiomyoma; malignancy and hyperplasia; coagulopathy; ovulatory dysfunction; endometrial; iatrogenic)
Source: Munro MG et al., 2011.

MECHANISMS OF INFERTILITY

Fibroids are seen in various sizes, different locations, and in variable numbers. Similarly, there are many mechanisms by which they may cause infertility.

TABLE 2: European Society of Gastrointestinal Endoscopy (ESGE)—classification of submucous myomas.

Type 0
- Entirely within the endometrial cavity
- No myometrial extension (pedunculated)

Type I
- <50% myometrial extension (sessile)
- <90° angle of myoma surface to the uterine wall

Type II
- ≥50% myometrial extension (sessile)
- ≥90° angle of myoma surface to the uterine wall

Source: Modified from Wamsteker K, Emanuel MH, de Kruif JH. Transcervical hysteroscopic resection of submucous fibroids for abnormal uterine bleeding: results regarding the degree of intramural extension. Obstet Gynecol. 1993;82(5):736-40.

Physical Impact of Fibroids and Perfusion of Fibroids

Fibroids, especially submucous fibroids are known to cause physical impedance to the transport of gametes as well as embryo. Blood flow to the uterine fibroids is less than that to the adjacent myometrium. This has been proved by perfusion studies.

Uterine Contractions and Infertility

Uterine contractions increase in frequency from fundus to the cervix in early follicular phase. In the perifollicular phase the direction of uterine contractions is reversed. It is from the cervix to the fundus.[14] Fibroids are known to have their effect on myometrial contractions. There is an increase in myometrial peristalsis in patients with intramural and submucosal fibroids.[12,15,16]

Yoshino et al with the cine model, MRI found that there is accelerated mid-luteal uterine peristalsis. It is defined as >2 movements in 3 minutes in the presence of uterine fibroids.[17]

In another prospective study, the author reported the impact of uterine peristalsis due to fibroid on the outcome of non-in vitro fertilization (IVF) fertility treatment.[18]

Increase myometrial contractility is due to cytokines, growth factors, neurotensin, neuropeptides, enkephalin, and oxytocin modulators in the fibroid capsule.[19]

Myomas alter uterine contractility. It probably interferes with sperm and ovum interaction and embryo migration.

Cytokine Factors

There was a significant reduction in the levels of cytokines mainly IL-10 and glycodelin in midluteal uterine washings of women with submucosal fibroids. This was reported by Ben-Nagi et al.[20]

Genetic Factors

HOXA 10, *HOXA 11*, and *BETB 1* gene expression modulate endometrial receptivity. The reduction or absence of *HOXA 10* in the uterine endometrium is the cause of implantation failure and infertility.[21]

Significant reduction in the concentration of these genes during the follicular phase of an infertile couple with submucosal fibroids has been demonstrated [The International Federation of Gynecology and Obstetrics (FIGO) L0–L2]—Rackow et al.[12]

A significant decrease in *HOXA 10* concentrations during the luteal phase in infertile women with intramural fibroids was noted by Matsuzaki et al.[22]

Alizadeh et al. reported an increase in endometrial *HOXA 1* gene expression following myomectomy.[23]

Endomyometrial Junctional Zone and Fibroids

The endomyometrial junctional zone (EMJ) is the inner one-third of the myometrium abutting the endometrium. EMJ contributes macrophages and uterine natural killer cells. They are essential for process of endometrial decidualization in the midluteal window of implantation. Kitaya et al. found a significant reduction in the concentration of both macrophages and uNK cells in the EMJ. This has a negative impact on fertility.[24,25]

DOES THE PRESENCE OF UTERINE FIBROIDS REDUCE IMPLANTATION RATES?

Submucosal fibroids are known to have a negative impact on implantation and early pregnancy. Pritts et al have shown that submucosal fibroids—FIGO L0–L2, resulted in decreased clinical pregnancy, implantation, and ongoing pregnancy rates. It is also associated with an increased risk of spontaneous abortions.[8]

WHAT ABOUT THE FIBROIDS THAT DO NOT CAUSE DISTORTION OF A CAVITY?

As far as subserosal fibroids are concerned, FIGO L5–L7, there is a clear finding that they do not decrease any measure of infertility.[26]

Even noncavity distorting intramural fibroids have an impact on fertility. 21% reduction in the live birth rate was found in such fibroids.[27] African women were found to have significantly high rates of miscarriage and fibroids are the contributing factor for this.[27]

TO REMOVE OR NOT TO REMOVE? THAT IS THE QUESTION

Myomectomy has definite benefits. Many studies have reported this. Babaknia et al way back in 1978 noted 38% term pregnancy following myomectomy in 34 women. They otherwise were cases of unexplained infertility.[28]

Casini et al. subjected all women with fibroids but otherwise, unexplained infertility to undergo myomectomy. Increased pregnancy rate was reported. This was irrespective of baseline fibroid staging. A statistically significant increase, however, was observed only in women with submucosal fibroid.[29] Beneficial effects of pre-IVF myomectomy in an adequately controlled trial were established. In this trial all patients were selected with one to five fibroids, with one measuring at least 5 cm and all with submucosal component, they found a 25% take-home baby rate in the myomectomy group as compared to 12% in the nonmyomectomy group.[7]

In the case of intramural or subserosal fibroids, Cochrane review of three randomized controlled trials (RCTs) concluded that there is insufficient evidence to recommend a myomectomy for the purpose of improving fertility outcomes.[30]

To summarize, there is a clear division between where the fibroids are located, and the benefit of myomectomy provides on reproductive outcomes. This was noted both in spontaneous pregnancy as well as IVF pregnancies. Subserosal fibroid and infertility have very little link as far as a cause is concerned. Therefore, myomectomy to remove subserosal fibroids for infertility is not evidence-based. On the other hand, submucosal fibroids are shown to lower fertility rates. It has been proved that when you remove such fibroids, you find improvement in both conceptions and live birth rates.

As far as intramural fibroids are concerned, both the evidence and consensus for myomectomy, purely for infertility, is weak. Such cases have to be managed on an individual basis, given the risk of significant morbidity of the surgery.

WHAT IS THE PRAGMATIC APPROACH TO MANAGEMENT?

Fibroid mapping is the crucial step in the management of fibroids and infertility. In fact, it is the first step after the diagnosis of fibroid which decides the plan of treatment. Ultrasound is the critical tool in this assessment. Transvaginal ultrasound and three-dimensional (3D) ultrasound are value addition to the diagnosis. Saline infusion sonography plays important role in the diagnosis of submucosal fibroids while MRI is gaining more and more importance in the exact location, myometrial invasion, and differentiation between fibroid and adenomyosis.

As far as infertility is concerned, it is equally important to ascertain the cause of infertility and this workup includes an assessment of ovarian reserve and ovulation, tubal patency, and semen analysis. Myomectomy is an opportunity to test tubal patency. **Flowchart 1** shows the treatment outline of infertility.[31]

Flowchart 1: Approach and management of infertile couple.[8]

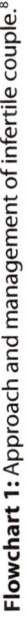

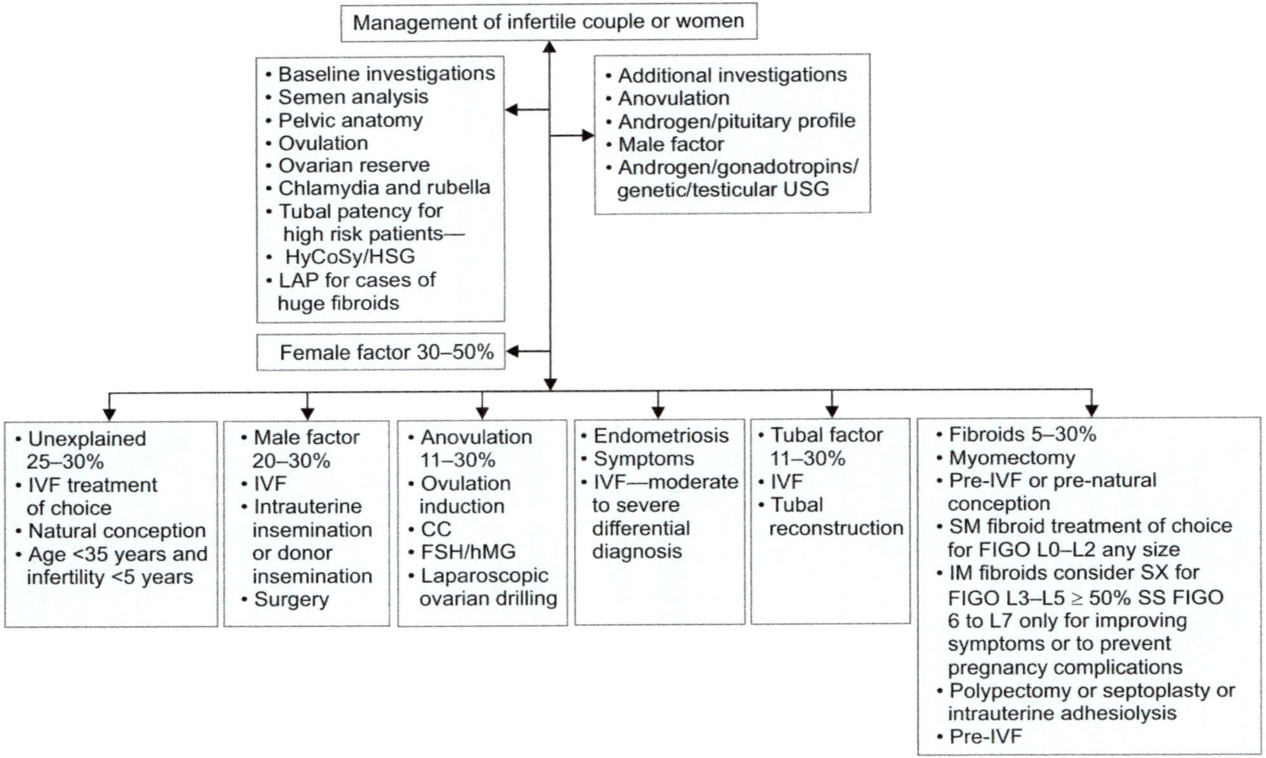

Management of infertile couple or women

Baseline investigations
- Semen analysis
- Pelvic anatomy
- Ovulation
- Ovarian reserve
- Chlamydia and rubella
- Tubal patency for high risk patients—HyCoSy/HSG
- LAP for cases of huge fibroids

Additional investigations
- Anovulation
- Androgen/pituitary profile
- Male factor
- Androgen/gonadotropins/ genetic/testicular USG

Unexplained 25–30%
- IVF treatment of choice
- Natural conception
- Age <35 years and infertility <5 years

Male factor 20–30%
- IVF
- Intrauterine insemination or donor insemination
- Surgery

Female factor 30–50%

- Anovulation 11–30%
- Ovulation induction
- CC
- FSH/hMG
- Laparoscopic ovarian drilling

- Endometriosis
- Symptoms
- IVF—moderate to severe
- differential diagnosis

- Tubal factor 11–30%
- IVF
- Tubal reconstruction

- Fibroids 5–30%
- Myomectomy
- Pre-IVF or pre-natural conception
- SM fibroid treatment of choice for FIGO L0–L2 any size
- IM fibroids consider SX for FIGO L3–L5 ≥ 50% SS FIGO 6 to L7 only for improving symptoms or to prevent pregnancy complications
- Polypectomy or septoplasty or intrauterine adhesiolysis
- Pre-IVF

(CC: clomiphene citrate; FIGO: The International Federation of Gynecology and Obstetrics; FSH: follicle-stimulating hormone; hMG: human menopausal gonadotropin; HSG: hysterosalpingography; HyCoSy: hysterosalpingo contrast sonography; IM: intramural; IVF: in vitro fertilization; LAP: laparoscopy fertility treatment; SM: submucosal)

DOES THE MEDICAL TREATMENT HAVE ANY ROLE IN THE MANAGEMENT OF FIBROIDS WITH INFERTILITY?

All the options available in the medical management of fibroids are contraceptives and hence do not have a direct role in the management. Combined oral contraceptive (OC) pills, levonorgestrel-releasing intrauterine system (LNG-IUS), progesterone-only pills, gonadotropin hormone-releasing hormone (GnRH) agonists, and ulipristal acetate have a role to play in the managing menstrual and pain symptoms. They, to some extent, help in reducing the size of fibroids, but do not play any direct role in infertility management. Promoting Empowerment And Risk Reduction (PEARL) clinical trials have proved the safety and efficacy of ulipristal in the management of fibroids. Ulipristal also helps in the reduction of size of fibroids. Luyckx et al. have reported first series. There are 18 pregnancies in 52 women participating in PEARL II and PEARL III studies. Of 21 women who wished to conceive after ulipristal therapy, myomectomy was done in 19 women. Fifteen women conceived total of 18 times, 12 of which were spontaneous and six were IVF conceptions. There were 13 live births and six miscarriages.[32]

SURGICAL TREATMENT

Hysteroscopic Myomectomy

Submucosal fibroids are treated with hysteroscopic myomectomy, and this is the best approach. Hysteroscopic myomectomy restores the cavity dimensions and improves implantation and fertility outcomes. The risk associated with the procedure includes difficulty in removing FIGO L2 or European Society of Gastrointestinal Endoscopy (ESGE) type 2 fibroids, the possibility of adhesions, and perforation. The dreadful complication of fluid overload and also Asherman's syndrome. All the possibilities should be discussed while counseling regarding the treatment modality.

Intrauterine adhesions have been reported by Valle et al. in 7.5% of hysteroscopic myomectomies.[33] To prevent further adhesions, postoperative adjuvant therapy such as estrogen therapy for 4–8 weeks or insertion of an intrauterine device, pediatric Foley catheter, or another balloon for 1 week postoperatively, have all been used.

The two-stage procedure may be required in FIGO L2 fibroids, with <50% fibroids located in the cavity. They are more difficult to resect, especially if a fibroid is >3 cm in size.[34]

Laparoscopy versus Laparotomy

Abdominal approach is the best in fibroids FIGO L3 and above and in some situations even large L2 fibroids. The improvement in reproductive outcome is the same by both approaches. The recovery with laparoscopic myomectomy is much better with less postoperative morbidity.[35]

In another study of 132 women with fibroids, though cumulative outcomes were similar within first 12 months, the per cycle outcomes such as pregnancy rate per cycle was significantly higher in laparoscopic as compared to the laparotomy group.[36]

Uterine Artery Embolization

Treatment option for women with large fibroids who no longer desire fertility is uterine artery embolization (UAE). This was described for the first time in 1995 by Ravina.[37]

The evaluation of UAE versus abdominal myomectomy in infertile patients was conducted in an RCT. The pregnancy rates were 50% and 78% respectively in UAE and myomectomy groups. Mean age was 32 years which may explain the overall high conception rate. The time to the conception period was longer for UAE (mean 18 months). This was much more as compared to myomectomy (mean 13 months). The reintervention rates were also higher in UAE arm (19 out of 58) as compared to myomectomy arm.[38]

35.2% rate of miscarriage in UAE conception as compared to 16.5% in fibroid was reported by Homer et al. in pregnancies matched for age and fibroid location.[39]

Thus, UAE is not a treatment of choice for women with infertility and for those who desire pregnancy in future as far as the current evidence base is concerned.

Magnetic Resonance-guided Focused Ultrasound Surgery

Promising early results are shown by this treatment modality. Magnetic resonance-guided focused ultrasound (MRgFUS) involves application of MRI-directed beams of ultrasound. They are capable of heating an area of fibroid tissue. This is done up to 70°C, causing destruction through coagulative necrosis.

All pregnancies following MRgFUS were reviewed by Rabinovici et al. Total number of 54 pregnancies were reported in 51 women. Mean age at procedure of 37.2 years and mean time to conception of 8 months. Miscarriage rate was 28%. Preliminary results are encouraging.[40] National Institute of Health and Care Excellence (NICE) encourages further research into the efficacy of MRgFUS.

SUMMARY

The evidence regarding the effect of fibroids on infertility is weak and inconclusive. The most important is proper evaluation and classification of fibroids, particularly those involving the cavity of the uterus.

There is no controversy as far as the treatment of submucosal fibroids, FIGO L0–L2 is concerned. They need to be treated hysteroscopically. In the case of large L2 fibroids, laparoscopic approach may work well rather than hysteroscopic approach. This improves the conception rate.

The management of intramural fibroids should be individualized on a case-to-case basis.

Subserosal fibroids do not have a major impact on infertility. All the systemic reviews and meta-analysis agreed on this point.

Conservative modalities such as UAE, MRgFUS, and drugs like ulipristal should not be offered as a part of the treatment in infertility with fibroids. There is no role for medical therapy as a standalone treatment for fibroids in an infertile population. This is due to a lack of good clinical trials on the subject as far as safety and effectiveness are concerned.

Society of Obstetricians and Gynaecologists of Canada (SOGC) have provided recommendations regarding the best management of fibroids in couples with infertility.[41]

They have made the following summary statements and recommendations:

Summary Statements

- Subserosal fibroids do not appear to have an impact on fertility, the effect of intramural fibroids remains unclear. If intramural fibroids do have an impact on fertility, it appears to be small and to be even less significant when the endometrium is not involved. (II-3)
- Because the current medical therapy for fibroids is associated with suppression of ovulation, reduction of estrogen production, or disruption of the target action of estrogen or progesterone at the receptor level, and it has the potential to interfere in endometrial development and implantation, there is no role for medical therapy as a standalone treatment for fibroids in the infertile population. (III)
- Preoperative assessment of submucosal fibroids is essential to the decision on the best approach for treatment. (III)
- There is little evidence on the use of Foley catheters, estrogen, or intrauterine devices for the prevention of intrauterine adhesions following hysteroscopic myomectomy. (II-3)
- In the infertile population, cumulative pregnancy rates by the laparoscopic and the minilaparotomy approaches are similar, but the laparoscopic approach is associated with a quicker recovery, less postoperative pain, and less febrile morbidity. (II-2)
- There are lower pregnancy rates, higher miscarriage rates, and more adverse pregnancy outcomes following uterine artery embolization than after myomectomy. (II-3) Studies also suggest that uterine artery embolization is associated with loss of ovarian reserve, especially in older patients. (III)

Recommendations

- In women with infertility, an effort should be made to adequately evaluate and classify fibroids, particularly those impinging on the endometrial cavity, using transvaginal ultrasound, hysteroscopy, hysterosonography, or magnetic resonance imaging. (III-A)
- Preoperative assessment of submucosal fibroids should include, in addition to an assessment of fibroid size and location within the uterine cavity, an evaluation of the degree of invasion of the cavity and thickness of residual myometrium to the serosa. A combination of hysteroscopy and transvaginal ultrasound or hysterosonography are the modalities of choice. (III-B)
- Submucosal fibroids are managed hysteroscopically. The fibroid size should be <5 cm, although larger fibroids have been managed hysteroscopically, but repeat procedures are often necessary. (III-B)
- A hysterosalpingogram is not an appropriate exam to evaluate and classify fibroids. (III-D)
- In women with otherwise unexplained infertility, submucosal fibroids should be removed in order to improve conception and pregnancy rates. (II-2A)
- The removal of subserosal fibroids is not recommended. (III-D)
- There is fair evidence to recommend against myomectomy in women with intramural fibroids (hysteroscopically confirmed intact endometrium) and otherwise unexplained infertility, regardless of their size. (II-2D) If the patient has no other options, the benefits of myomectomy should be weighed against the risks, and the management of intramural fibroids should be individualized. (III-C)
- If fibroids are removed abdominally, efforts should be made to use an anterior uterine incision to minimize the formation of postoperative adhesions. (II-2A)
- The widespread use of the laparoscopic approach to myomectomy may be limited by the technical difficulty of this procedure. The patient selection should be individualized based on the number, size, and location of uterine fibroids and the skill of the surgeon. (III-A)
- Women, fertile or infertile, seeking future pregnancy should not generally be offered uterine artery embolization as a treatment option for uterine fibroids. (II-3E)

So, to summarize, treatment of fibroids should be individualized, and symptomatology may be a decisive factor in whether or not fibroid is removed. Myomectomy remains the gold standard for treatment.

REFERENCES

1. Walker CL, Stewart EA. Uterine fibroids: the elephant in the room. Science. 2005;308(5728):1589-92.

2. Cramer SF, Patel A. The frequency of uterine leiomyomas. Am J Clin Pathol. 1990;94(4):435-8.
3. Baird DD, Dunson DB, Hill MC, Cousins D, Schectman JM. High Cumulative incidence of uterine leiomyoma in black and white women: ultrasound evidence. Am J Obstet Gynecol. 2003;188(1):100-7.
4. Ezzati M, Norian JM, Segars JM. Management of uterine fibroids in the patient pursuing assisted reproductive technologies. Women's Health (Lond Engl). 2009;5:413-21.
5. Cook H, Ezzati M, Segars J, McCarthy K. The impact of uterine leiomyomas on reproductive outcomes. Minerva Ginecol. 2010;62:225-36.
6. Donnez J, Jadoul P. What are the implications of myomas on fertility? A need for a debate? Hum Reprod. 2002;17:1424-30.
7. Bulletti C, De Ziegler D, Polli V, Flamigni C. The role of leiomyomas in infertility. J Am Assoc Gynecol Laparosc. 1999;6:441-5.
8. Pritts EA, Parker WH, Olive DL. Fibroids and infertility: an updated systematic review of the evidence. Fertil Steril. 2009;91(4):1215-23.
9. Olive DL, Pritts EA. Fibroids and Reproduction. Semin Reprod Med. 2010;28:218-27.
10. Somigliana E, Vercellini P, Daguati R, Pasin R, De Giorgi O, Crosignani PG. Fibroids and female reproduction: a critical analysis of the evidence. Hum Reprod Update. 2007;13:465-76.
11. Benecke C, Kruger TF, Siebert TI, Van der Merwe JP, Steyn DW. Effect of fibroids on fertility in patients undergoing assisted reproduction. A structured literature review. Gynecol Obstet Invest. 2005;59(4):225-30.
12. Rackow BW, Taylor HS. Submucosal uterine leiomyomas have a global effect on molecular determinants of endometrial receptivity. Fertil Steril. 2010;93(6):2027-34.
13. Sinclair DC, Mastroyannis A, Taylor HS. Leiomyoma simultaneously impair endometrial BMP-2-mediated decidualization and anticoagulant expression through secretion of TFG-β3. J Clin Endocrinol Metab. 2011;96:412-21.
14. Lyons EA, Taylor PJ, Zheng XH, Ballard G, Levi CS, Kredentser JV. Characterization of subendometrial myometrial contractions throughout the menstrual cycle in normal fertile women. Fertil Steril. 1991;55(4):771-4.
15. Richards PA, Richards PD, Tiltman AJ. The ultrastructure of fibromyomatous myometrium and its relationship to infertility. Hum Reprod Update. 1998;4(5):520-5.
16. Kido A, Ascher SM, Hahn W, Kishimoto K, Kashitani N, Jha RC, et al. 3T-MRI uterine peristalsis: comparison of symptomatic fibroid patients versus controls. Clin Radiol. 2014;69(5):468-72.
17. Yoshino O, Nishii O, Osuga Y, Asada H, Okuda S, Orisaka M, et al. Myomectomy decreases abnormal uterine peristalsis and increases pregnancy rate. J Minim Invasive Gynecol. 2012;19(1):63-7.
18. Yoshino O, Hayashi T, Osuga Y, Orisaka M, Asada H, Okuda S, et al. Decreased pregnancy rate is linked to abnormal uterine peristalsis caused by intramural fibroids. Hum Reprod. 2010;25(10):2475-9.
19. Malvasi A, Cavallotti C, Nicolardi G, Pellegrino M, Dell'Edera D, Vergara D, et al. NT, NPY and PGP 9.5 presence in myomeytrium and in fibroid pseudocapsule and their possible impact on muscular physiology. Gynecol Endocrinol. 2013;29:177-81.
20. Ben-Nagi J, Miell J, Mavrelos D, Naftalin J, Lee C, Jurkovic D. Endometrial implantation factors in women with submucous uterine fibroids. Reprod Biomed Online. 2010;21(5):610-5.
21. Cakmak H, Taylor HS. Implantation failure: molecular mechanisms and clinical treatment. Hum Reprod Update. 2011;17(2):242-53.
22. Matsuzaki S, Canis M, Darcha C, Pouly JL, Mage G. HOXA-10 expression in the mid-secretory endometrium of infertile patients with either endometriosis, uterine fibromas or unexplained infertility. Hum Reprod. 2009;24(12):3180-7.

23. Alizadeh Z, Faramarzi S, Saidijam M, Alizamir T, Esna-Ashari F, Shabab N, et al. Effect of intramural myomectomy on endometrial HOXA10 and HOXA11 mRNA expression at the time of implantation window. Iran J Reprod Med. 2013;11(12):983-8.
24. Kitaya K, Yasuo T. Leukocyte density and composition in human cycling endometrium with uterine fibroids. Hum Immunol. 2010;71(2):158-63.
25. Tocci A, Greco E, Ubaldi FM. Adenomyosis and endometrial-subendometrial myometrium unit disruption disease are two different entities. Reprod Biomed Online. 2008;17(2):281-91.
26. Sunkara SK, Khairy M, El-Toukhy T, Khalaf Y, Coomarasamy A. The effect of intramural fibroids without uterine cavity involvement on the outcome of IVF treatment: a systematic review and meta-analysis. Hum Reprod. 2010;25(2):418-29.
27. Feinberg EC, Larsen FW, Catherino WH, Zhang J, Armstrong AY. Comparison of assisted reproductive technology utilization and outcomes between Caucasian and African American patients in an equal-access-to-care setting. Fertil Steril. 2006;85(4):888-94.
28. Babaknia A, Rock JA, Jones Jr HW. Pregnancy success following abdominal myomectomy for infertility. Fertil Steril. 1978;30(6):644-7.
29. Casini ML, Rossi F, Agostini R, Unfer V. Effects of position of fibroids on fertility. Gynecol Endocrinol. 2006;22(2):106-9.
30. Metwally M, Cheong YC, Horne AW. Surgical treatment of fibroids for subfertility. Cochrane Database Syst Rev. 2012;11:CD003857.
31. Suresh YN, Narvekar NN. The role of tubal patency tests and tubal surgery in the era of assisted reproductive techniques. Obstet Gynaecol. 2014;16:37-45.
32. Luyckx M, Squifflet JL, Jadoul P, Votino R, Dolmans MM, Donnez J. First series of 18 pregnancies after ulipristal acetate treatment for uterine fibroids. Fertil Steril. 2014;102(5):1404-9.
33. Valle RF, Sciarra JJ. Intrauterine adhesions: hysteroscopic diagnosis, classification, treatment, and reproductive outcome. Am J Obstet Gynecol. 1988;158(6 Pt 1):1459-70.
34. Camanni M, Bonino L, Delpiano EM, Ferrero B, Migliaretti G, Deltetto F. Hysteroscopic management of large symptomatic submucous uterine myomas. J Minim Invasive Gynecol. 2010;17(1):59-65.
35. Seracchioli R, Rossi S, Govoni F, Rossi E, Venturoli S, Bulletti C, et al. Fertility and obstetric outcome after laparoscopic myomectomy of large myomata: a randomized comparison with abdominal myomectomy. Hum Reprod. 2000;15(12):2663-8.
36. Palomba S, Zupi E, Falbo A, Russo T, Marconi D, Tolino A, et al. A multicenter randomized, controlled study comparing laparoscopic versus minilaparotomic myomectomy: reproductive outcomes. Fertil Steril. 2007;88(4):933-41.
37. Ravina JH, Herbreteau D, Ciraru-Vigneron N, Bouret JM, Houdart E, Aymard A, et al. Arterial embolisation to treat uterine myomata. Lancet. 1995;346(8976):671-2.
38. Mara M, Maskova J, Fucikova Z, Kuzel D, Belsan T, Sosna O. Midterm clinical and first reproductive results of a randomized controlled trial comparing uterine fibroid embolization and myomectomy. Cardiovasc Intervent Radiol. 2008;31(1):73-85.
39. Homer H, Saridogan E. Uterine artery embolization for fibroids is associated with an increased risk of miscarriage. Fertil Steril. 2010;94(1):324-30.
40. Rabinovici J, David M, Fukunishi H, Morita Y, Gostout BS, Stewart EA, et al. Pregnancy outcome after magnetic resonance-guided focused ultrasound surgery (MRgFUS) for conservative treatment of uterine fibroids. Fertil Steril. 2010;93(1):199-209.
41. Carranza-Mamane B, Havelock J, Hemmings R, Reproductive Endocrinology and Infertility Committee; Special Contributor. The Management of Uterine Fibroids in Women with Otherwise Unexplained Infertility. J Obstet Gynaecol Can. 2015;37(3):277-85.

CHAPTER 15 | Infections in Infertility

Jyotsana Daule, Anil Bendre

INTRODUCTION

Pelvic infection is one of the most common cause of infertility in female and male. In female, *Neisseria gonorrhoeae* and *Chlamydia trachomatis* account for 14–35% cases and tuberculosis also very common about 2–19% in developing countries, such as India and other Asian and African countries. Urogenital tuberculosis is the third most common form of extrapulmonary TB. Incidence of female genital TB (FGTB) is very common around 24% in patients seeking assisted reproductive technology (ART) treatment.

INFECTIONS CAUSING INFERTILITY IN MALE AND FEMALE

- Female
  - Lower genital tract infection
  - Upper genital tract infection
- Male
  - Acute genital tract infection
    - Acute orchitis
    - Acute epididymitis
  - Chronic genital tract infection, chronic prostatitis.

Factors Associated with Infection

- Effect of sexual promiscuity
- Less use of barrier contraceptives
- Changing multiple sexual partners
- Past history of sexually transmitted disease (STD) in any partner.

Common Organisms causing Lower Genital Tract Infection

Bacterial vaginosis: *Trichomonas vaginalis* and *Candida albicans*. *Chlamydia trachomatis* accounts for 14–35% of cases of genital tract infection.

Organisms associated with Upper Genital Tract Infection

Tuberculosis and *Chlamydia trachomatis*.

Upper Genital Tract Infection and Pelvic Inflammatory Disease

- Factors associated with sexual habits of patient as mention earlier.
- Inflammatory complication such as insertion of intrauterine device, termination of pregnancy, hysterosalpingography (HSG), puerperal sepsis or appendicular rupture, hysteroscopy or procedures for treatment of infertility as intrauterine insemination (IUI) or in vitro fertilization (IVF).
- Blood-borne infection also cause infertility as tuberculosis and mixed aerobic or anaerobic infections.
- Genital tuberculosis is very common in India and in developing countries. There is hematogenous spread from primary focus such as lungs.

Tuberculosis

Female genital TB is caused by *Mycobacterium tuberculosis* and rarely by *Mycobacterium bovis* or atypical mycobacteria. A TB affects commonly the fallopian tubes, endometrium and ovaries. FGTB can cause both primary as well as secondary infertility.

Genital tuberculosis and various pelvic infections leading to infertility are as follows:

- *Tubal factors*
  - Blockage of fallopian tubes due to endosalpingitis
  - Loss of tubal function due to ciliary damage
  - Perisalpingitis leading to adhesions and tubo-ovarian (TO) masses
  - Tubal hydrosalpinx formation has adverse effect on embryo implantation due to harmful cytokine factors leaking into endometrial cavity **(Table 1)**.

TABLE 1: Factors influencing the frequency of tubal occlusion after salpingitis.

Clinical findings	Tubal occlusion
Degree of infection at laparoscopy	
• Mild	6%
• Moderate	13%
• Severe	30%
Number of episodes of PID	
• One	11%
• Two	23%
• Three or more	54%
Types of salpingitis	
• Gonococcal	9%
• Nongonococcal	16%
• Tubercular	80–90%

- *Endometrial factors*
    - Decreased endometrial receptivity due to adverse effect on endometrial markers
    - Defective vascularization leading to reduced subendometrial blood flow
    - Defective implantation due to harmful cytokines and activated killer cells
    - Antigonadotrophic effect of infections on endometrium requiring more gonadotropins in IVF cycles
    - Destruction of endometrium leading to Asherman's syndrome formation.

Endometritis: Endometritis classified as acute, chronic, and fibrotic. It may be due to acute or chronic non-tubercular or tubercular infections.

- *Acute:* Due to foreign bodies, retained products of conception (RPOC), postpartum infection, postsurgical or after invasive procedures of genital tract such as HSG, IUI or IVF.
- *Chronic: Chlamydia trachomatis,* bacterial, tubercular, mycoplasma, toxoplasmosis, etc.
- *Fibrotic intrauterine (Asherman's syndrome):* Symptoms are chronic lower abdominal pain, amenorrhea hypomenorrhea, abnormal vaginal discharge, etc.

Symptoms related to infertility are spontaneous abortion, recurrent abortions, recurrent implantation failure (RIF), etc.

But intrauterine adhesions, which are caused by tuberculer endometritis or due to trauma, severely affects the fertility.

It causes RIF, abortion, premature deliveries and problems with separation of placenta.

- *Ovarian factors*
    - Ovaries get affected in 20–30% cases of infertility due to PID.
    - There may be adhesion, caseation, cyst formation or may be TO masses.
    - This leads to disruption of follicular maturation, luteinized unovulatory follicle (LUF) or difficulty in ovum pick-up by fimbria.
    - Infections also reduce ovarian reserve and so premature aging of ovaries, impair fertilization and affect the embryo quality and ultimately cause infertility.
    - *Abdomen and pelvis:* There may be flimsy or dense adhesion in pelvis, frozen pelvis in case of tuberculosis, perihepatic synechiae (Fitz-Hugh-Curtis syndrome), colonic adhesions, etc.
    - *Common organisms/infections*
        - *Gonococcal infection: N. gonorrhoeae* recovered from almost 30% of patients of tubal and endometrial cause of infertility. It affects nonciliated tubal cells and cilia.

Chlamydial Infections

The spectrum of disease is urethritis, endometritis, and salpingitis. Salpingitis is more common and it causes more tubal damage than *Trichomonas*.

The damage or occlusion of tubes is more because of proinflammatory response to the organism.

Symptoms:
- Asymptomatic (up to 10%)
  - *General symptoms:* Low grade fever, loss of weight, anorexia, malaise, heavy menses
  - *Menstrual symptoms:* Menorrhagia (in early stages due to ulcerative lesions)
    - Oligomenorrhea (in late stages)
    - Hypomenorrhea (in late stages)
    - Amenorrhea (primary and secondary due to endometrial involvement)
  - Primary or secondary infertility
  - Abdominal lump
  - Dyspareunia
  - Abdominal pain
  - Chronic pelvic pain
  - Acute abdomen (due to rupture or torsion of TO mass)
  - Unhealthy vaginal discharge.

Signs:
- No physical signs (common)
- *Systemic examination:* Raised temperature, lymphadenopathy, crackles on chest
- *Adnominal examination:* Mass in abdomen (vague or definite), doughy feel of abdomen, ascites
- *Vaginal examination:* Uterine enlargement (Pyometra), tenderness and induration in fornices, fullness in pouch of Douglas (POD), tender adnexal masses, small uterus (shrunken endometrial TB), per speculum examination, cervical ulcerative lesions, vulval ulcerative lesions

INVESTIGATIONS

When patient comes with infertility following investigations are done.
- Complete blood count
- C-reactive protein (CRP)
- Erythrocyte sedimentation rate (ESR)
- Human immunodeficiency virus (HIV)
- Blood sugar
- Urine analysis/culture
- *Vaginal wet mount:* For Chlamydia and gonorrhea

- *Mantoux (Tuberculin) test and interferon gamma released assays:* Sensitivity up to 55% and specificity up to 80%.
- *X-ray chest:* To rule old lesions or to exclude coexisting pulmonary TB.

Imaging Methods

- *Ultrasonography (USG):* It can diagnose adnexal masses and hydrosalpinges in advanced cases
- *Computed tomography (CT) scan:* It can aid diagnosis of USG
- *Magnetic resonance imaging (MRI):* Better resolution than CT scan
- *Positron emission tomography (PET) scan:* Increased glucose uptake by TB lesions can be helpful to differentiate from CA ovary
- *HSG:* It is contraindicated in diagnosed case of FGTB as it can flare up the disease. But if done as a infertility workup it shows tubal blocks either corneal or terminal, hydrosalpinges or venous intravasation of dye.

Uterine features seen are uterine synechiae formation, uterine contour distortion, obliteration of the uterine cavity, venous and lymphatic intravasation.

Chronic infections may result in complete destruction of endometrium and narrowing of cavity.

In patients of tuberculosis following tests are done.

Endometrial Biopsy (or Endometrial Aspirates or Menstrual Blood in Unmarried Girls)

It is done in premenstrual phase, sample is collected can be used for—
- Histopathological examination (HPE) to see epithelioid granulomas
- Smear on slide examination for acid-fast bacilli (AFB) using Ziehl-Neelsen (ZN) staining or fluorescent staining (at least 100–105 bacilli are needed per mL of specimen for *positive* results)
- Culture using Lowenstein-Jensen (LJ) medium or BACTEC culture: BACTEC culture has higher sensitivity and results are quick
- MGIT (Mycobacteria Growth Indicator Tube) 960 tube: Used for culture
- Polymerase chain reaction (PCR): DNA PCR can detect as low as 1–10 organisms/mL sample, but false positive and negative rates are high so PCR alone should not be used for either starting or stopping antituberculous therapy (ATT) in FGTB
- GeneXpert MTB/RIF assay: It gives very rapid results within 2 hours (against culture which requires at least 14 days). This test has very high specificity and furthermore it also gives information about susceptibility of the strain to rifampicin.

Laparoscopy

Laparoscopy is advised in patients who do not conceive even after regular treatment. USG showing free fluid in pelvic cavity or consistent thin endometrium or evidence of hydrosalpinx or pyosalpinx.

In FGTB, lesions can be identified as tubercles on peritoneum and ovary, caseous nodules, TO masses, hydrosalpinx, tubal blockage with beaded tubes, abdominal, pelvic and perihepatic adhesions (Fitz-Hugh-Curtis syndrome), encysted ascites, etc.

TREATMENT

Early treatment of upper genital tract infection is mandatory as it may cause tubal damage or endometrial scaring and ultimately causes infertility.

Mild cases of cervicitis and endometritis are managed on outpatient basis with different antibiotics regimens.

Severe cases of PID need hospitalization. Good hydration with intravenous fluids and intravenous antibiotics are given till the clinical improvements and then oral therapy started. If anemia is associated, it should be corrected.

Antibiotics

Mild Disease/Moderate Disease

- Tablet doxycycline for 7–14 days
- Or tablet azithromycin for 10 days
- Or combination of tablet ofloxacin and tablet metronidazole for 14 days.

Severe Disease

Regimen A:
- Injection ceftriaxone, IV/IM daily one plus
- Tablet doxycycline for 7 to 14 days
- Or tablet azithromycin for 10 days
- Or combination of tablet ofloxacin and tablet metronidazole for 14 days.

Regimen B:
- Injection clindamycin 900 mg 8 hourly plus
- Injection gentamicin 1.5 mg/kg body weight 8 hourly
- This is followed by tablet clindamycin 450 mg 6 hourly for 14 days or
- Tablet doxycycline 100 mg twice daily for 14 days plus
- Tablet metronidazole 400 mg twice daily for 14 days.

Treatment of Female Genital TB

- The drug treatment of drug sensitive FGTB is given in **Table 2**.
- Isoniazid resistant but rifampicin sensitive FGTB
- LREZ-(Levofloxacin + REZ) is given orally for 6 months as uniphasic pill

Multidrug-resistant FGTB (Flowchart 1)

Treatment should not be started by gynecologist on himself and patient should be referred to DOT center. For these patients, the treatment is usually given for 18–20 months. Drugs such as bedaquiline, levofloxacin or

TABLE 2: Drug treatment of drug sensitive FGTB.

Weight category	Intensive phase (HRZE) (75/150/400/275 mg) Orally daily for 2 months	Continuation phase (HRE) (75/150/275 mg) Orally daily for 4 months	Streptomycin (g)
Daily dose for adults [Number of tablets of fixed drug combination (FDC)]			
25–39 kg	2	2	0.5
40–54 kg	3	3	0.75
55–69 kg	4	4	1
≥70 kg	5	5	1

(H: isoniazid; R: rifampicin; Z: pyrizinamide; E: ethambutol, streptomycin is given only when there is an adverse drug reaction like hepatitis to HRZ)

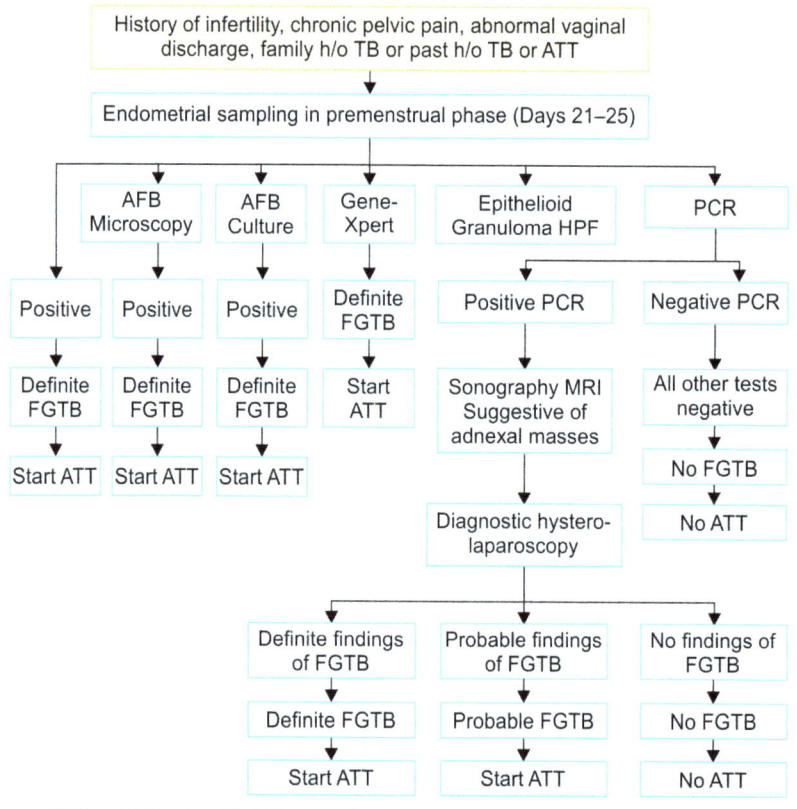

Flowchart 1: Diagnosis and treatment algorithm of female genital tuberculosis (FGTB) to be used in clinical practice.

(AFB: acid-fast bacilli; ATT: antituberculous therapy; HPE: histopathological examination; PCR: polymerase chain reaction; MRI: magnetic resonance imaging)

moxifloxacin, linezolid, cycloserine, clofazimine, and ethionamide are used to treat such patients.

TABLE 3: Common male genital tract infections.

Orchitis	Mumps, tuberculosis, syphilis
Epididymitis	Gonorrhea, tuberculosis, Chlamydia, Ureaplasma
Seminal vesiculitis	Tuberculosis, trichomoniasis and other bacteria
Urethritis	Gonorrhea, Chlamydia and trichomoniasis

MALE INFERTILITY

Infections may be acute or chronic. These infections may cause acute orchitis or epididymitis responsible for damage to testes and obstructions in ejaculatory ducts **(Table 3)**.

These infections associated with leukocytosis in semen and formation of antisperm antibodies which causes agglutination.

Treatment

Antibiotics such as ofloxacin, doxycycline can be given for 14 days. Azithromycin can be added for 14 days.

SUGGESTED READING

1. Bustos Lopez HH, Barron Valloyo J, Garcia Malvaez B, Ambe AK, Zelaya HC. Use of a diagnostic prospective algorithm for patients with recurrent miscarriage. Ginecol Obstet Mex. 1995;63:96-101.
2. Cates JrW, Wasserheit JN. Genital chlamydia infection, epidemiology and reproductive sequelae. Am J Obstet Gynecol. 1991;164(6 Pt 2):1771-81.
3. Das P, Ahuja A, Gupta SD. Incidence, etiopathogenesis and pathological aspects of genitourinary tuberculosis in India: a journey revisited. Indian J Urol. 2008;24(3):356-61.
4. Eschenbach DA. Infertility caused by infection. Contemp Obstet Gynecol. 1984;64:256.
5. Hurry DJ, Larsen B, Charles D. Effects of postcesarean section febrile morbidity on subsequent fertility. Obstet Gynecol. 1984;64(2):256-60.
6. Jindal UN, Verma S, Bala Y. Favourable infertility outcomes following anti-tubercular treatment prescribed on the sole basis of a positive polymerase chain reaction test for endometrial tuberculosis. Hum Reprod. 2012;27(5):1368-74.
7. Jones RB, Ardery BR, Hui SL, Cleary RE. Correlation between serum antichlamydial antibodies and tubal factor as a cause of infertility. Fertil Steril. 1982;38(5):553-8.
8. Lee JY. Diagnosis and treatment of extrapulmonary tuberculosis. Tuberc Respir Dis (Seoul). 2015;78(2):47-55.
9. Mccormack WM, Rosner B, Alpert S, Evrard JR, Crockett VA, Zinner SH. Vaginal colonization with *Mycoplasma hominis* and *Ureaplasma urealyticum*. Sex Transm Dis. 1986;13(2):67-70.
10. Merchant SA, Bharati AH, Badhe PB. Female genital tract tuberculosis: a review of hysterosalphingraphic appearances part 2-the uterus. J Women Imag. 2004;6(4):153-9.
11. Ministry of Health & Family Welfare. Standards for TB case in India. New Delhi: Ministry of Health & Family Welfare; 2016.
12. Novy MJ. Tubal surgery or IVF making the best choice in the 1990s. Int J Fertil Menopausal Stud. 1995;40(6):292-7.

13. Schaaf HS, Zumla AI. Tuberculosis Comprehensive Clinical Reference, 1st edition. St.Louis (MD): Saunders; 2009.
14. Sharma JB. Current diagnosis and management of female genital tuberculosis. J Obstet Gynaecol India. 2015;65(6):362-71.
15. Sweet RL, Gibbs RS. Infectious diseases of the female genital tract. In: Sweet RL, Gibbs RS (Eds). Genital Infections and Infertility, 3rd edition. Baltimore: Williams & Wilkins; 1995. pp. 399.
16. Sweet SL, Mills J, Hadley KW, Blumenstock E, Schachter J, Robbie MO, et al. Use of laparoscopy to determine the microbiologic etiology of acute salpingitis. Amj Obstet Gynecol. 1979;134(1):68-74.
17. Witkin SS, Viti D, David SS, Stangel J, Rosenwaks Z. Relation between antisperm antibodies and rate of fertilization of human oocyte in vitro. J Assist Reprod Genet. 1992;9(1):9-13.
18. Wolff H. The Biological significance of white blood cells in semen. Fertil Steril. 1995;63(6):1143-57.

CHAPTER 16: Unexplained Infertility

Chaitanya Shembekar, Parul Saoji

INTRODUCTION

Explaining the unexplained is the most difficult task. Counseling couples with unexplained infertility is not easy. Incidence of unexplained infertility is as high as 30%.[1,2]

Unexplained infertility is the diagnosis of exclusion after a standard evaluation which includes normal semen analysis, documentation of ovulation, and at least one patent Fallopian tube.

Further evaluation of a patient with unexplained infertility includes sperm function tests in male partner like DNA fragmentation and analysis of genetic causes, fertilization defects, and coital factors.

In female partner we need to rule out endometriosis, undiagnosed tubal and immunological factors, ovarian reserve testing, and endometrial factors such as polyps and Asherman syndrome.

The cause for infertility will remain unexplained if the investigations done are superficial and with increasing number of investigations which would help to frame the diagnosis in these infertile couples. Immunological causes are hardly ever investigated and premature ovarian aging is becoming a cause of concern for all of us **(Tables 1 and 2)**.[3]

TABLE 1: Causes of male and female unexplained infertility.

Causes of female unexplained infertility	Causes of male unexplained infertility
Endometriosis	Sperm DNA damage
Undiagnosed tubal factor	Immune infertility
Premature ovarian aging	Oxidative stress
Immune infertility	Genetic defects
Oxidative stress	Fertilization defects
Poor oocyte quality	Coital factors
Uterine cavity abnormalities like synechiae, polyps, and chronic endometritis	Inappropriate timing of intercourse, erectile dysfunction, and anejaculation

TABLE 2: Investigations for male and female infertility.

Investigations for female infertility	Investigations for male infertility
Hormonal assays: FSH, LH, AMH, S. prolactin, S. TSH, FT4	Semen analysis
Ovulation studies: Follicular monitoring, S. progesterone	Antisperm antibodies
Tubal patency tests: HSG and LAP	Test for reactive oxygen species (ROS) like chemiluminescence
Uterine cavity assessment: TVS, 3D, hysteroscopy	Sperm DNA damage assays: • Comet • SCSA • Acridine orange test • TUNEL • SCD

(AMH: anti-Müllerian hormone; FSH: follicle-stimulating hormone; HSG: hysterosalpingogram; LH: luteinizing hormone; SCD: sperm chromatin dispersion; SCSA: sperm chromatin structure assay; TSH: thyroid-stimulating hormone; TUNEL: terminal deoxynucleotidyl transferase dUTP nick end labeling; TVS: transvaginal sonography)

LAPAROSCOPIC SURGERY IN UNEXPLAINED INFERTILITY

According to American Society for Reproductive Medicine (ASRM) guidelines 2015 there is no role of laparoscopy in cases of unexplained infertility (UEI) where the initial tests are not performed like hysterosalpingogram (HSG) to rule out any tubal or other pelvic pathology. However, diagnostic laparoscopy can be done in cases of unexplained infertility where duration of infertility exceeds a period of 3 years.[4]

Canadian Fertility and Andrology Society recommends no laparoscopy in UEI especially in cases where no confirmation of tubal or other pelvic pathologies are stated (Level II-2B).[5]

Treatment—spontaneous pregnancy rate is 15% in 1 year and 35% in 2 years.[6]

So, initially expectant management is advised where in couples are given advice on lifestyle and fertile period. They are asked to report after few months. This period is utilized for preconception counseling and starting folic acid tablets.

Age plays an important role in further management of such cases. Age above 35 years is associated with falling fertility and hence poor prognosis.[6]

Steures and colleagues published a multicenter trial of 253 good-prognosis couples (mean age 33 years, median duration of infertility 2 years): 127 underwent immediate treatment and 126 expectant management. The probability of live birth without intervention after 6 months was around 27% implying that there was no delay in time to conception if expectant management was tried.[7]

Bhattacharya et al. published a randomized controlled trial (RCT) 580 couples in which three treatment modalities were offered and plotted against a graph.

First 193 people were offered expectant management, 194—oral cc and 193 unstimulated intrauterine insemination (IUI) × 6 months and live birth rates of each were compared 17%, 14%, 23%, respectively which were not significantly different.

Both the studies, Stresses and Bhattacharya, were reviewed and for the Steureus study patients were more convinced with expectant management whereas with Bhattacharya's study they wanted the treatment modality over the expectant management.

Canadian Fertility and Andrology Society recommends expectant management in patients of unexplained infertility. Considering the age and duration of infertility expectant management may be advocated as these patients have good prognosis (Level 1A).[8]

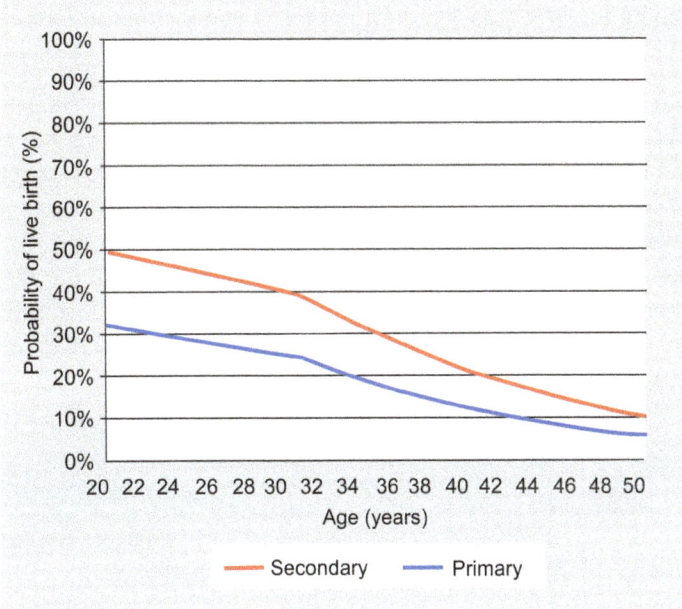

Since we need to have proper direction in the management of unexplained infertility, it would be better to discuss the latest guidelines given by ASRM in the year 2020.

ASRM has suggested ovarian stimulation followed by IUI as the first-line treatment. However, natural cycle of IUI has no role and stimulated cycles give better results and hence preferred over natural cycle IUI.

Natural cycle of IUI is not recommended in treatment of unexplained infertility.[9,10]

Ovarian stimulation with clomiphene citrate or letrozole and timed intercourse (TI) is not recommended for the treatment of unexplained infertility as per ASRM guidelines.

Clomiphene citrate with IUI gives the best results with almost 19 RCTs, 4 systemic reviews, and 3 cohort studies recommending ovarian stimulation with clomiphene citrate and IUI.[11]

This study has shown significant increase—31% versus 9%—in live birth rate with clomiphene citrate and IUI combination.[11]

ASRM guidelines have given strong recommendation for clomiphene citrate and IUI combination. Similar strong recommendation is given for letrozole and IUI combination.

Gonadotropins alone or in combination with oral ovulogens give high pregnancy rate in unexplained infertility. However, ASRM does not recommend gonadotropins because of high chance of multiple pregnancy rate.

When to plan in vitro fertilization (IVF) in unexplained infertility?
There are 12 RCTs suggesting IVF as the next treatment option after unsuccessful attempts of IUI **(Table 3)**.

Latest guidelines say that IUI should be tried over the period of 6 months before going for IVF. This 6-month period includes three to four cycles of IUI.[12]

Canadian society Recommendations:[5]
IVF should be planned for the patients who have undergone three cycles of ovulation induction (OI) or have had previous failed IUI cycles (Level 1A).

Age has an important role to play as far as management of unexplained infertility is concerned.

There are two interesting clinical trials which mention about the role of age of female partner in the management of unexplained infertility—fast track and standard treatment (FASTT) trial and the Forty and Over Treatment Trial (FORT-T) trial.[13]

TABLE 3: Published randomized controlled trials comparing gonadotropin/IUI with IVF for the treatment of unexplained infertility.

Reference	Number of subjects[a]	Clinical pregnancy rate	Gonadotropin/IUI with IVF
Goverde et al., 2000	172	7.8% per cycle	12.2% per cycle
Reindollar et al., 2010	503	21.4% after three cycles	52% after three cycles
van Rumste et al., 2014	116	17.2% after three cycles	22.4% per cycle
Bensdorp et al., 2015	602	56.0% after six cycles	58.7% after three cycles
Goldman et al., 2014[b]	154	17.3% after two cycles	49% after two cycles
Nandi et al., 2017	207	28.7% after three cycles	33.1% per cycle

[a]Number of couples randomized to either treatment strategy.
[b]This study specifically assessed couples in which the woman's age was 38–42 years.
(IUI: intrauterine insemination; IVF: in vitro fertilization)

In FASTT trial patients with unexplained infertility with age <40 years were divided into two groups, one with six cycles of IUI—three with clomiphene and three with FSH and in second arm the three cycles of FSH with IUI were omitted and patients were directly taken for IVF. It has been suggested that elimination of FSH with IUI gives best results and saves time as well.[14]

FORT-T trial typically includes patients with age of 40 years and above and they have recommended direct and immediate IVF treatment in such situations.

Follow the latest guidelines.

Ref: ASRM guidelines about unexplained infertility 2020

- For the treatment of UI the results are almost the same when it is the expectant management compared to clomiphene citrate/letrozole with TI.
- In natural cycles, IUI should not be done for UI.
- For TI, gonadotropins should not be used.

So, how do we go ahead?

Expectant management for 2 years is not pragmatic as the patients are anxious.

The way forward is to do IUI with clomiphene citrate or letrozole (Moderate evidence) and IUI with combination of oral agents along with gonadotropins is associated with higher multiple births though the pregnancy rates are higher, hence not recommended by ASRM.

IVF is not recommended as the first line of treatment for UI and has not been approved over expectant management for at least 6 months or OS with IUI for women below 38 years of age.

In nutshell, age, duration of marriage, and anxiety associated with UI decide the line of management in these patients.

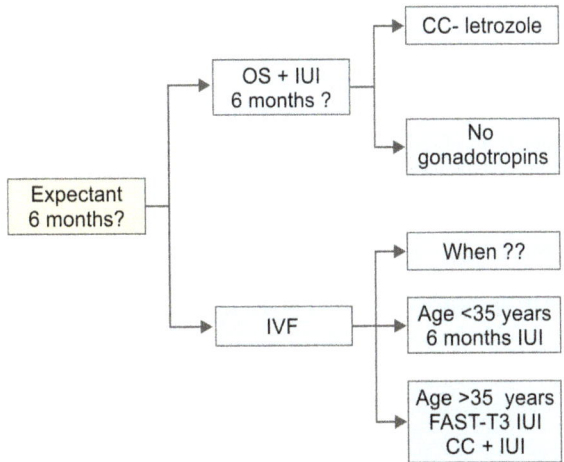

(CC: clomiphene citrate; FASTT: fast track and standard treatment; FORT-T: the Forty and Over Treatment Trial; IUI: intrauterine insemination; IVF: in vitro fertilization; OS: ovarian stimulation)

REFERENCES

1. Aboulghar MA, Mansour RT, Serour GI, Al-Inany1-Aboulghar HG. Diagnosis and management of unexplained infertility: an update. Arch Gynecol Obstet. 2003;267(4):177-88.
2. Isaksson R, Tiitinen A. Present concept of unexplained infertility. Gynecol Endocrinol. 2004;18(5):278-90.
3. Gleicher N, Kuhnir VA, Barad DH. Unexplained infertility. Lancet. 2018;392:1516-7.
4. Medscape. (2015). American Society for Reproductive Medicine (ASRM) 2015 Annual Meeting October 17 - 21, 2015; Baltimore, Maryland. [online] Available from https://www.medscape.com/viewcollection/33513 [Last accessed April, 2022].
5. Buckett W, Sierra S. The management of unexplained infertility: an evidence-based guideline from the Canadian Fertility and Andrology Society. Reprod Biomed Online. 2019;39(4):633-40.
6. Isaksson R, Tiitinen A. Obstetric outcome in patients with unexplained infertility: comparison of treatment-related and spontaneous pregnancies. Acta Obstet Gynecol Scand. 1998;77(8):849-53.
7. Steures P, van der Steeg JW, Hompes PGA, Habbema JDF, Eijkemans MJC, Broekmans FJ, et al. Collaborative Effort on the Clinical Evaluation in Reproductive Medicine Intrauterine insemination with controlled ovarian hyperstimulation versus expectant management for couples with unexplained subfertility and an intermediate prognosis: a randomised clinical trial. Lancet. 2006;368(9531):216-21.
8. Bhattacharya S, Harrild K, Mollison J, Wordsworth S, Tay C, Harrold A, et al. Clomifene citrate or unstimulated intrauterine insemination compared with expectant management for unexplained infertility: pragmatic randomised controlled trial.BMJ. 2008;337:a716.
9. Guzick DS, Carson SA, Coutifaris C, Overstreet JW, Factor-Litvak P, Steinkampf MP, et al. Efficacy of superovulation and intrauterine insemination in the treatment of infertility. National Cooperative Reproductive Medicine Network. N Engl J Med. 1999;340(3):177-83.
10. Evans-Hoeker EA, Eisenberg E, Diamond MP, Legro RS, Alvero R, Coutifaris C, et al. Major depression, antidepressant use, and male and female fertility. Fertil Steril. 2018;109(5):879-87.
11. Farquhar CM, Liu E, Armstrong S, Arroll N, Lensen S, Brown J. Intrauterine insemination with ovarian stimulation versus expectant management for unexplained infertility (TUI): a pragmatic, open-label, randomised, controlled, two-centre trial. Lancet. 2018;391(10119):441-50.
12. Custers IM, van Rumste MM, van der Steeg JW, van Wely M, Hompes PG, Bossuyt P, et al. Long-term outcome in couples with unexplained subfertility and an intermediate prognosis initially randomized between expectant management and immediate treatment. Hum Reprod. 2012;27(2):444-50.
13. Reindollar RH, Regan MM, Neumann PJ, Levine BS, Thornton KL, Alper MM, et al. A randomized clinical trial to evaluate optimal treatment for unexplained infertility: the fast track and standard treatment (FASTT) trial. Fertile Sterile. 2010;94(3):888-99.
14. Goldman MB, Thornton KL, Ryley D, Fung JL, Hornstein MD, Reindollar RH, et al. A randomized clinical trial to determine optimal infertility treatment in older couples: the Forty and Over Treatment Trial (FORT-T). Fertil Steril. 2014;101:1574-81.

CHAPTER 17: Step by Step Management of Infertility

Aditi Tandon, Sadhana Desai

INTRODUCTION

- *Definition:* Inability of a couple to conceive naturally after 1 year of regular unprotected sexual intercourse.
- Incidence worldwide is 10–14%, with higher rates in urban population.
- Prevalence is less in developed countries and more in developing countries due to limited resources for investigation and treatment options available[1]
- Evaluation is indicated after 12 months; however, it may be started earlier in women over 35 years of age.

EPIDEMIOLOGY OF INFERTILITY

- Probability of getting pregnancy per a reproductive cycle:
  - Young healthy couples: 20–25%
- Cumulative probabilities of conception
  - 60% within the first 6 months
  - 84% within the first year and
  - 92% within the second year
- Common causes of infertility[2-4] **(Fig. 1)**
- Lifestyle factors are considered risk factors for infertility, such as excess alcohol intake[5] and cigarette smoking.[6]

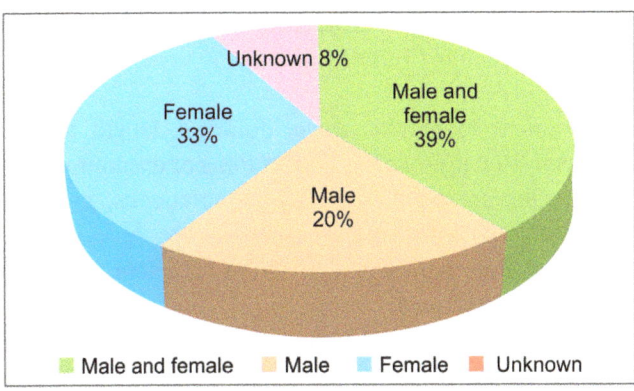

Fig. 1: Causes of infertility.

The American College of Obstetricians and Gynecologists (ACOG) and the American Society for Reproductive Medicine (ASRM) make the following recommendations and conclusions:
- An infertility evaluation may be offered to any patient who by definition has infertility or is at high risk of infertility.
- Women <35 years should receive an expedited evaluation and undergo treatment after 6 months of failed attempts to become pregnant or earlier, if clinically indicated. In women <40 years, more immediate evaluation and treatment are warranted. If a woman has a condition known to cause infertility, the obstetrician–gynecologist should offer immediate evaluation.
- A comprehensive medical history, including items relevant to the potential etiologies of infertility, should be obtained from the patient and partner, should one exist.
- A targeted physical examination of the female partner should be performed with a focus on vital signs and include a thyroid, breast, and pelvic examination.
- For the female partner, tests will focus on ovarian reserve, ovulatory function, and structural abnormalities.
- Imaging of the reproductive organs provides valuable information on conditions that affect fertility. Imaging modalities can detect tubal patency and pelvic pathology and assess ovarian reserve.
- A women's health specialist may reasonably obtain the male partner's medical history and order the semen analysis. Alternatively, it is also reasonable to refer all male infertility patients to a health care specialist with expertise in male reproductive medicine.

EVALUATION AND WORKUP FOR INFERTILE COUPLES

History Taking and Physical Examination
- Male and female partners both must be thoroughly evaluated, counseled, and included in the therapeutic decision-making processes, as infertility is a two-person problem (**Tables 1 and 2**).
- Timing of puberty
- *Menstrual history:* Menarche, cycle, duration, length and amount of bleeding, associated premenstrual symptoms or dysmenorrhea
- Ovulatory cycles are usually regular, spontaneous, cyclic with mild dysmenorrhea
- Anovulatory cycles are irregular, often painless, with history of amenorrhea, unpredictable
- A history of galactorrhea may indicate high prolactin levels which may lead to oligomenorrhea

TABLE 1: Summary of relevant history and physical examination findings for determining female factors in the infertile couple.

History	Physical examination
• Duration of infertility • Menstrual history • Pregnancy history • Previous methods of contraception • Coital frequency and sexual dysfunction • Past surgery (procedures, indications) • Hospitalizations (illnesses or injuries) • Pelvic inflammatory disease (sexually transmitted diseases) • Thyroid disease, galactorrhea, hirsutism • Abnormal pap smears or cervical surgeries • Current medications and allergies • Family reproductive history • Exposure environmental hazards • Use of tobacco, alcohol or illicit drugs	• Weight, body mass index, blood pressure, and pulse • Thyroid enlargement and presence of any nodules or tenderness • Breast secretions and their character • Signs of androgen excess • Vaginal or cervical abnormality or discharge • Pelvic or abdominal tenderness, organ size, or masses • Uterine size, shape, position, and mobility • Adnexal masses or tenderness • Cul-de-sac masses, tenderness, or nodularity

Source: Adapted from Practice Committee of the American Society for Reproductive Medicine. Diagnostic evaluation of the infertile female: a committee opinion. Fertil Steril. 2012;98(2):302-7; with permission.

TABLE 2: Summary of relevant history and physical examination findings for determining male factors in the infertile couple.

History	Physical examination
• A history of prior fertility • Coital frequency and timing • Duration of infertility and prior fertility • Childhood illnesses • Developmental history • Systemic medical illnesses (e.g., diabetes mellitus and upper respiratory diseases) • Previous surgery • Medications • Sexual history (including sexually transmitted infections) • Exposures to gonadal toxins (including environmental and chemical toxins and heat)	• Examination of the penis, noting the location of the urethral meatus • Palpation and measurement of the testes • Presence and consistency of both the vasa and epididymides • Presence or absence of a varicocele • Body habitus • Hair distribution • Breast development

Source: Adapted from Practice Committee of the American Society for Reproductive Medicine. Diagnostic evaluation of the infertile male: a committee opinion. Fertil Steril. 2012;98(2):294-301; with permission.

- A history of onset of progressive hirsutism in puberty along with oligomenorrhea may indicate polycystic ovarian syndrome or other disorders of androgen excess hallmarked by chronic anovulation.
- Extremes of weight loss or weight gain, elevated stress or extreme exercise is often associated with hypogonadotropic hypogonadism ovulatory disorders.
- *Uterine pathology:* Abnormal menstrual bleeding
- *Endometriosis:* Dyspareunia, severe dysmenorrhea
- A history of pelvic inflammatory disease, sexually transmitted infection, ruptured appendix or any other abdominal surgery, and the history of use of an intrauterine device may be associated with tubal disease.
- Sexual, social, and psychological issues should be evaluated.
- Any prior infertility evaluation, treatment records, films, or intraoperative findings and photographs should be sought and re-evaluated.

Male

- *Diabetes:* Increased risk for retrograde ejaculation
- Hypogonadism due to serious debilitating disease, adult mumps orchitis, or pituitary problems
- Some surgical procedures may impair fertility such as herniorrhaphy, varicocele, and bladder neck suspension.

The process of evaluation for female and male partner is shown in **Flowcharts 1 and 2**.

Diminished Ovarian Reserve

The ovarian reserve represents the number of oocytes available for at that point in time. Poor ovarian reserve predicts future response to gonadotropins but does not necessarily predict inability to achieve a pregnancy and a live birth.[7]

The following values can be considered as poor ovarian reserve:
- Anti-Müllerian hormone (AMH) value <1 ng/mL
- Antral follicle count (AFC) <5–7
- Follicle-stimulating hormone (FSH) >10 IU/L[9]
- A history of poor response to in vitro fertilization stimulation (fewer than four oocytes at time of egg retrieval).
- FSH and estradiol between cycle days 2 and 5
- Estradiol basal levels <60–80 pg/mL; elevated estradiol are indicative of decreased ovarian reserve levels as it may have a suppressive effect on FSH levels.[8]

If a woman has unexplained ovarian insufficiency or failure or an elevated FSH level before age 40 years and fragile X carrier screening is recommended to evaluate whether she has an *FMR1* premutation.[9]

Flowchart 1: Evaluation of female partner.

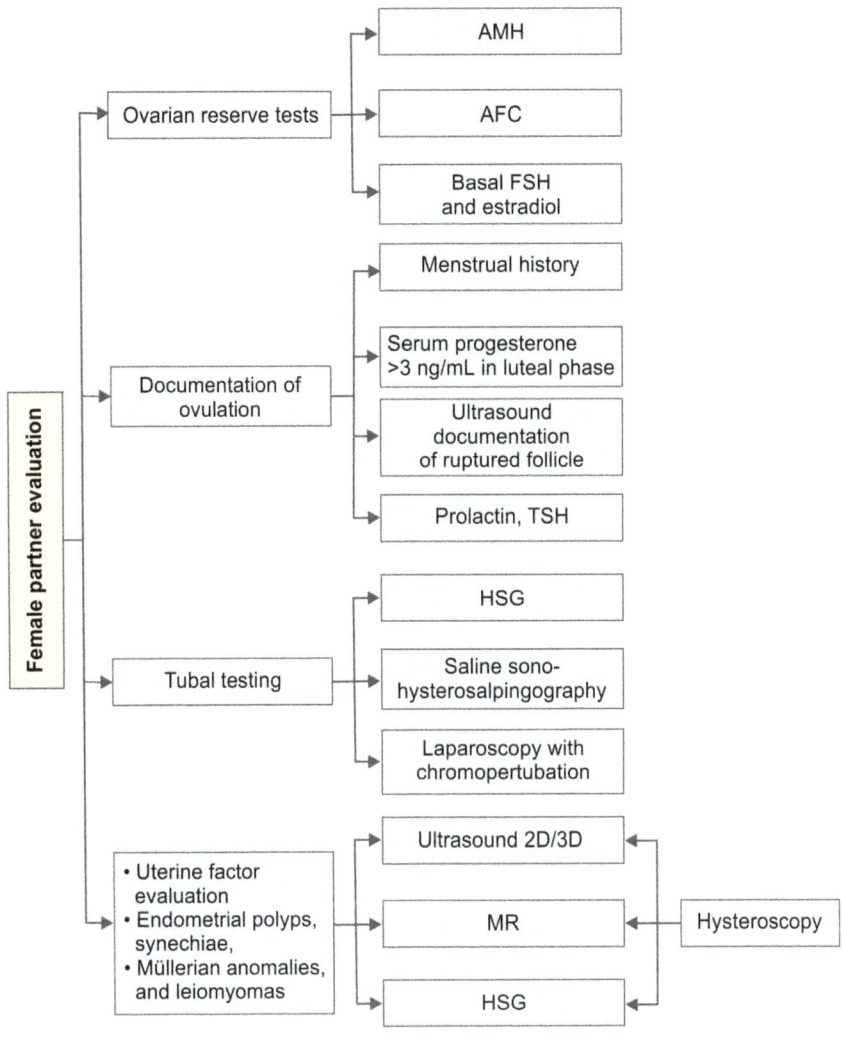

(AFC: antral follicular count; AMH: anti-Müllerian hormone; FSH: follicle-stimulating hormone; HSG: hysterosalpingography; TSH: thyroid-stimulating hormone)

Antral follicle counts may be high in women with polycystic ovary syndrome (PCOS) or reduces in those women on long-term hormonal contraceptives or with hypothalamic amenorrhea.[10]

Male Factor Infertility

Evaluation of Male Infertility

History and physical examination focusing on previous fertility, pelvic or inguinal surgeries, systemic diseases, and exposures.

Flowchart 2: Evaluation of male partner.

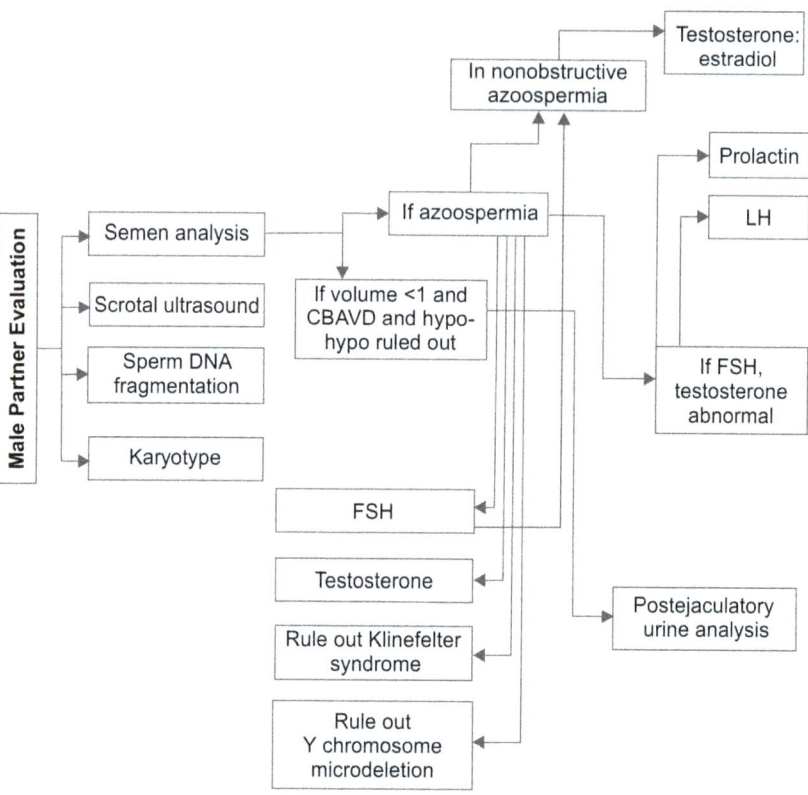

(CBAVD: congenital bilateral absence of the vas deferens; FSH: follicle-stimulating hormone; LH: luteinizing hormone)

Semen analysis: It is recommended to wait 3 months before repeat sampling because sperm generation time is just over 2 months.[8]

A normal sample according to the 2010 World Health Organization (WHO) guidelines is described in **Table 3**.[11] If abnormal, further evaluation is indicated **(Table 4)**.[12-17]

Suspect hypogonadism if oligospermia or azoospermia is present. Check morning levels of total testosterone [normal range = 240–950 ng per dL (8.3–33.0 nmol per L)] and FSH [normal range = 1.5–12.4 mIU per mL (1.5–12.4 IU per L)]. A decreased testosterone level with an increased FSH level suggests primary hypogonadism. A low testosterone level with a low FSH level indicates a secondary cause. Other causes, such as hyperprolactinemia, are reversible with treatment. Other testing may be needed including testicular biopsy, genetic testing, and imaging **(Table 4)**,[12-17] *as per case.* Postcoital testing and antisperm antibody (ASA) testing are no longer considered important.[18,19]

TABLE 3: The World Health Organization's accepted reference values for semen analysis, 2010.

Parameter (Units)	Reference value (lower limits, 5th centile)
Semen volume (mL)	1.5
pH	≥7.2
Sperm concentration (10⁶ per mL)	15
Total sperm number (10⁶ per ejaculate)	39
Total motility (%)	40
Progressive motility (PR, %)	32
Sperm agglutination	Absent*
Sperm morphology (normal forms, %)	• *World Health Organization criteria:* Lower reference limit for normal forms is 4% • *Tygerberg strict criteria:* Excellent prognosis (>14% morphologically normal spermatozoa), good prognosis (4–14%) and poor prognosis (<4%)†

*Diagnostic evaluation of the infertile male: a committee opinion. Practice Committee of the American Society for Reproductive Medicine. Fertil Steril. 2015;103:e18-25.
†Kruger TF, Acosta AA. Simmons KF, Swanson RJ, Matta JF. Oehninger S. Predictive value of abnormal sperm morphology in in vitro fertilization. Fertil Steril. 1988:49:112-7.
Source: Modified from WHO laboratory manual for the examination and processing of human semen (Appendix 1), 5th edition. Geneva: WHO; 2010. p. 225. Also Available at http;//www.vvho.int/reproductivehealth/ publications/infertility/9789241547789/en/.

TABLE 4: Etiology and evaluation of infertility.

Condition	History and physical examination	Laboratory and radiologic testing
Female		
Endometriosis or pelvic adhesions	History of abdominal or pelvic surgery; history consistent with endometriosis	Rarely helpful
Hypothalamic amenorrhea	Amenorrhea or oligomenorrhea; low body mass index	Low to normal FSH level; low estradiol level
Ovarian failure/insufficiency	Amenorrhea or oligomenorrhea; menopausal symptoms; family history of early menopause; single ovary; chemotherapy or radiation therapy; previous ovarian surgery; history of autoimmune disease	Elevated FSH level; low estradiol level

Contd...

Contd...

Condition	History and physical examination	Laboratory and radiologic testing
Ovulatory disorder	Irregular menses; hirsutism; obesity (polycystic ovary syndrome); galactorrhea (hyperprolactinemia); fatigue; hair loss (hypothyroidism)	Progesterone level <5 ng per mL (15.9 nmol per L); elevated prolactin level; low TSH level
Tubal blockage	History of pelvic infections or endometriosis	Abnormal hysterosalpingography result
Uterine abnormalities	Dyspareunia; dysmenorrhea; history of anatomic developmental abnormalities; family history of uterine fibroids; abnormal palpation and inspection	Abnormal hysterosalpingography or ultrasonography result

Male

Condition	History and physical examination	Laboratory and radiologic testing
Genetic etiology: Y deletions XXY (Klinefelter syndrome)	Y deletions: small testes Klinefelter phenotype: small testes, tall, gynecomastia, learning disabilities	• Both syndromes result in normal semen volume but low sperm count • Y deletions may present as normal hormone levels or have an elevated FSH level • Klinefelter syndrome typically results in low testosterone level and an elevated FSH level
Other genetics: CFTR gene (cystic fibrosis) 5T allele (cystic fibrosis)	Absence of the vas deferens	Low volume semen analysis
• Obstruction of the vas deferens or epididymis • Ejaculatory dysfunction	History of infection, trauma, or vasectomy; normal testicular examination	Low volume semen analysis; transrectal ultrasonography can identify obstruction
Systemic disease (not all-inclusive): • Hemochromatosis • Kallmann syndrome • Pituitary tumor • Sarcoidosis		Low FSH level; low testosterone level; check prolactin level and, if elevated, perform imaging for pituitary tumor
Unclear etiology	Normal testicular examination	Normal FSH level; normal semen volume; low sperm count

Endocrine Evaluation

Hypothalamic-pituitary-testicular axis abnormalities are well-recognized, but uncommon as a cause of male infertility. Endocrine disorders are highly uncommon in men with normal semen analysis.

An endocrine evaluation is indicated for men having:
- Abnormal semen parameters, particularly when the sperm concentration is <10 million/mL
- Impaired sexual function; or
- Other clinical findings that suggest a specific endocrinopathy.

It should include measurement of serum FSH and total testosterone (T). If the total T level is low (<300 ng/mL), further evaluation is indicated including a second early morning measurement of total T and measurements of serum free testosterone, LH, and prolactin (PRL). A single measurement of serum gonadotropin usually is sufficient to determine the clinical endocrine status even though concentrations vary because they are secreted in a pulsatile manner. The relationships among serum T, LH, FSH, and PRL concentrations help to provide an understanding of abnormal total T levels **(Table 5)**. A markedly elevated serum FSH concentration indicates an abnormal spermatogenesis. Measurement of the thyroid-stimulating hormone (TSH) concentration should also be obtained in men who require a more thorough endocrine evaluation.

Postejaculatory Urinalysis

Differential diagnosis of a low-volume or absent antegrade ejaculate suggests incomplete semen collection, retrograde ejaculation, absent emission, hypogonadism, obstruction of ejaculatory duct or congenital bilateral absence of the vas deferens (CBAVD). A postejaculatory urinalysis should be performed in men with ejaculate volume <1.0 mL, to exclude retrograde

TABLE 5: Basal hormone levels in various clinical states.

Clinical condition	FSH	LH	T	PRL
Normal spermatogenesis	Normal	Normal	Normal	Normal
Hypogonadotropic hypogonadism	Low	Low	Low	Normal
Abnormal spermatogenesis	High/normal	Normal	Normal	Normal
Complete testicular failure/ hypergonadotropic hypogonadism	High	High	Normal/low	Normal
PRL-secreting pituitary tumor	Normal/low	Normal/low	Low	High

ejaculation, other than those diagnosed with hypogonadism or CBAVD. Exclude an improper or incomplete collection or a very short abstinence interval (<1 day).

The postejaculatory urine is centrifuged for 10 minutes at 300 g, followed by microscopic examination of the pellet at X400 magnification. In men with retrograde ejaculation with azoospermia or aspermia, there will be presence of sperm in the postejaculatory urine. In case of low ejaculate volume and oligozoospermia, "significant numbers" of sperm must be observed to suggest the diagnosis of retrograde ejaculation; but there is not any consensus on the minimum number required.[20,21]

Ultrasonography

Ultrasonography is a useful imaging tool for detecting abnormalities of the male genital tract that may negatively affect fertility but is indicated for only a few number of infertile male patients.

Transrectal Ultrasonography

Transrectal ultrasonography (TRUS) suggesting dilated seminal vesicles or ejaculatory ducts and/or midline cystic prostatic structures points to, but does not confirm, the diagnosis of ejaculatory duct obstruction, complete or partial. Normal seminal vesicles are usually <1.5 cm anteroposteriorly.[22]

Affected men classically produce a low-volume acidic ejaculate with no sperm or fructose. Men with CBAVD may present similarly because they often have absent or atrophic seminal vesicles. Men with partial ejaculatory duct obstruction may also present with low semen volume, oligoasthenospermia, and low progressive motility.

Scrotal Ultrasonography

Physical examination can palpate most scrotal pathology, including varicoceles, spermatoceles, epididymal induration, absent vasa, and testicular masses. Scrotal ultrasonography is needed for small varicoceles that are not palpable, but such lesions do not have any documented clinical significance.[23] Scrotal ultrasonography is helpful when there are ambiguous examination findings (including apparent masses) and is useful in men having testes located in the upper scrotum, a small scrotal sac, or other anatomy that prevents physical examination. Consider it for men presenting with infertility and risk factors for testicular cancer, such as cryptorchidism or a previous testicular neoplasm, but not routinely as a screening.

Specialized Clinical Tests on Semen and Sperm

When a semen analyses has failed to predict fertility accurately, specialized clinical tests should be reserved for circumstances where results would clearly help to guide treatment.

Quantification of Leukocytes in Semen

Men with true pyospermia (>1 million leukocytes/mL) should be evaluated to rule out genital tract infection or inflammation.

Tests for Antisperm Antibodies

Antisperm antibodies are an unusual cause of male subfertility that are often managed with the use of intracytoplasmic sperm injection (ICSI), and do not require routine testing. One study suggested that detection of serum ASA correlates with the presence of spermatogenesis in men with azoospermia and can negate the need for diagnostic testicular biopsy to help determine whether obstruction is present.[24] Men with azoospermia and ASA are likely to have reproductive tract obstruction. Otherwise, routine testing for ASA is not indicated.

Sperm Viability Tests

The viability of sperm can be assessed by mixing fresh semen with a supravital dye, such as eosin Y or trypan blue, or by the hypoosmotic swelling (HOS) test.[25] Nonmotile sperms that are viable have intact cell membranes. In the HOS test, viable nonmotile sperm, which swell when incubated in a hypoosmotic solution, can be used successfully for ICSI.[26] Viable nonmotile sperm can also be identified by incubation in pentoxifylline and these develop motility after exposure to pentoxifylline.[27]

Sperm Deoxyribonucleic Acid Fragmentation Tests

For an embryo to grow, its deoxyribonucleic acid (DNA) integrity is important. The DNA integrity of sperm is maintained in part by the effect of disulfide cross-links between protamines that facilitate the compaction of chromatin in the nucleus. Intrinsic factors, such as protamine deficiency and mutations affecting DNA compaction, or extrinsic factors, such as heat, radiation, and gonadotoxins can negatively impact sperm DNA integrity. The term "DNA fragmentation" is the denatured or damaged sperm DNA that cannot be repaired. There are various clinical tests developed to measure sperm DNA fragmentation rates. Direct methods, such as the single-cell gel electrophoresis assay (Comet) and terminal deoxynucleotidyl transferase-mediated dUTP nick-end labeling (TUNEL) assays analyze the number of breaks in the DNA. Indirect tests, such as the sperm chromatin structure assay (SCSA), define abnormal chromatin structure as an increased susceptibility of sperm DNA to acid-induced denaturation in situ.[28] Threshold values used to define an abnormal test are ≥25–27% for the SCSA[29] and ≥36% for TUNEL assays.[30]

Infertile men have higher sperm DNA damage and this may lead to poor reproductive performance such as spontaneous recurrent miscarriage. However, existing data regarding the relationship between abnormal DNA integrity and reproductive outcomes are too sparse to routinely recommend these tests, but the effect of abnormal sperm DNA fragmentation on the success rates of intrauterine insemination (IUI) or in vitro fertilization (IVF) and ICSI may be clinically informative.[31] Varicocele repair and use of antioxidants may improve sperm DNA integrity. Albeit, no treatment for abnormal DNA integrity has been proven to have clinical value. In men with high DNA fragmentation, sperm retrieved from the testes often have better sperm DNA quality.[32] The routine use of DNA integrity tests in the clinical evaluation of male-factor infertility is not established, because the prognostic clinical value of DNA integrity testing may not affect the treatment of couples.[33]

Less Commonly Used Specialized Tests

- Sperm penetration assays
- Measurements of sperm creatine kinase and reactive oxygen species (ROS)
- Genetic screening

Infertility can be due to genetic abnormalities due to sperm production or sperm transport being affected. Men with nonobstructive azoospermia or severe oligozoospermia with a sperm count <5 million/mL are known to be at an increased risk for having a genetic abnormality when compared to men with normal sperm parameters.[34] The most common genetic abnormalities found are numeric and structural chromosomal aberrations that impair testicular function and Y-chromosome microdeletions that are associated with isolated defects in spermatogenesis. In addition, most men with CBAVD can be presumed to have a cystic fibrosis transmembrane conductance regulator *(CFTR)* gene mutation. Efforts should be made to identify genetic causes for infertility, when indicated.

Cystic Fibrosis Gene Mutations

There is a strong association between CBAVD and *CFTR* gene mutations, which is located on chromosome 7.[35] Most men with clinical cystic fibrosis exhibit CBAVD. Additionally, up to 80% of men with CBAVD may have documented mutations of the *CFTR* gene. Inability to detect a *CFTR* abnormality in men with CBAVD does not exclude the presence of a mutation that cannot be identified with the methods presently available. Therefore, most men with CBAVD should be assumed to have a *CFTR* gene mutation unless they have renal anomalies. It is important to test the female partner of an affected man to determine the risk of conceiving a child affected with cystic fibrosis. Even if the female partner is negative with the currently available testing, the couple does remains at some risk because some of the uncommon mutations may be missed unless the entire gene is sequenced.

The prevalence of *CFTR* mutations is also increased among men with azoospermia related to congenital bilateral obstruction of the epididymides and those with unilateral vasa agenesis. Consequently, genetic evaluation must be considered for those having either of those abnormalities. Some men present with either unilateral or bilateral vasal agenesis and unilateral renal agenesis and have the mesonephric duct abnormalities associated with hereditary renal adysplasia. This is inherited in an autosomal dominant fashion with incomplete penetrance and variable expression. These patients have no CFTR mutations and require genetic counseling before IVF.[36,37] Karyotypic chromosomal abnormalities.

Chromosomal abnormalities are increasingly seen in infertile men and inversely proportional to sperm count; with prevalence of 10-15% in azoospermic men,[38] ~5% in severe oligozoospermia (<5 million/mL), and <1% in men with normal sperm concentrations.[39] The other common anomaly is sex chromosomal aneuploidy (Klinefelter syndrome; 47,XXY) which accounts for about two-thirds of all chromosomal abnormalities observed in infertile men.[40] Structural autosomal abnormalities, such as inversions and balanced translocations, are also seen higher in infertile men than others.[41] Rare azoospermic men may be found to have the 46,XX disorder of sexual development resulting from translocation of sex-determining region Y (SRY) to one of their X chromosomes. Couples with the male partner having a gross karyotypic abnormality are at increased risk for miscarriages and for conceiving children with chromosomal and congenital defects. Therefore, before using their sperm to perform ICSI, men with nonobstructive azoospermia or severe oligozoospermia should be evaluated with a high-resolution karyotype.

Y-chromosome Microdeletions

Microdeletions of regions of the Y chromosome that are clinically relevant have been found in 7% of infertile men with severely impaired spermatogenesis. They are found in 2% of normal men. However, this percentage of Y chromosome microdeletions increases to 16% in men with azoospermia or severe oligozoospermia.[42] Such microdeletions can be identified with the use of polymerase chain reaction techniques to analyze sequence-tagged sites that have been mapped along the full length of the Y chromosome. They are too small to be detected by standard karyotyping.

Most deletions causing azoospermia or oligozoospermia occur in regions of the long arm of the Y chromosome (Yq11) known as the azoospermia factor (AZF) regions, designated as AZFa (proximal), AZFb (central), and AZFc (distal). AZFa, b and c, and possibly other regions of the Y chromosome, contain multiple genes necessary for spermatogenesis. The DAZ (deleted in azoospermia) gene, for example, encodes a transcription factor usually present in men with normal fertility, is located in the AZFc region.

The exact location of the deletion along the Y chromosome has an influence on its effect on spermatogenesis. A microdeletion in the AZFc region of the Y chromosome may lead to severe oligozoospermia. Others with AZFc region deletions are azoospermic but may still produce sufficient numbers of sperm, with a favorable result in testicular sperm extraction. The AZFc deletion does not adversely affect the results of ICSI and sperm production in such men appears to be stable over time.[43] But, deletions involving the entire AZFb and AZFa region predict an unfavorable prognosis for sperm retrieval.[44,45]

The Y-chromosome microdeletions are inheritable by the male offspring who, therefore, may also be infertile.[46] A microdeletion of the Y chromosome is not known to be associated with other health problems, but few data suggests that some men with Y-chromosome microdeletions had abnormalities of the pseudoautosomal regions (PARs) of the Y chromosome. Most of these men had some sperm production, 16% of men had genetic aberrations of the short-stature-homeo-box *(SHOX)* gene, the most known gene in PAR1. *SHOX* gene abnormalities are also associated with mental retardation, short stature and arm and wrist deformities.[47] More importantly, a negative Y-chromosome microdeletion test result does not exclude a genetic abnormality, because there may be other, gene sequences on the Y or other chromosomes that also might be required for normal spermatogenesis, that are not currently known. Conversely, some Y-chromosome microdeletions are rarely found in men who are fertile or subfertile.[48] So before performing ICSI with their sperm, Y-chromosome analysis should be offered to men who have nonobstructive azoospermia or severe oligozoospermia.

SPERM CHROMOSOME ANEUPLOIDY

Sperm DNA aneuploidy can be studied by fluorescent in situ hybridization technology.[49] One study has reported that up to 6% of men presenting with infertility may have a normal karyotype but have an increased frequency of meiotic alterations detectable in their sperm DNA.[50] Men with the highest risk of sperm aneuploidy are those with karyotypic abnormalities, severely abnormal sperm morphology, and nonobstructive azoospermia.[49] Couples that present with recurrent IVF failure and recurrent pregnancy loss may benefit from sperm aneuploidy testing.[51,52] Currently, limitations to the routine use of this technology are cost, inability to screen the actual sperm used in ICSI, and difficulty of assigning a risk assessment to couples based on the test results that is meaningful.[53]

UNEXPLAINED INFERTILITY

Unexplained infertility may be evident in as many as 30% of infertile couples.[54] When all the tests results are normal and these couples should have evidence of ovulation, tubal patency, and a normal semen analysis.[54] Endometrial biopsy should be performed only in women with suspected chronic endometritis or neoplasia.

Management of Infertility

After evaluation, when the cause of infertility is known, the management depends on male or female factor infertility **(Flowcharts 3 to 6)**.

Flowchart 3: Female factor infertility management.

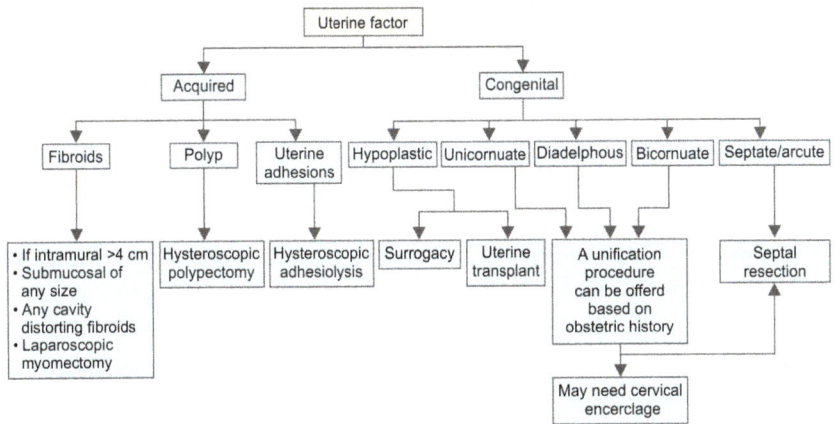

(IUI: intrauterine insemination; IVF: in vitro fertilization; ICSI: intracytoplasmic sperm injection)

Flowchart 4: Female factor infertility management: Uterine factor.

Flowchart 5: Female factor infertility management: Tubal factor.

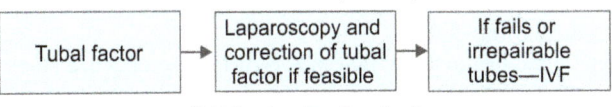

(IVF: in vitro fertilization)

Flowchart 6: Male factor infertility management.

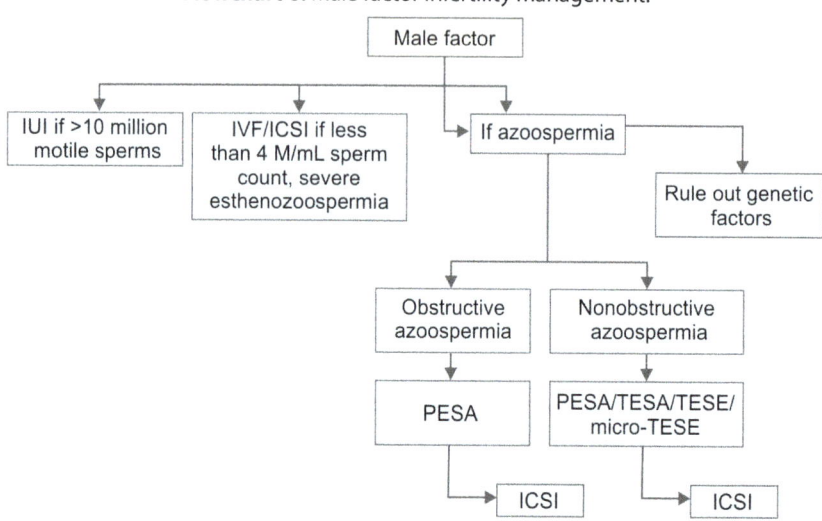

(TESA: testicular sperm aspiration; TESE: testicular sperm extraction; PESA: percutaneous epididymal sperm aspiration; IUI: intrauterine insemination; IVF: in vitro fertilization; ICSI: intracytoplasmic sperm injection)

SUMMARY

Men with nonobstructive azoospermia or severe oligozoospermia (<5 million/mL) are at increased risk for having a genetic abnormality and should surely be offered karyotype and Y-chromosome analysis before ICSI is performed with their sperm. Genetic counseling should be offered when a genetic abnormality is suspected in either the female or the male partner.

REFERENCES

1. Cates W, Farley TM, Rowe PJ. Worldwide patterns of infertility: is Africa different? Lancet. 1985;2(8455):596-8.
2. Poppe K, Velkeniers B. Thyroid and infertility. Verh K Acad Geneeskd Belg. 2002;64(6):389-99.
3. Razzak AH, Wais SA. The infertile couple: A cohort study in Duhok, Iraq. East Mediterr Health J. 2002;8(2-3):234-8.
4. Ikechebelu JI, Adinma JIB, Orie EF, Ikegwuonu SO. High prevalence of male infertility in Southeastern Nigeria. J Obstet Gynecol. 2003;23(6):657-9.
5. Tolstrup JS, Kjaer SK, Holst C, Sharif H, Munk C, Osler M, et al. Alcohol use as predictor for infertility in a representative population of Danish women. Acta Obstet gynecol Scand. 2003;82(8):744-9.
6. Saleh RA, Agarwal A, Sharma RK, Nelson DR, Thomas AJ Jr. Effect of cigarette smoking on levels of seminal oxidative stress in infertile men: A prospective study. Fertil Steril. 2002;78(3):491-9.
7. Practice Committee of the American Society for Reproductive Medicine. Testing and interpreting measures of ovarian reserve: a committee opinion. Fertil Steril. 2015;103:e9-17.

8. Practice Committee of the American Society for Reproductive Medicine. Diagnostic evaluation of the infertile female: a committee opinion. Fertil Steril. 2015;103:e44-50.
9. Committee Opinion No. 691. American College of Obstetricians and Gynecologists. Obstet Gynecol. 2017;129:e41-e55.
10. D'Arpe S, Di Feliciantonio M, Candelieri M, Franceschetti S, Piccioni MG, Bastianelli C. Ovarian function during hormonal contraception assessed by endocrine and sonographic markers: a systematic review. Reprod Biomed Online. 2016;33:436-48.
11. Cooper TG, Noonan E, von Eckardstein S, Auger J, Baker HWG, Behre HM, et al. World Health Organization reference values for human semen characteristics. Hum Reprod Update. 2010;16(3):231-45.
12. Practice Committee of American Society for Reproductive Medicine. Diagnostic evaluation of the infertile female: a committee opinion. Fertil Steril. 2012;98(2):302-7.
13. Thonneau P, Marchand S, Tallec A, Ferial ML, Ducot B, Lansac J, et al. Incidence and main causes of infertility in a resident population (1,850,000) of three French regions (1988-1989). Hum Reprod. 1991;6(6):811-6.
14. National Collaborating Centre for Women's and Children's Health (UK). Fertility: assessment and treatment for people with fertility problems: (Clinical guideline no. CG156). London, United Kingdom: National Institute for Health and Clinical Excellence (NICE);2013: pp.1-63.
15. Anderson K, Norman RJ, Middleton P. Preconception lifestyle advice for people with subfertility. Cochrane Database Syst Rev. 2010;(4):CD008189.
16. American Urological Association Education and Research, Inc. The evaluation of the azoospermic male: AUA best practice statement. Linthicum, Md: American Urological Association, Inc.; 2010. p. 38.
17. Hofherr SE, Wiktor AE, Kipp BR, Dawson DB, Van Dyke DL. Clinical diagnostic testing for the cytogenetic and molecular causes of male infertility: the Mayo Clinic experience. J Assist Reprod Genet. 2011;28(11):1091-8.
18. Kamel RM. Management of the infertile couple: an evidence-based protocol. Reprod Biol Endocrinol. 2010;8:21.
19. Oei SG, Helmerhorst FM, Bloemenkamp KW, Hollants FA, Meerpoel DE, Keirse MJ. Effectiveness of the postcoital test: randomised controlled trial. BMJ. 1998;317(7157):502-5.
20. Kumanov P, Nandipati K, Tomova A, Agarwal A. Inhibin B is a better marker of spermatogenesis than other hormones in the evaluation of male factor infertility. Fertil Steril. 2006;86(2):332-8.
21. Mehta A, Jarow JP, Maples P, Sigman M. Defining the "normal" postejaculate urinalysis. J Androl. 2012;33:917-20.
22. Carter SS, Shinohara K, Lipshultz LI. Transrectal ultrasonography in disorders of the seminal vesicles and ejaculatory ducts. Urol Clin North Am. 1989;16:773-90.
23. Practice Committee of the American Society for Reproductive Medicine. Report on varicocele and infertility. Fertil Steril. 2014;102:1556-60.
24. Lee R, Goldstein M, Ullery BW, Ehrlich J, Soares M, Razzano RA, et al. Value of serum antisperm antibodies in diagnosing obstructive azoospermia. J Urol. 2009;181:264-9.
25. World Health Organization. (2010). WHO laboratory manual for the examination and processing of human semen. [online] Available from http://whqlibdoc.who.int/publications/2010/9789241547789_eng.pdf. [Last accessed June, 2022].
26. Liu J, Tsai YL, Katz E, Compton G, Garcia JE, Baramki TA. High fertilization rate obtained after intracytoplasmic sperm injection with 100% nonmotile spermatozoa selected by using a simple modified hypo-osmotic swelling test. Fertil Steril. 1997;68:373-5.
27. de Mendoza MV, Gonzalez-Utor AL, Cruz N, Gutierrez P, Cascales F, Sillero JM. In situ use of pentoxifylline to assess sperm vitality in intracytoplasmic sperm injection for treatment of patients with total lack of sperm movement. Fertil Steril. 2000;74(1):176-7.

28. Evenson DP, Jost LK, Marshall D, Zinaman MJ, Clegg E, Purvis K, et al. Utility of the sperm chromatin structure assay as a diagnostic and prognostic tool in the human fertility clinic. Hum Reprod. 1999;14:1039-49.
29. Larson-Cook KL, Brannian JD, Hansen KA, Kasperson KM, Aamold ET, Evenson DP. Relationship between the outcomes of assisted reproductive techniques and sperm DNA fragmentation as measured by the sperm chromatin structure assay. Fertil Steril. 2003;80:895-902.
30. Henkel R, Hajimohammad M, Stalf T, Hoogendijk C, Mehnert C, Menkveld R, et al. Influence of deoxyribonucleic acid damage on fertilization and pregnancy. Fertil Steril. 2004;81(4):965-72.
31. Collins JA, Barnhart KT, Schlegel PN, Do sperm DNA integrity tests predict pregnancy with in vitro fertilization? Fertil Steril. 2008;89:823-31.
32. Greco E, Scarselli F, Iacobelli M, Rienzi L, Ubaldi F, Ferrero S, et al. Efficient treatment of infertility due to sperm DNA damage by ICSI with testicular spermatozoa. Hum Reprod. 2005;20:226-30.
33. Practice Committee of the American Society for Reproductive Medicine. The clinical utility of sperm DNA integrity testing: a guideline. Fertil Steril. 2013;99(3):673-7.
34. Foresta C, Garolla A, Bartoloni L, Bettella A, Ferlin A. Genetic abnormalities among severely oligospermic men who are candidates for intracytoplasmic sperm injection. J Clin Endocrinol Metab. 2005;90(1):152-6.
35. Anguiano A, Oates RD, Amos JA, Dean M, Gerrard B, Stewart C, et al. Congenital bilateral absence of the vas deferens. A primarily genital form of cystic fibrosis. JAMA. 1992;267(13):1794-7.
36. McCallum T, Milunsky J, Munarriz R, Carson R, Sadeghi-Nejad H, Oates R. Unilateral renal agenesis associated with congenital bilateral absence of the vas deferens: phenotypic findings and genetic considerations. Hum Reprod. 2001;16(2):282-8.
37. McPherson E, Carey J, Kramer A, Hall JG, Pauli RM, Schimke RN, et al. Dominantly inherited renal adysplasia. Am J Med Genet. 1987;26(4):863-72.
38. van Assche E, Bonduelle M, Tournaye H, Joris H, Verheyen G, Devroey P, et al. Cytogenetics of infertile men. Hum Reprod. 1996;11:1-25.
39. Ravel C, Berthaut I, Bresson JL, Siffroi JP, Genetics Commission of the French Federation of CECOS. Prevalence of chromosomal abnormalities in phenotypically normal and fertile adult males: large-scale survey of over 10,000 sperm donor karyotypes. Hum Reprod. 2006;21(6):1484-9.
40. de Braekeleer M, Dao TN. Cytogenetic studies in male infertility: a review. Hum Reprod. 1991;6:245-50.
41. Debiec-Rychter M, Jakubowski L, Truszczak B, Moruzgala T, Kaluzewski B. Two familial 9;17 translocations with variable effect on male carriers' fertility. Fertil Steril. 1992;57:933-5.
42. Pryor JL, Kent-First M, Muallem A, Van Bergen AH, Nolten WE, Meisner L, et al. Microdeletions in the Y chromosome of infertile men. N Engl J Med. 1997;336:534-9.
43. Oates RD, Silber S, Brown LG, Page DC. Clinical characterization of 42 oligospermic or azoospermic men with microdeletion of the AZFc region of the Y chromosome, and of 18 children conceived via ICSI. Hum Reprod. 2002;7:2813-24.
44. Brandell RA, Mielnik A, Liotta D, Ye Z, Veeck LL, Palermo GD, et al. AZFb deletions predict the absence of spermatozoa with testicular sperm extraction: preliminary report of a prognostic genetic test. Hum Reprod. 1998;13(1O):2812-15.
45. Krausz C, Quintana-Murci L, McElreavey K. Prognostic value of Y deletion analysis: what is the clinical prognostic value of Y chromosome microdeletion analysis? Hum Reprod. 2000;15(7):1431-4.
46. Kent-First MG, Kol S, Muallem A, Ofir R, Manor D, Blazer S, et al. The incidence and possible relevance of Y-linked microdeletions in babies born after intracytoplasmic sperm injection and their infertile fathers. Mol Hum Reprod. 1996;2(12):943-50.

47. Jorgez CJ, Weedin JW, Sahin A, Tannour-Louet M. Han S, Bournat JC, et al. Aberrations in pseudoautosomal regions (PARs) found in infertile men with Y-chromosome microdeletions. J Clin Endocrinol Metab. 2011;96(94):E674-E9.
48. Kent-First M, Muallem A, Shultz J, Pryor J, Roberts K, Nolten W, et al. Defining regions of the Y-chromosome responsible for male infertility and identification of a fourth AZF region (AZFd) by Y-chromosome microdeletion detection. Mol Reprod Dev. 1999;53(1):27-41.
49. Carrell DT. The clinical implementation of sperm chromosome aneuploidy testing: pitfalls and promises. J Androl. 2008;29:124-33.
50. Egozcue S, Blanco J, Vendrell JM, Garcia F, Veiga A, Aran B, et al. Human male infertility: chromosome anomalies, meiotic disorders, abnormal spermatozoa and recurrent abortion. Hum Reprod Update. 2000;6(1):93-105.
51. Carrell DT, Wilcox AL, Lowy L, Peterson CM, Jones KP, Erickson L, et al. Elevated sperm chromosome aneuploidy and apoptosis in patients with unexplained recurrent pregnancy loss. Obstet Gynecol. 2003;101(6):1229-35.
52. Petit FM, Frydman N, Benkhalifa M, Le Du A, Aboura A, Fanchin R, et al. Could sperm aneuploidy rate determination be used as a predictive test before intracytoplasmic sperm injection? J Androl. 2005;26:235-41.
53. Tempest HG, Martin RH. Cytogenetic risks in chromosomally normal infertile men. Curr Opin Obstet Gynecol. 2009;21(3):223-7.
54. Practice Committee of the American Society for Reproductive Medicine. Effectiveness and treatment for unexplained infertility. Fertil Steril. 2006;86(5 Suppl 1):S111-4.

CHAPTER 18

Intrauterine Insemination: Indications and Protocol

Unnati Mamtora, Parzan Mistry

INTRODUCTION

Intrauterine insemination (IUI) is the procedure in which the highly processed sperm's sample is introduced high up in the cavity of the uterus by using husband semen sample or the donor semen sample in the periovulatory period with the aim to achieve better fertilization by bringing the sperm closer to the egg. It is one of the most common first-line management in the treatment of infertility.

INDICATIONS OF INTRAUTERINE INSEMINATION

- Unexplained infertility
- Minimal to mild endometriosis
- Mild male factor infertility
- Erectile dysfunction/ejaculatory dysfunction
- Vaginismus
- Cervical factor
- Serodiscordant couples
- Inability to have intercourse
- Hypospadias
- Donor insemination
- Ovulatory dysfunction
- Unilateral tubal block.

FACTORS INFLUENCING IUI SUCCESS RATES

- Age of wife and husband
- Indications of IUI
- Semen parameters
- Number of mature follicles.

PREREQUISITE FOR INTRAUTERINE INSEMINATION

- At least one fallopian tube should be patent with good tube ovarian relationship.

- A good access to uterine cavity with easy negotiation through the cervical canal
- Post wash semen sample should be at least 5 million/mL.

PROTOCOL FOR INTRAUTERINE INSEMINATION

- The process of IUI can be done in a natural cycle with follicular monitoring or with the addition of ovulation induction drugs in combination with follicular monitoring.
- When used in combination with the ovulation induction drugs, intrauterine insemination helps achieve higher pregnancy rates (10–15%) as compared to planned relation alone.[1-3]

Drugs used in Ovulation Induction

- Oral ovulogens
- Only gonadotropin
- Combined—oral ovulogens and gonadotropins.

Clomiphene Citrate/Letrozole Only

- Clomiphene citrate (CC) 100 mg once a day or Letrozole 2.5 mg once/twice a day from day 2 to day 6 **(Table 1 and Fig. 1)**
- Serial follicular monitoring from day 8 onward
- Injection human chorionic gonadotropin (hCG) 5,000/10,000 IU IM when leading follicle is 18–20 mm and endometrial thickness is ≥7–9 mm
- IUI > 36–40 hours of hCG administration
- Luteal support with oral or micronized vaginal progesterone.

TABLE 1: Clomiphene citrate and letrozole.

Clomiphene citrate	Letrozole
Normoresponders and poor responders preferably	Preferred in PCOS patients as a first drug of choice
Mechanism of action: Anti-estrogenic (two isomers—enclomiphene and zuclomiphene) Both central and peripheral action (endocervix and cervical mucus)	Aromatase inhibitor
Multifollicular growth	Monofollicular growth
Dose: 100 mg once a day for 5 days	2.5 mg once/twice a day for 5 days
Side effects: Antiestrogenic effect (thin endometrium)	No antiestrogenic effects
Associated with reduced blood flow	Blood flow is increased hence associated with better implantation rates
(PCOS: polycystic ovary syndrome)	

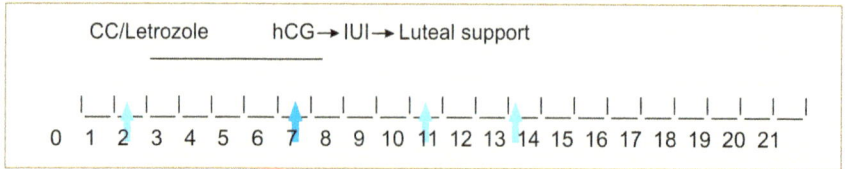

Fig. 1: Clomiphene citrate (CC)/Letrozole dose protocol.

Letrozole Step-up Protocol

Step-up protocol consists of one, two, three, and four tablets of letrozole (2.5 mg) daily on menstrual cycle days 2, 3, 4, and 5. Higher pregnancy rates were reported in a study by using this protocol in comparison to clomiphene citrate.[4] The step-up letrozole protocol is associated with multifollicular development due to prolonged suppression of estrogen levels. More randomized controlled trials are required.

Extended letrozole therapy: Extended letrozole for 10 days instead of 5 days in previous clomiphene-resistant polycystic ovary syndrome (PCOS) patients, achieved better ovulation rates though statistically insignificant. The pregnancy rates were reported to be higher in the extended protocol due to increase in the follicle-stimulating hormone (FSH) window.[5]

Clomiphene Resistance and Clomiphene Failure

CC resistance: Patients who fail to ovulate after induction with 150 mg of CC for three consecutive cycles are classified as CC resistant patients.

CC failure: Patients who ovulate but fail to achieve pregnancy or pregnancy ends in miscarriage are classified as CC failure patients.

As per guidelines of Royal College of Obstetricians and Gynaecologists (RCOG) and American College of Obstetricians and Gynecologists (ACOG), clomiphene citrate should be used for a maximum of 12 months in lifetime and maximum of 6 months continuously.

Follicular monitoring is done from day 2 of periods preferably to rule out cyst from previous cycle, to see the antral follicle count in both the ovaries.

Ovulation induction drugs are then started and patient is called for monitoring from day 8 onward gain on alternate days till the follicle is around 18–20 mm in size.

This is then followed by **trigger injection (hCG 5,000 units intramuscular or injection ovitrelle 250 units subcutaneously) followed by IUI**.

TIMING OF INTRAUTERINE INSEMINATION

Intrauterine insemination is done 36–40 hours after trigger injection (after the follicular rupture) or 24 hours after the LH surge.

Serum hCG levels are assessed 14 days after trigger injection or LH surge detection, and ultrasonography confirmation of pregnancy is obtained in all pregnant patients. Clinical pregnancy is defined as the presence of an intrauterine gestation with fetal cardiac activity.

ROLE OF DOUBLE INTRAUTERINE INSEMINATION

In double insemination, first insemination is done at 12–24 hours and second one is done at 36 hours.

Studies in the past have not shown any additional benefit of double IUI over single IUI.[6-9]

Frozen thawed donor sample cycles: However, some studies have demonstrated higher pregnancy rates with double IUI using frozen thawed donor samples.[10,11]

GONADOTROPINS AND INTRAUTERINE INSEMINATION

Gonadotropins are highly effective for ovulation induction. Gonadotropins may be used in conjunction with the ovulogens on alternate days or sequentially. But there is always an increased risk of multiple gestation and increase in the overall cost of the treatment. Usage of gonadotropins in IUI cycles either alone or in addition to the ovulogens, in cases of unexplained infertility, increased the live birth rates only when the gonadotropins were used in higher doses with the risk of increase in number of multiple gestations as well. It was reported in the systemic review that the benefits were minimal without the risk for cancellation of cycle (>3 follicles) with increased multiple gestation.[12]

The Fast Track and Standard Treatment (FASTT) trial also concluded that gonadotropin use was not an ideal intermediate step between oral OS medication and IUI or IVF. The other drawback reported in the studies was increased cost and time to pregnancy in unsuccessful IUI treatments.[13]

Addition of antagonist injection to prevent premature luteinization and avoid rupture of the growing follicle was found to demonstrate good pregnancy rates in a study in PCOS patients and has suggested more randomized systemic reviews may be done to evaluate further.[14,15]

Progesterone support in the luteal phase is beneficial to the patients undergoing ovulation induction with gonadotropins and IUI.[16]

Indications of gonadotropin use:
- In WHO class 1 patients, human menopausal gonadotropin (hMG) is used as a substitution therapy
- In cases of clomiphene resistance or clomiphene failure.

Gonadotropin Therapy

Conventional Therapy
- Baseline ultrasonography (USG) to rule out ovarian cyst
- *Day 3:* Luteinizing hormone (LH)/FSH/estradiol (E2)

- In patient of <35 years, starting dose of 75/150 mIU/mL (from day 2 to 3) onward; if patient >35 years or poor respondent, starting dose of 150/225 mIU/mL (from 2 to 3 day onward) **(Fig. 2)**
- *Serial USG:* Day 8 onward
- *Serum E2 (Day 8/9):* If serum E2 >200 pg/mL and follicle >10 mm, same dose should be given; if serum E2 <200 pg/mL and number of follicles <10 mm, dose increased by 75 IU/day
- Injection hCG is given when leading follicle ≥16–18 mm.

Step-up regime:
- Starting dose of 75 units given for 7 days
- If day 8 serum E2 >200 pg/mL and follicle >10 mm, dose maintained
- If not, dose increased by 37.5 or 75 IU
- hCG—leading follicle ≥18 mm or endometrium ≥7 mm.

Step-down protocol: Starting with initial higher dose of gonadotropin and decreasing the dose stepwise once follicle of 10 mm is achieved on transvaginal sonography **(Fig. 3)**.

Combination protocol:
- Combination of oral ovulogens with gonadotropins: Gonadotropins may be added on alternate days or daily or sequentially along with oral ovulogens.

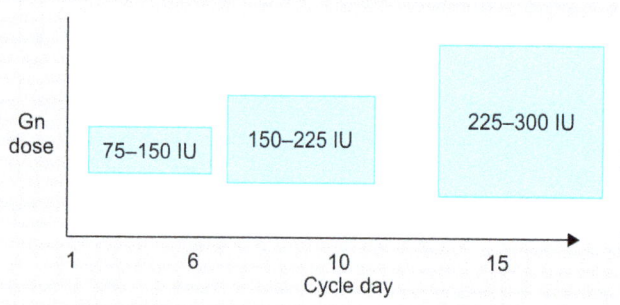

Fig. 2: Conventional therapy. (Gn: gonadotropin)

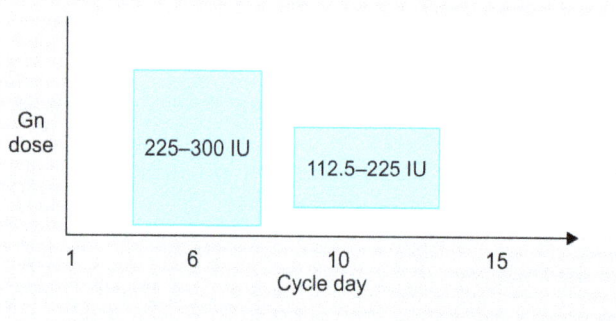

Fig. 3: Step-down protocol. (Gn: gonadotropin)

ADJUVANTS IN OVULATION INDUCTION

Adjuvant therapy may be defined as the usage of medicines, in addition to the ovulation inducing agents, to receive better ovarian response and results.

Dexamethasone: Dexamethasone therapy may be useful in CC failure cases associated with hyperandrogenemia (with high DHEA-S levels). It is also documented to be helpful in CC failure cases with normal levels of DHEA-S. It is given in the dose of 0.25–5 mg daily at bedtime from Day 1 of stimulation protocol, till day 11.

Metformin: It is useful as an adjuvant especially in cases of PCOS women with mild to moderate obesity, insulin resistance and mild hyperandrogenemia with hirsutism. Metformin is given in doses of 500–2,000 mg in PCOS patients for 3–6 months increases the live birth rates.

Myoinositol: It is used as an alternative to metformin in the PCOS patients. It potentiates the action of insulin. In obese PCOS patients, myoinositol and D-chiroinositol should be used in the ratio of 40:1. Dose of myoinositol is 2,000–4,000 mg once daily before breakfast for PCOS women for 3–6 months. At least 3 months are required for proper insulin sensitivity.

Thyroxine: Levothyroxine is useful in patients with subclinical hypothyroidism which present with elevated levels of serum thyroid-stimulating hormone (TSH: >2.5 mIU/mL). Elevated serum TSH levels are associated with increased serum sex hormone-binding globulin (SHBG) levels.

Bromocriptine and cabergoline: This is useful in patients with hyperprolactinemia without any space occupying lesion in the hypothalamus.

REFERENCES

1. Veltman-Verhulst SM, Cohlen BJ, Hughes E, Heineman MJ. Intra-uterine insemination for unexplained subfertility. Cochrane Database Syst Rev. 2012:CD001838.
2. Cohlen BJ, Vandekerckhove P, te Velde ER, Habbema JD. Timed intercourse versus intra-uterine insemination with or without ovarian hyperstimulation for subfertility in men. Cochrane Database Syst Rev. 2000:CD000360.
3. Goverde AJ, McDonnell J, Vermeiden JP, Schats R, Rutten FF, Schoemaker J. Intrauterine insemination or in-vitro fertilisation in idiopathic subfertility and male subfertility: a randomised trial and cost-effectiveness analysis. Lancet. 2000;355:13-8.
4. Mitwally MF, Said T, Galal A, Chan S, Cohen M, Casper RF, et al. Reproductive Medicine and Fertility Center of Colorado and New Mexico; Toronto Center for Advanced Reproductive Technology, Toronto, Canada. Letrozole step-up protocol: a successful superovulation protocol. Fertil Steril; 2008. pp. s23-24.
5. Badawy A, Mosbah A, Tharwat A, Eid M. Extended letrozole therapy for ovulation induction in clomiphene-resistant women with polycystic ovary syndrome: a novel protocol. Fertil Steril. 2009;92(1):236-9.
6. Randall GW, Gantt PA. Double vs. single intrauterine insemination per cycle: use in gonadotropin cycles and in diagnostic categories of ovulatory dysfunction and male factor infertility. J Reprod Med. 2008;53:196-202.

7. Zavos A, Daponte A, Garas A, Verykouki C, Papanikolaou E, Anifandis G, et al. Double versus single homologous intrauterine insemination for male factor infertility: a systematic review and meta-analysis. Asian J Androl. 2013;15:533-8.
8. Polyzos NP, Tzioras S, Mauri D, Tatsioni A. Double versus single intrauterine insemination for unexplained infertility: a meta-analysis of randomized trials. Fertil Steril. 2010;94:1261-6.
9. Cantineau AE, Heineman MJ, Cohlen BJ. Single versus double intrauterine insemination in stimulated cycles for subfertile couples: a systematic review based on a Cochrane review. Hum Reprod. 2003;18:941-6.
10. Matilsky M, Geslevich Y, Ben-Ami M, Ben-Shlomo I, Weiner-Megnagi T, Shalev E. Two-day IUI treatment cycles are more successful than one-day IUI cycles when using frozen-thawed donor sperm. J Androl. 1998;19:603-7.
11. Chavkin DE, Molinaro TA, Roe AH, Sammel MD, Dokras A. Donor sperm insemination cycles: are two inseminations better than one? J Androl. 2012;33:375-80.
12. Zolton JR, Lindner PG, Terry N, DeCherney AH, Hill MJ. Gonadotropins versus oral ovarian stimulation agents for unexplained infertility: a systematic review and meta-analysis. Fertil Steril; 2020. pp. 417-25.
13. Reindollar RH, Regan MM, Neumann PJ, Levine BS, Thornton KL, Alper MM, et al. A randomized clinical trial to evaluate optimal treatment for unexplained infertility: the Fast Track and Standard Treatment (FASTT) trial. Fertil Steril. 2010;94:888-99.
14. Winkler N, Plosker SM. Outcome of gonadotropin superovulation/intrauterine insemination (SO-IUI) using 3 mg cetrorelix acetate. Women and Infants Hospital, Providence, RI. Fertil Steril. 2004;07:370.
15. Beydoun SH, Bocca S, Pultz B, Oehninger S. Jones Institute for Reproductive Medicine, Eastern Virginia Medical School, Norfolk, VA. Randomized Controlled Trial Evaluating The Effect of a GnRH-Antagonist In Women With PCOS Undergoing Ovulation Induction With Gonadotropins And Intrauterine Insemination (IUI). Fertil Steril. 2009;3:92.
16. Green KA, Zolton JR, Schermerhorn SM, Lewis TD, Healy MW, Terry N, et al. Progesterone luteal support after ovulation induction and intrauterine insemination: an updated systematic review and meta-analysis. Fertil Steril. 2017;107(4):924-33.e5.

19. Ovulation Induction

Parag Hitnalikar, Anil Chittake, Rahul Patil

INTRODUCTION

Disorders of ovulation accounts for almost 20% of the causes for subfertility.[1] Diagnosing the cause of anovulation and classifying it is the first step toward making an appropriate treatment plan for the patient. In all patients having disorders of ovulation, the ultimate aim should be development of single follicle and subsequent ovulation to assist her in conception. Various treatment modalities including lifestyle modifications, pharmacological agents and surgical methods are available. The choice of treatment depends upon diagnosis, response to treatment and counseling of patient regarding treatment modality and its probable outcome. The World Health Organization (WHO) classification of anovulation is given in **Table 1**.

Apart from above classification, hyperprolactinemia can be considered separately as it has distinct characteristics and specific treatment options.

HYPERPROLACTINEMIA

Hyperprolactinemia is found in 15% of women with anovulation and in 75% of women with anovulation and galactorrhea.[2] It interferes with normal pulsatile secretion of gonadotropin releasing hormone (GnRH). It can be caused by prolactin producing adenoma, pituitary tumor, and hypothyroidism.

Treatment (Flowchart 1)

- Asymptomatic patients only require observation and follow-up
- Symptomatic patients or those who want to conceive require treatment
- Bromocriptine is given in dose of 2.5–5 mg twice daily for 12 weeks
- Cabergoline is given in dose of 0.5 mg twice weekly for 12 weeks.

Lifestyle Modification

First line of treatment is lifestyle modifications, which is aimed at weight loss and overcoming insulin resistance (IR).

Weight loss can be achieved by any hypocaloric diet (*reduction of caloric intake by 500 kcal/day*) and physical activity for at least 60 min/day continued for 3 months.

TABLE 1: World Health Organization (WHO) classification of anovulation.

WHO category	Name	Features	Examples
I (5–10%)	Hypogonadotropic hypogonadism	Hypothalamic pituitary failure	• *Congenital:* Kallmann's syndrome • *Acquired:* Hyperprolactinemia, pituitary tumor, Cushing syndrome, acromegaly, iatrogenic (steroids, opiates), anorexia nervosa, Sheehan syndrome, cerebral radiotherapy
II (85%)	Normogonadotropic anovulation	Hypothalamic pituitary dysfunction	Polycystic ovarian syndrome (PCOS)
III (5–10%)	Hypergonadotropic hypogonadism	Premature ovarian failure	• *Genetic:* Turner syndrome, other X chromosome abnormalities (Xq deletions, trisomy X), Fragile X syndrome, familial autoimmune disorders • Infectious diseases • *Surgical:* Ovarian surgery, uterine artery embolization • *Toxic:* Chemo/radiotherapy

Flowchart 1: Diagnosis and treatment of hyperprolactinemia.

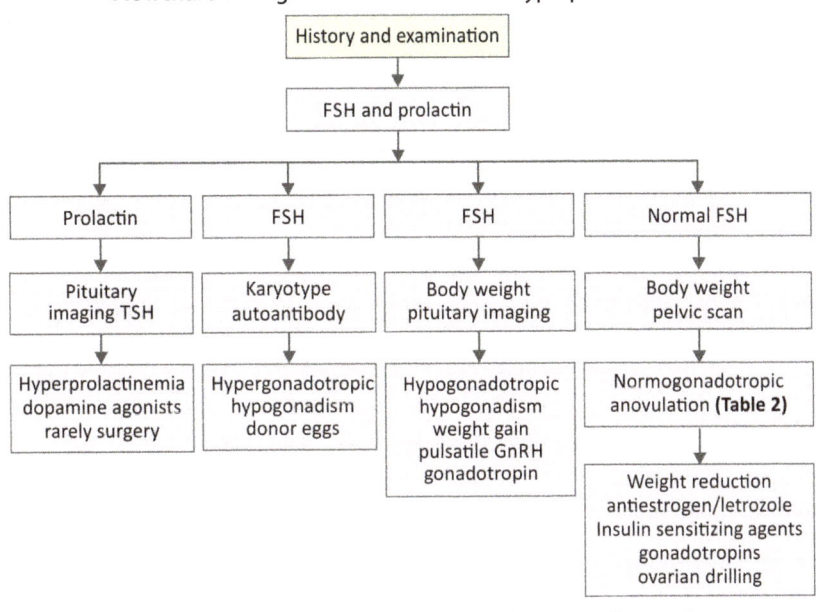

(FSH: follicle-stimulating hormone; GnRH: gonadotropin releasing hormone; TSH: thyroid-stimulating hormone)

TABLE 2: Treatment of normogonadotropic anovulation [polycystic ovarian syndrome (PCOS)].

Rotterdam Consensus Diagnostic Criteria for PCOS		
Oligo/amenorrhea (cycle length >35 days)	PCOS (2 out of 3) • Oligo- or amenorrhea • Hyperandrogenism (clinical/biochemical) • PCOM	After exclusion of: • Hyperprolactinemia • Nonclassic adrenal hyperplasia (NCAH) • Cushing syndrome • Androgen secreting tumor • Acromegaly
Hyperandrogenism (Hirsutism and/or FAI > 4.5)		
Polycystic ovarian morphology (PCOM: >12 follicles, 2–9 mm, in one ovary and/or ovarian volume >10 mL)		

(FAI: free androgen index)

Evidences also suggest Yoga as an effective adjuvant in management of polycystic ovarian syndrome (PCOS).

Orlistat, which affects intestinal absorption of fat and sibutramine, which is an appetite suppressant, can be used for weight loss. But these are not to be used as first-line drugs and used in obese patients who are not responding to lifestyle modifications.

Clomiphene Citrate

It is a selective estrogen receptor (ER) modulator and having estrogenic as well as antiestrogenic properties.

Mechanism of action: Reduction in negative feedback of endogenous estrogen by prolonged depletion of hypothalamic and pituitary ERs, which leads to release of GnRH from hypothalamus leading to increase in release of pituitary gonadotropins **(Fig. 1)**.

It is first-line treatment for ovulation induction in PCOS patients. Starting dose is 50 mg daily from day 2 or 3 of cycle for 5 days. Dose can be increased up to 150 mg in subsequent cycles if there is no response.[3] Doses >150 mg are not helpful and patient is labeled as CC resistant if no response with 150 mg dose.

If no pregnancy is achieved after 6 cycles, it is labeled as *CC failure.* In any case CC should not be given for >12 cycles in lifetime of a patient. CC is effective in achieving ovulation in 60–85% with a pregnancy rate of 30–50%.[4]

Side effects: Hot flushes (10%), abdominal distension, bloating or discomfort (5%), breast discomfort (2%), visual symptoms and headache (1.5%).

Insulin Sensitizing Agents

Insulin resistance is an important factor in pathogenesis of PCOS. Insulin sensitizers are given in an attempt to reduce IR and resume ovulation.

Metformin is the drug of choice in this category. Other drugs in this category are rosiglitazone and pioglitazone, which are used only in special circumstances.

Benefits: Increase in ovulatory frequency, reduction in body mass index (BMI), testosterone and insulin resistance.

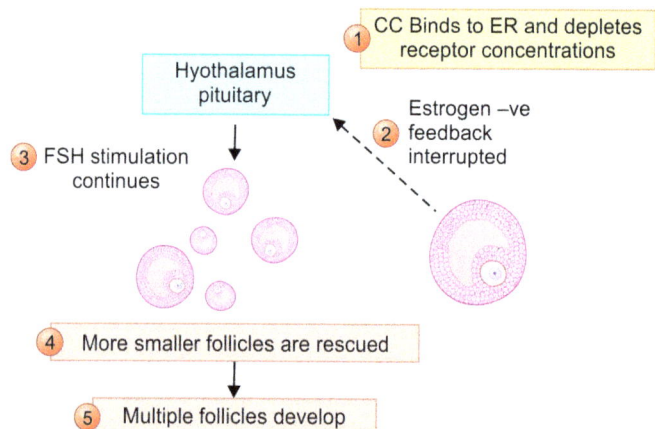

Fig. 1: Mechanism of action in clomiphene citrate (CC).

Indications for metformin use are:
- CC resistance
- CC failure
- As an adjuvant to CC
- PCOS patients with impaired glucose tolerance
- Patients at high risk for ovarian hyperstimulation syndrome (OHSS)
- Recommended dose of metformin is 1,500 mg to 2,550 mg.[5] It should be started with a dose of 500 mg daily and increase every 1–2 weeks till therapeutic dose is achieved.
- *Combination therapy with CC:* Significantly higher ovulation rate, increase in pregnancy and live birth rates.
- *Side effects and safety:* Diarrhea (53%), nausea and vomiting (25%), flatulence (12%), asthenia (9%), indigestion (7.1%), abdominal discomfort and headache.

Aromatase Inhibitors

Aromatase inhibitors (AIs) are the class of drugs, which inhibit estrogen biosynthesis thereby preventing the negative feedback by estrogen on pituitary gland. This increases follicle-stimulating hormone (FSH) secretion and hence folliculogenesis.

Benefits: Reduced dose required for ovarian stimulation, no antiestrogenic side effects on endometrium, high rates of monofollicular development.

Letrozole and anastrozole are the two AIs commonly used for ovulation induction **(Fig. 2)**.

Letrozole is widely studied as an ovulation induction drug. Many studies have found it to be superior or at least as effective as CC as far as ovulation rate, pregnancy rate, live birth rate and miscarriage rate is concerned.

Few studies have found letrozole having higher risk for congenital cardiac and bone anomalies. But at least two subsequent studies have found no increased risk for the same.[6] Although it is recommended that the patients should be informed about its risk before starting ovulation induction.

Letrozole could achieve 70–84% ovulation rate and 20–27% pregnancy rate in women who were CC resistant.[7]

Recommended dose for letrozole is 2.5–7.5 mg/day for 5 days starting from day 3 of cycle. This protocol achieves monofollicular growth.

Prolong dose protocol in which letrozole is started on day 3 with 2.5 mg dose and continued for 10 days was studied. It produced more number of follicles and higher pregnancy rate.[8]

Gonadotropins

Gonadotropins are used in patients with either CC resistance or CC failure. Various preparations such as human menopausal gonadotropins (hMG), urinary or recombinant FSH can be used with almost similar efficacy **(Fig. 3)**.

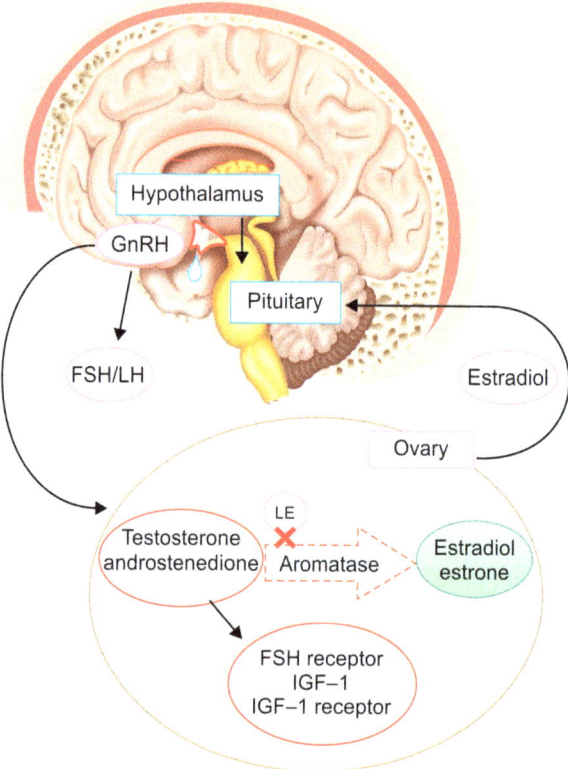

Fig. 2: Mechanisms of letrozole for ovarian induction.

All patients planned for gonadotropin use should be counseled regarding need for strict monitoring and high incidence of multifollicular development and OHSS along with high multiple pregnancy rate.

Regimens used for gonadotropins are discussed here.

Chronic step-up protocol: In this protocol, gonadotropins are started from day 2 or 3 of cycle with a dose of 37.5 or 50 IU/day depending upon BMI and antral follicle count. It is continued for 7–10 days and if no response, dose increased by 50% of starting or previous dose till follicle is 18 mm size when trigger is given **(Fig. 4)**.

Step-down protocol: This protocol is generally used in older women with low ovarian reserve. Starting dose is 150 IU daily till lead follicle is 10–12 mm and then dose is tapered to 112.5 and then 75 IU every 3–4 days till follicle is 18 mm **(Fig. 5)**.

Combined CC and gonadotropin protocol: CC is given in a dose of 100 mg daily for 5 days followed by gonadotropin 75–150 IU daily till lead follicle is 18 mm. This protocol is used in patients who have endogenous gonadotropins secretion and it reduces gonadotropin dose significantly **(Fig. 6)**.

Ovulation Induction

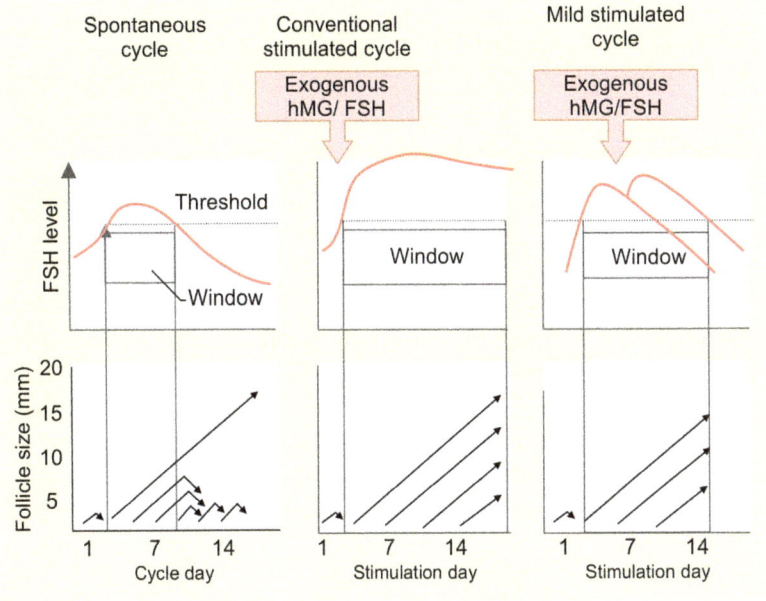

Fig. 3: Follicle-stimulating hormone (FSH) threshold and window of stimulation.

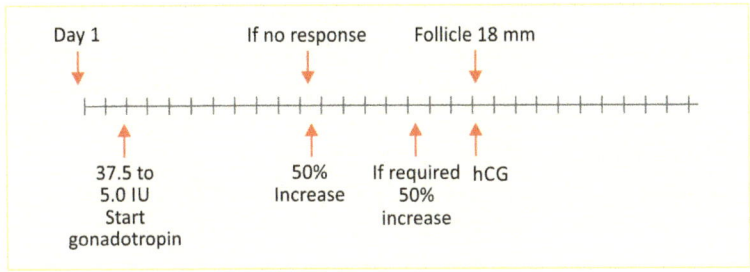

Fig. 4: Chronic step-up protocol.

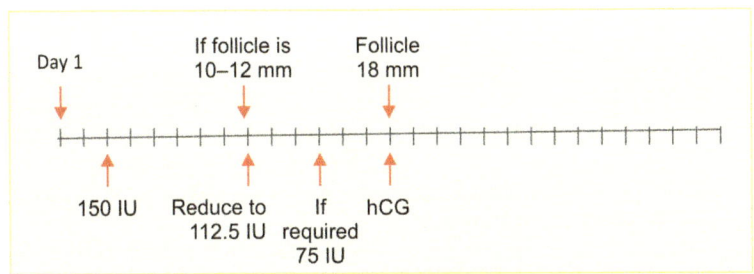

Fig. 5: Step-down protocol.

Gonadotropin-releasing Hormones

Gonadotropin-releasing hormone stimulation is used in women with hypogonadotropic hypogonadism where pituitary ovarian axis is intact but GnRH secretion is not there.

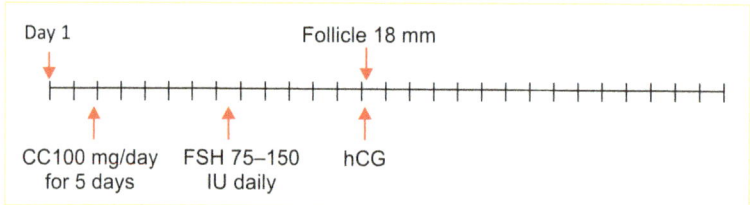

Fig. 6: Combined protocol.

Gonadotropin-releasing hormone is administered by subcutaneous or intravenous route with a small butterfly cannula and a battery operated pump. This system delivers GnRH at a dose 2.5–20 μg every 60–120 minutes interval.[9]

Treatment is monitored by regular estradiol measurement and pelvic ultrasound. Luteal phase has to be supported by continuing GnRH in pulsatile fashion or by administering exogenous human chorionic gonadotropin (hCG) injections.

Surgical Induction of Ovulation

Laparoscopic ovarian drilling (LOD) is a preferred surgical method for ovulation induction over wedge resection because of its less invasive nature and less chances of postoperative adhesion formation.

This method is more suitable for the women who are CC resistant or for whom frequent monitoring and follow-ups are difficult.

Most commonly four puncture method is used in which four electrocautery penetrations are made in ovarian capsule with a setting of 30 Watts for 5 seconds in each ovary.

Surgical methods work by reducing ovarian androgen producing tissue and reducing conversion of peripheral androgens to estrogen.

Ovulation rate of 52–67% can be achieved in CC-resistant cases with a pregnancy rate of 67%.[10]

REFERENCES

1. Hull MG, Glazener CM, Kelly NJ, Conway DI, Foster PA, Hinton RA, et al. Population study of causes, treatment, and outcome of infertility. BMJ. 1985;291:1693-7.
2. Greer ME, Moraczewski T, Rakoff JS. Prevalence of hyperprolactinemia in anovulatory women. Obstet Gynecol. 1980;56:65-9.
3. Thessaloniki ESHRE/ASRM-Sponsored PCOS Consensus Workshop Group. Consensus on infertility treatment related to polycystic ovary syndrome. Hum Reprod. 2008;23:462-77.
4. Homburg R. Clomiphene citrate – End of an era? A mini-review. Hum Reprod. 2005;20:2043-51.
5. Hoeger K, Davidson K, Kochman L, Cherry T, Kopin L, Guzick DS. The impact of metformin, oral contraceptives, and lifestyle modification on polycystic ovary syndrome in obese adolescent women in two randomized, placebo-controlled clinical trials. J Clin Endocrinol Metab. 2008;93:4299-306.

6. Forman R, Gill S, Moretti M, Tulandi T, Koren G, Casper R. Fetal safety of letrozole and clomiphene citrate for ovulation induction. J Obstet Gynaecol Can. 2007;29:668-71.
7. Mitwally MF, Biljan MM, Casper RF. Pregnancy outcome after the use of an aromatase inhibitor for ovarian stimulation. Am J Obstet Gynecol. 2005;192:381-6.
8. Badawy A, Mosbah A, Tharwat A, Eid M. Extended letrozole therapy for ovulation induction in clomiphene-resistant women with polycystic ovary syndrome: a novel protocol. Fertil Steril. 2009;92:236-9.
9. Bobde JA, Bhosle D, Kadam R, Shelke S. Comparison of efficacy and safety of metformin, oral contraceptive combination of ethinyl estradiol and drospirenone alone or in combination in polycystic ovarian syndrome. J Obes Metab Res. 2014;1:112-7.
10. Farquhar C, Lilford R, Marjoribanks J, Vanderkerchove P. Laparoscopic "drilling" by diathermy or laser for ovulation induction in anovulatory polycystic ovary syndrome. Cochrane Database Syst Rev. 2007;3:CD001122.

CHAPTER 20 | Adjuvants in Polycystic Ovarian Syndrome

Rajeev Dabade, Meenal Chidgupkar

INTRODUCTION

Polycystic ovarian syndrome (PCOS) is the most common endocrinopathy affecting, 6-10% of women of reproductive age.[1] Even though the incidence varies based on the diagnostic criteria used, PCOS is undisputedly the most prevalent cause of female anovulatory infertility affecting women across their lifespan.

Anovulatory disorders account for about 30-40% of female infertility, with PCOS accounting for 80-90% of World Health Organization group 2 normogonadotropic normoestrogenic anovulation (hypothalamic-pituitary-ovarian dysfunction).[2]

Due to varying diagnostic criteria issues have been raised about compatibility in PCOS research worldwide and confusion within clinical practice. Therefore, the National Institutes of Health (NIH) in 2012 undertook an evidence-based methodology PCOS workshop to address the "benefits and drawbacks" of existing diagnostic criteria.[3] The panel then recommended the use of broader European Society of Human Reproduction and Embryology (ESHRE) or American Society for Reproduction Medicine (ASRM) 2003 criteria but with description of the PCOS phenotype as proposed by Azziz et al. **(Table 1)**.[4]

Four phenotypes have been identified, which may be influenced by genes—(1) nutrient, (2) physical activity, (3) pollutants, (4) psychological stress and androgen excess act to program and modify epigenome leading to PCOS **(Table 2)**.[5]

RATIONALE FOR USE OF ADJUVANTS

Insulin resistance plays a central role in the pathogenesis of PCOS. An estimated prevalence of 60-70% in PCOS patients has been reported.[11]

The adjuvants used in PCOS aim at decreasing the insulin resistance, balancing the oxidative stress and thus subsequently reduce the hyperandrogenic environment finally achieving ovulation.

TABLE 1: Defining polycystic ovarian syndrome (PCOS) evolution of the diagnostic criteria.

Parameter	NIH Consensus 1990[6]	ESHRE/ASRM/ Rotterdam Consensus 2003[7]	AEPCOS definition 2009[8]	NIH 2012 extension of ESHRE/ASRM 2003[3]
Criteria	• Clinical and/or biochemical HA • Oligo/ amenorrhea, anovulation	• Clinical and/or biochemical HA • Oligo/ amenorrhea, anovulation • PCO appearance on ultrasound	• Clinical and/or biochemical HA • Oligo/ amenorrhea, anovulation • PCO appearance on ultrasound	• Clinical and/or biochemical HA • Oligo/ amenorrhea, anovulation • PCO appearance on ultrasound
Limitations	Two of two criteria required	Two of three criteria required	Androgen excess and one other criterion	Two of three criteria required; and identification of specific phenotypes **(Table 2)**

(AEPCOS: Androgen Excess and Polycystic Ovary Syndrome Society; ASRM: American Society for Reproduction Medicine; ESHRE: European Society of Human Reproduction and Embryology; HA: hyperandrogenism; NIH: National Institutes of Health; PCO: polycystic ovaries)

TABLE 2: Classification of polycystic ovarian syndrome (PCOS) phenotypes.[4,9,10]

Parameter	Phenotype A	Phenotype B	Phenotype C	Phenotype D
PCOS features	HA/OD/PCOM	HA/OD	HA/PCOM	OD/PCOM
HA	+	+	+	−
OD	+	+	−	+
PCOM	+	−	+	+
NIH 1990 criteria	×	×		
Rotterdam 2003 criteria	×	×	×	×
AEPCOS 2006 criteria	×	×	×	

(AEPCOS: Androgen Excess and PCOS Society; HA; hyperandrogenism; NIH: National Institutes of Health; OD; ovulatory dysfunction; PCOM: polycystic ovarian morphology)
Source: Lizneva D, Suturina L, Walker W, Brakta S, Gavrilova-Jordan L, Azziz R. Criteria, prevalence, and phenotypes, and phenotypes of polycystic ovary syndrome. Fertil Steril. 2016;106(1):6-15.

ADJUVANTS

Insulin-sensitizing Agents

Metformin

Metformin is an oral biguanide that lowers blood glucose level in hyperglycemic individuals with type 2 diabetes mellitus but has no effect on glucose levels in normal subjects.

Mechanism of action:[11]
- Inhibits hepatic glucose production
- Improves insulin stimulated peripheral glucose up take by liver, skeletal muscle and adipose tissue
- Reduces absorption of glucose update from the gastrointestinal (GI) tract
- Reduces substrate availability for gluconeogenesis by lowering serum lipid levels.

Dosage: Orally in the dose of 500 mg/day and then increased gradually every week up to a total dose of 1,500 mg/day after confirming normal renal and liver function test.

It is category B drug in pregnancy.

Advantages: Metformin has been shown to increase the frequency of ovulation in PCOS, although this may be because of weight loss, because slight anorectic effect and with some evidence of benefit on parameters of metabolic syndrome.[11]

Metformin has been observed to reduce serum testosterone concentration and free androgen index.[12]

Usage of metformin for 12 weeks prior to IVF reduces risk of moderate to severe ovarian hyperstimulation syndrome (OHSS) by decreasing the expression of "vascular endothelial growth factor (VEGF)".[13]

Metformin in combination with clomiphene citrate (CC) had better ovulation versus CC or metformin alone (60.4% vs. 49.0% vs. 29.0%) as shown by Legro et al., in a multicentric RCT.[14]

Evidence:
- ASRM 2017:[11]
  - Metformin alone versus placebo increases the ovulation rate in PCOS (Gr A).
  - Metformin in combination with CC improves ovulation and clinical pregnancy rate but does not improve life birth rates compared with CC alone (Gr A).
- Cochrane 2017:[15]
  - Improvement in clinical pregnancy and ovulation suggest that CC remains preferable to metformin for ovulation induction in obese women with PCOS.

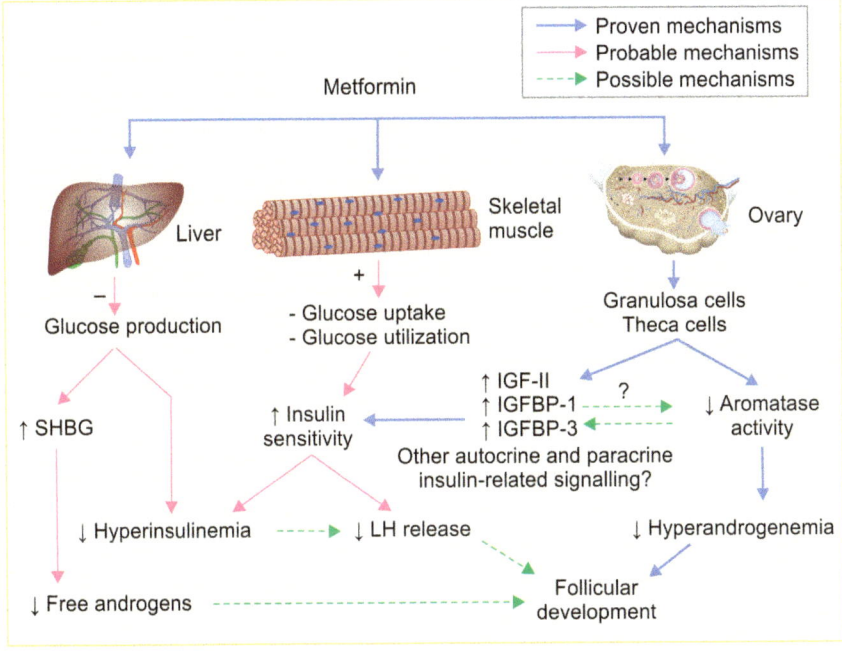

Fig. 1: Effect of metformin.

- It suggests that combined therapy (metformin and clomiphene citrate) may be useful in improving clinical pregnancy and ovulation rate but it is not known whether this translates into increased live birth.
- Women taking metformin alone or with combined therapy should be advised that there is no evidence of miscarriage but GI side effects are more likely.

- Cochrane 2019:[16]
    - Review suggests that metformin may be beneficial over placebo for live birth, however more women probably experience GI side effects.
    - When metformin was compared with CC, data for live birth were inconclusive and the findings were limited by lack of evidence.
    - Due to low quality of the evidence, we are uncertain of the effect of metformin (**Fig. 1**) on miscarriage in all comparisons.

Inositol: Myo-inositol (MI) is an insulin sensitizer and acts at the level of ovary to reduce hyperandrogenemia, regularizes cycle with spontaneous ovulation improve ovarian response, including nucleus and cytoplasmic maturation thereby improving oocyte competence.[17]

D-chiro-inositol (DCI) acts at the level of periphery to reduce insulin resistance (IR), improves glucose metabolism, improves lipid profile and thereby reduces cardiovascular and metabolic complication.

Hence, administration of both MI and DCI in the physiological plasma ratio (40:1) ensures better clinical results.

Dose: 2–4 g/day

Cochrane 2018[18]: In the light of available evidence of low quality, we are uncertain whether MI improves live birth rate or clinical pregnancy in subfertile women with PCOS undergoing IVF pretreatment taking MI compared to standard treatment.

No pooled evidence is available for use of MI in women undergoing ovulation induction.

Meta-analysis 2017[19]: The current meta-analysis highlight the beneficial effect of inositol supplementation namely MI in improving the metabolic profile of PCOS patient.

Vitamin D

Supplementation with vitamin D_3 (400 IU/day) and calcium (1,000 mg/day) for 3 months can reduce the androgens with positive effect on follicle maturation and menstrual disorder.[20]

Evidence from the current meta-analysis result suggested that the use of vitamin D as a treatment for patient with PCOS could improve IR, hyperandrogenism and a number of the lipid metabolic parameters in PCOS patients in the short-term follow-up intervention.[21]

L-methylfolate

2017 Meta-analysis[22]

In conclusion, the meta-analysis suggests that MTHFR C6677 variant can increase or decrease or have no effect on the PCOS depending on the ethnicity.

Antioxidant

N-acetyl Cysteine

- N-acetyl cysteine (NAC)—precursor of glutathione is an antioxidant.
- It has effect on Insulin receptor action and insulin secretion and thereby increases glucose utility.
- Total cholesterol, LOL, homocysteine, oxidative stress and increases HDL level.
- Combination of NAC and CC enhances ovulation and pregnancy rates in CC resistant PCOS.[23]
- Dose 600 mg BD for 6 weeks.

Melatonin

Melatonin administration reduces intrafollicular oxidative damage, prevents DNA damage, lipid peroxidation and acts as a free radical scavenger, reduces reactive oxygen species, thereby improving follicular growth and maturation and pregnancy rates. However, there needs more clarity regarding the benefit of adding melatonin in all PCOS.[24]

L-carnitine

Administration of 3 g/day over 8–12 weeks reduces the IR with improvement in lipid profile.

In CC-resistant cases, use of L-carnitine throughout the cycle was shown to improve the ovulation and pregnancy rates.[25]

Omega 3 Fatty Acids

In the dose of 4 g/day for 8 weeks reduces IR, total cholesterol, triglycerides LDL, TC/HDL, LDL/HDL ratios and malondialdehyde levels.[26]

Multiple Micronutrients and Minerals

These supplementation in PCOS undergoing OI reduces the ROS levels and maintains the cellular oxidant-antioxidant balance trace and thereby improves the reproductive outcome.[27]

Corticosteroids

Indication: PCOS with high DHEAS levels which is seen in about 20–33% and in CC-resistant cases along with CC.

Addition of 2 mg of dexamethasone in CC-resistant cases from day 5 to 14 was shown to be associated with a higher ovulation rate and cumulative pregnancy rate.[28]

However, prolonged use should be discouraged.

Oral Contraceptive Pill Pretreatment

For many decades oral contraceptive pills (OCPs) have been standard therapy for women with PCOS not seeking pregnancy. There have been several advantages of treatment with OCP, including immediate regularization of menses, amelioration of hirsutism and acne and foremost protection from the development of endometrial carcinoma.

In PCOS women with OC-induced menses in an antagonist protocol cycle resulted in a significantly lower clinical pregnancy rate and live birth rates as compared to spontaneous menses or progestin-induced menses. In an antagonist cycle where freeze-all policy was adopted and frozen embryo transfer (FET) done where OCP was used to induce menstrual bleeding resulted in significantly higher rates of conception, clinical pregnancy, and live birth compared with fresh embryo transfer.[29]

Pretreatment with oral contraceptives in infertile anovulatory patients with PCOS who receive gonadotropins for controlled ovarian stimulation was carried out in 2008 and study published in Fertility Sterility and conclusion was no effect was observed in rates of cycle cancellation, pregnancy, abortion, live birth, multiple pregnancies, and OHSS.[30]

It is clear that PCOS is an enigma. Its pathophysiology still remains to be fully understood. No treatment is a panacea as the treatment so far has been directed at the symptoms but not at the syndrome itself.

With understanding of these drugs as adjuvants to PCOS treatment, it is important for us that the extensive efforts should be directed toward more successful therapy and avoiding the serious long-term effects of the disease on patient's health.

REFERENCES

1. Konchenhauer ES, Key TJ, Kahsar-Miller M, Waggoner W, Boots LR, Azziz R. Prevalence of the polycystic ovary syndrome in unselected black and white women of the south eastern United States: a prospective study. J Clin Endocrinol Metab. 1998;83(9):3078-82.
2. Broekmans FJ, Knauff EAH, Valkenburg O, Laven JS, Eijkemans MJ, Fauser BCJM. PCOS according to the Rotterdam consensus criteria: change in prevalence among WHO-II anovulation and association with metabolic factors. BJOG. 2006;113(110):1210-7.
3. National Institutes of Health. (2012). Evidence-based methodology workshop on polycystic ovary syndrome. Executive summary. [Online] Available at https://prevention.nih.gov/docs/programs/pcos/FinalReport.pdf. [Last Accessed July, 2022].
4. Azziz R. Carmina E, Dewailly D, Diamanti-Kandarakis E, Escobar-Morreale HF, Futterweit W. Positions statement: criteria for defining polycystic ovary syndrome as a predominantly hyperandrogenic syndrome: an Androgen Excess Society guideline. J Clin Endocrinol Metab. 2006;91(11):4237-45.
5. Azziz R. Woods KS, Reyna R, Key TJ, Knochenhauer ES, Yildiz BO. The prevalence and features of the polycystic ovary syndrome in an unselected population. J Clin Endocrinol Metab. 2004;89(6):2745-9.
6. Zawadzki JK, Dunaif A. Diagnostic criteria for polycystic ovary syndrome: towards a rational approach. In: Dunaif A, Givens JR, Haseltine F, Merriam GR (Eds). Polycystic ovary syndrome. Massachusetts: Blackwell Scientific Publications; 1992. pp. 377-84.
7. Rotterd ESHRE-ASRM Sponsored PCOS Consensus Workshop Group. Revised 2003 consensus on diagnostic criteria and long-term health risks related to polycystic ovary syndrome. Fertil Steril. 2004;81(1):19-25.
8. Azziz R, Carmina E, Dewailly D, Diamanti-Kandarakis E, Escobar-Morreale HF, Futterweit W, et al. The Androgen Excess and PCOS Society Criteria for the polycystic ovary syndrome: the complete task force report. Fertil Steril. 2009;91(2):456-88.
9. Lizneva D, Suturina L, Walker W, Brakta S, Gavrilova-Jordan L, Azziz R. Criteria, prevalence, and phenotypes of polycystic ovary syndrome. Fertil Steril. 2016;106(1):6-15.
10. Ciaraldi TP, el-Roeiy A, Madar Z, Reichart D, Olefsky JM, Yen SS. Cellular mechanisms of insulin resistance in polycystic ovarian syndrome. J Clin Endocrinol Metab. 1992;75(2):577-83.
11. Practice committee of the American Society for Reproductive Medicine. Role of metformin for ovulation induction in infertile patients with polycystic ovary syndrome (PCOS): a guideline. Fertil Steril. 2017;108(3):426-41.
12. Tang T, Glanville J, Orsi N, Barth JH, Balen AH. The use of metformin for women with PCOS undergoing IVF treatment. Hum Reprod. 2006;21(6):1416-25.
13. Tso LO, Costello MF, Albuquerque LET, Andriolo RB, Macedo CR. Metformin treatment before and during IVF or ICSI in women with polycystic ovary syndrome. Cochrane Database Syst Rev. 2014;2014(11):CD006105.

14. Legro RS, Barnhart HX, Schlaff WD, Carr BR, Diamond MP, Carson SA, et al. Clomiphene, metformin, or both for infertility in the polycystic ovary syndrome. N Engl J Med. 2007;356(6):551-66.
15. Bordewijk EM, Nahuis M, Costello MF, Van der Veen F, Tso LO, Molet BWJ. Metformin during ovulation induction with gonadotropins followed by timed intercourse or intrauterine insemination for subfertility associated with polycystic ovary syndrome. Cochrane Database Syst Rev. 2017;1(1):CD009090.
16. Sharpe A, Morley LC, Tang T, Norman RJ, Balen AH. Metformin for ovulation induction (excluding gonadotrophins) in women with polycystic ovary syndrome. Cochrane Database Syst Rev. 2019;12(12):CD013505.
17. Tang T, Lord JM, Norman RJ, Yasmin E, Balen AH. Insulin-sensitizing drugs (metformin, rosiglitazone, pioglitazone, D-chiro-inositol) for women with polycystic ovary syndrome, oligo amenorrhea and subfertility. Cochrane Database Syst Rev. 2012;(5):CD003053.
18. Showell MG, Mackenzie-Proctor R, Jordan V, Hodgson R, Farquhar C. Inositol for subfertile women with polycystic ovary syndrome. Cochrane Database Syst Rev. 2018;12(12):CD012378.
19. Mojaverrostami S, Asghari N, Khamisabadi M, Khoei HH. The role of melatonin in polycystic ovary syndrome: A review. International Journal of Reproductive BioMedicine. 2019;17:865-82.
20. Amini L, Tehranian N, Movahedin M, Tehrani FR, Ziaee S. Antioxidants and management of polycystic ovary syndrome in Iran: A systematic review of clinical trials. Iran J Reprod Med. 2015;13(1):1-8.
21. Miao CY, Fang XJ, Chen Y, Zhang Q. Effect of vitamin D supplementation on polycystic ovary syndrome: A meta-analysis. Exp Ther Med. 2020;19(4):2641-9.
22. Wang L, Xu W, Wang C, Tang M, Zhou Y. Methylenetetrahydrofolate reductase C677T polymorphism and the risks of polycystic ovary syndrome: an updated meta-analysis of 14 studies. Oncotarget. 2017;8(35):59509-17.
23. Badawy A, State O, Abdelgawad S. N-Acetyl cysteine and clomiphene citrate for induction of ovulation in polycystic ovary syndrome: a cross-over trial. Acta Obstet Gynecol Scand. 2007;86(2):218-22.
24. Seko LMD, Moroni RM, Leitao VMS, Teixeira DM, Nastri CO, Martins WP. Melatonin supplementation during controlled ovarian stimulation for women undergoing assisted reproductive technology: systematic review and meta-analysis of randomized controlled trials. Fertil steril. 2014;101(1):154-61.
25. Ismail AM, Hamed AH, Saso S, Thabet HH. Adding L-carmitine to clomiphene resistant PCOS women improves the quality of ovulation and the pregnancy rate. A randomized clinical trial. Eur Obstet Gynecol Reprod Biol. 2014;180:148-52.
26. Samy N, Hashim M, Sayed M, Said M. Clinical significance of inflammatory markers in polycystic ovary syndrome: their relationship to insulin resistance and body mass index. Dis Markers, 2009;26(4):163-70.
27. Günalan E, Yaba A, Yılmaz B. The effect of nutrient supplementation in the management of polycystic ovary syndrome-associated metabolic dysfunctions: A critical review. J Turk Ger Gynecol Assoc. 2018;19(4):220-32.
28. Parsanezhad ME, Alborzi S, Motazedian S, Omrani G. Use of dexamethasone and clomiphene citrate in the treatment of clomiphene citrate-resistant patients with polycystic ovary syndrome and normal dehydroeplandrosterone sulphate levels: a prosepective, double–blind, placebo-controlled trial. Fertil Steril. 2002;78(5):1001-4.
29. Wei D, Shi Y, Li J, Wang Z, Zhang L, Sun Y, et al. Effect of pretreatment with oral contraceptives and progestins on IVF outcomes in women with polycystic ovary syndrome. Hum Reprod. 2017;32:354-61.
30. Palomba S, Falbo A, Orio F Jr, Russo T, Tolino A, Zullo F. Pretreatment with oral contraceptives in infertile anovulatory patients with polycystic ovary syndrome who receive gonadotropins for controlled ovarian stimulation. Fertil Steril. 2008;89:1838-42.

CHAPTER 21: Adjuvants in Diminished Ovarian Reserve

Shilpi Sood, Chaitanya Shembekar, Laxmi Shrikhande

INTRODUCTION

Diminished ovarian reserve (DOR), the quantitative decline in the oocyte pool, is one of the main reasons that negatively impact female fertility **(Fig. 1)**.[1]

It has been long debated whether the decrease in number of viable oocytes, also is accompanied by a qualitative decline,[3,4] recurrent pregnancy loss in women with DOR may favor the hypothesis.[5] Though most of the cases of DOR are thought to be idiopathic, age,[6] genetics,[3,7] and environmental variables may play an important role in pathogenesis.

Evaluation of ovarian reserve (ovarian reserve testing) can help to confirm the diagnosis of DOR and individualize treatment protocols in cases of infertility.[8,9] Multiple tests are available of which both antral follicle count (AFC) and anti-Müllerian hormone (AMH) have good predictive value.[10] An AFC <5 on ultrasound, AMH <0.5–1 ng/mL, or raised levels of follicle-stimulating hormone (FSH) (>10 IU/L on cycle day 2–4) are indicative of abnormal ovarian reserve.[3]

The European Society of Human Reproduction and Embryology (ESHRE) proposed Bologna's criteria to represent DOR. It consists of the following components:[11]
- Old age
- Abnormal ovarian reserve tests
- Prior suboptimal response to stimulation

The POSEIDON (**P**atient-**O**riented **S**trategies **E**ncompassing **I**ndividualize**D** **O**ocyte **N**umber) criteria for "low prognosis" has replaced the Bologna's criteria and is being widely used to assess outcomes in patients undergoing assisted reproductive technology (ART).[12]

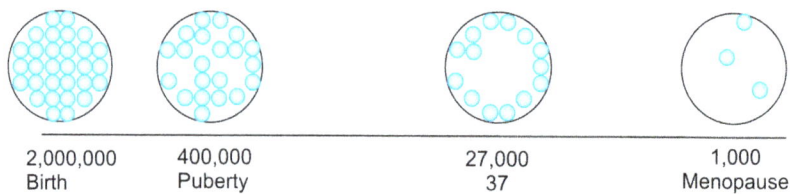

| 2,000,000 | 400,000 | 27,000 | 1,000 |
| Birth | Puberty | 37 | Menopause |

Fig. 1: Age-related decline in follicular number.[2]

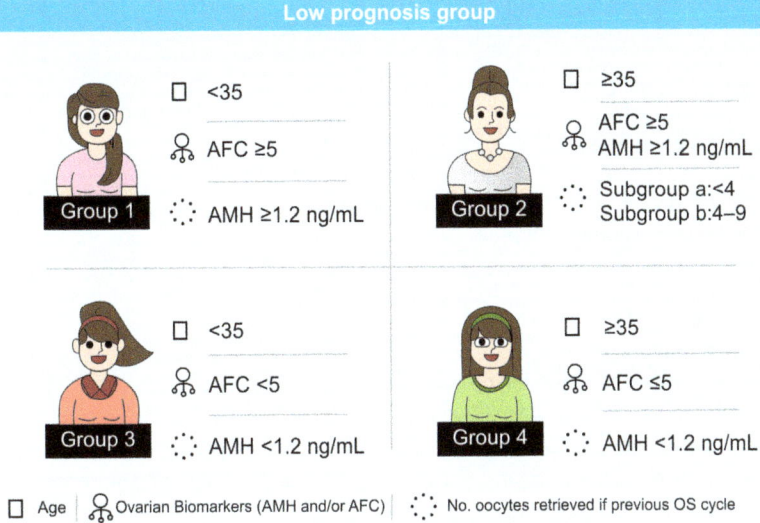

Fig. 2: POSEIDON criteria for low prognosis groups.

The POSEIDON groups 1 and 2[13] include patients who respond poorly (<4 oocytes retrieved) or suboptimally (4-9 oocytes retrieved) to gonadotropin stimulation despite the presence of adequate ovarian parameters whereas groups 3 and 4[14] are patients with history of poor ovarian reserve and inadequate ovarian parameters **(Fig. 2)**.

MANAGEMENT OF DIMINISHED OVARIAN RESERVE

Patients with DOR often face issues such as poor follicular response, premature luteinizing hormone (LH) surge, and poor embryo quality and may require ART for conception. DOR is also associated with poor ovarian response to controlled ovarian hyperstimulation (COH) while managing the cases of infertility.[3] Management of these patients is thus challenging and lack of specific guidelines further adds to the difficulties of attending physicians. Furthermore, the traditional controlled ovarian stimulation (COS) protocols used in ART have their own limitations.[15] Patients with DOR may need careful monitoring and tailor-made approaches to overcome these issues. Literature evidence supports minimal use and mild doses of gonadotropins, avoiding severe pituitary suppression, luteal phase stimulation, and a "freeze all" approach for patients who have failed traditional COS **(Box 1)**.

ROLE OF ADJUVANTS IN DIMINISHED OVARIAN RESERVE

The adjuvants (synonyms: treatment add-ons, adjuncts) are additional, optional, and therapeutic agents that may be combined with the standard protocols with an objective of improving treatment outcomes.[17] Through

BOX 1: Management protocols of DOR.[16]

Protocols
- High doses of gonadotropins
- Recombinant FSH
- Luteal initiation of FSH
- LH
- GnRH agonists—luteal onset of GnRH agonists
- "Stop" GnRH agonist protocols
- GnRHa—"flare" regimens
- Microdose GnRH agonist flare regimen
- Short protocol
- GnRH antagonists
- Natural cycle or modified natural cycle
- Low level hCG in early stimulation phase

(DOR: diminished ovarian reserve; FSH: follicle-stimulating hormone; GnRH: gonadotropin-releasing hormone; hCG: human chorionic gonadotropin; LH: luteinizing hormone)

TABLE 1: Adjuvants in management of diminished ovarian reserve (DOR).[20]

Androgens	Other hormones	Other
Dehydroepiandrosterone (DHEA)	Growth hormone	Vasoactive substances
Androstenedione	Recombinant luteinizing hormone (LH)	Steroids
Testosterone	Addition of estradiol in the luteal phase	

different mechanisms of action, they are intended to improve the ovarian yield, embryo quality thus increasing the chance of live birth. They are generally prescribed as add-on therapy for improving In vitro fertilization (IVF) outcomes, especially in cases where the previous cycles have failed. However, there are not enough evidences that support the choice of adjuvants as the reasons of failure themselves are difficult to diagnose.[18] Transdermal testosterone, dehydroepiandrosterone (DHEA), and growth hormone (GH) have often been used as pre- and co-treatment adjuvants based on the clinical experience in patients with DOR to improve the pregnancy rate in IVF **(Table 1)**.[19]

Dehydroepiandrosterone

Dehydroepiandrosterone, a C19 androgenic steroid with proinflammatory immune function, when administered as an adjuvant, increases insulin-like growth factor-1 (IGF-1) levels. As a consequence of this improvements in the oocytes yield and oocyte/embryo quality have been noted.[21,22] DHEA also improves the Th1 immune response and regulate the balance of the

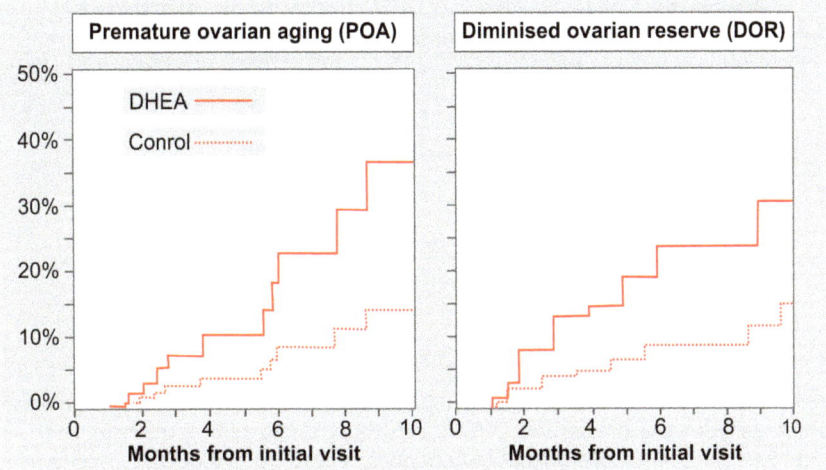

Fig. 3: Cumulative pregnancy rates in women with DOR with and without dehydroepiandrosterone (DHEA) supplementation.

Th1/Th2 response.[23] The increase in cumulative pregnancy rates after initiation of DHEA provides enough evidence of its efficacy **(Fig. 3)**.[22,24] DHEA may act as a testosterone precursor in the follicular fluid; it has been observed that 75 mg/day of DHEA results in improvement in AMH concentration, AFC, peak estradiol, number of oocytes retrieved, number of metaphase II oocytes, and high-quality embryos during assisted reproductive techniques.[20,25,26] Thus, 75 mg/day is the recommended dose which can be consumed as a whole or in three divided doses.

A prospective clinical trial conducted in India, treated 30 DOR patients with DHEA 25 mg thrice a day for 4 months and found significant increase ($p < 0.05$) in the serum AMH in all age groups (35, 36–38, and >38 years) resulting in a pregnancy rate of 16.7%.[27] DHEA is one of the most commonly used adjuvant constituting nearly 25% share in all of the IVF programs.[28]

Androstenedione

Androstenedione is an androgen precursor that intermediates in the synthesis pathway of testosterone from cholesterol **(Flowchart 1)**.[29] The role of androstenedione in the treatment of DOR is being explored.

Testosterone

Under normal physiological conditions, serum testosterone concentration steadily declines in women with increasing age, this is thought to be one of the factors leading to age-related decline in reproductive ability. Low basal testosterone levels are associated with poor IVF rates even in women with normal ovarian reserve.[30] Thus, use of testosterone supplementation in patients with DOR is thought to have more favourable outcomes, thought

Flowchart 1: Path for conversion of DHEA to other downstream steroids.[16]

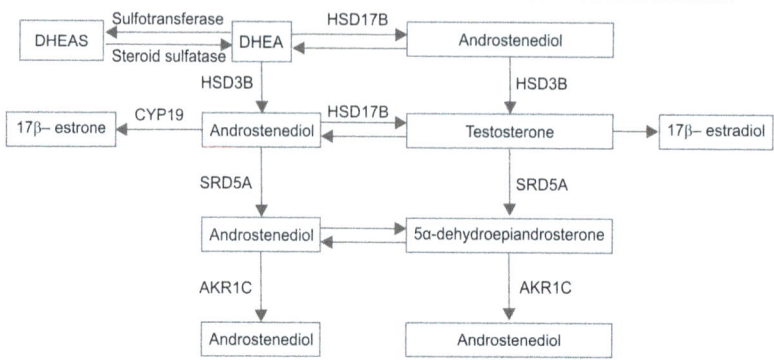

(AKR1C: 3α-hydroxysteroid dehydrogenase isoenzymes; CYP19A1: P450 aromatase; DHEA: dehydroepiandrosterone; DHEAS: dehydroepiandrosterone sulphate; HSD17B: 17β-hydroxysteroid dehydrogenase isoenzymes; HSD3B: 3β-hydrogenase isoenzymes; SRD5A: 5α-reductase isoenzymes)

supporting evidence are limited. Testosterone gel (strength 10 mg) may be applied on external side of thigh for 21 days starting from first day of menstruation prior to initiation of ovarian stimulation.[20] Literature evidences are conflicting and while few suggest mprovement in live birth rate with 3 and 4 weeks testosterone pretreatment[31] other study reported no significant difference in live birth rate in women who received testosterone for 2 weeks as a pretreatment as compared with the control group.[32] Therefore, the ESHRE guidelines do not recommend the use of adjuvant testosterone prior to ovarian stimulation in poor responders.[10]

Growth Hormone

Growth hormone works through the somatotropic axis (GH, IGF-1, IGF-2, and their binding proteins and receptors) and through its direct or indirect action on IGF-1, it affects follicular recruitment.[33] The hormone binds to the GH receptor in theca cells, granular cells, and oocytes, resulting in enhanced ovarian response and improved oocyte quality.[34] It further elevates the concentration of FSH receptors in granulosa cells and increases the mitochondrial quantity in human oocytes, which may enhance the ovarian response. There is no consensus on the dosage of GH, the reported dosage varying from 1 IU every other day to 10 IU daily.[35] A study reported that GH pretreatment is advantageous by elevating ovarian response and correlated with an improved live birth rate and reduced miscarriage rate in POSEIDON poor ovarian reserve patients older than 35 years.[35] Adjuvant GH is thought to be associated with decreased cycle cancellation rate, which consequently shortens the IVF treatment time.[36] However, the ESHRE guidelines do not recommend the use of adjuvant GH before and/or during ovarian stimulation for poor responders.[10]

Recombinant Luteinizing Hormone

Luteinizing hormone maintains the concentrations of intraovarian androgens and promotes steroidogenesis and follicular growth.[20] Recombinant human LH (r-hLH) supplementation may be beneficial in women with satisfactory prestimulation ovarian reserve parameters and an unexpected hyporesponse to recombinant human FSH (r-hFSH) monotherapy or women who are in between 36 and 39 years of age.[37] The addition of r-hLH to assisted reproduction technology cycles can improve implantation and clinical pregnancy rates in these patients.[38] The combination of r-hLH and r-hFSH also results in higher pregnancy rate versus r-hFSH alone in women with low-serum testosterone levels[39] and poor ovarian reserve.[40] In comparison with menopausal gonadotropins, numbers of eggs retrieved and embryos formed were higher with r-hLH while using less FSH.[41]

Letrozole

Letrozole is a selective and nonsteroidal aromatase inhibitor (AI) that blocks androgen conversion to estrogen causing reduction in serum estrogen levels thus enhancing the FSH receptors affinity and antral follicles growth.[42,43] There is also a temporary rise in intraovarian androgen concentrations which cause prolongation of the follicular phase.[44,45] Letrozole co-treatment might therefore improves ovarian response and IVF outcomes in poor/suboptimal responders.[46] A double-blind randomized clinical trial demonstrated that addition of 5 mg of letrozole to recombinant follicle-stimulating hormone/human menopausal gonadotropin (rFSH/hMG) antagonist protocol may result in improvement of outcome of IVF/intracytoplasmic sperm injection cycle in DOR patients.[47] However, in another double-blinded randomized control trial, use of letrozole in GnRH antagonist cycles does not improve clinical outcomes in these patients. Hence, further studies are essential to derive conclusions regarding its efficacy.[48]

Other Drugs that have been Used as Adjuvants

Due to lack of sufficient evidence and clinical experience with the above therapies, several other drugs are being studied for use as adjuvants. Aspirin, indomethacin, and sildenafil are being used to explore their role in improving ovarian reserve. The ESHRE guidelines do not recommend the use of these therapeutic interventions prior to ovarian stimulation in poor responders.[10] Platelet-rich plasma injection in the ovaries, mitochondrial replacement therapy (spindle transfer), melatonin, and mitochondrial deoxyribonucleic acid (DNA) load measurement are the other options that are being investigated and may provide hope for the future.[17]

Flowchart 2: Best practices based on POSEIDON groups.

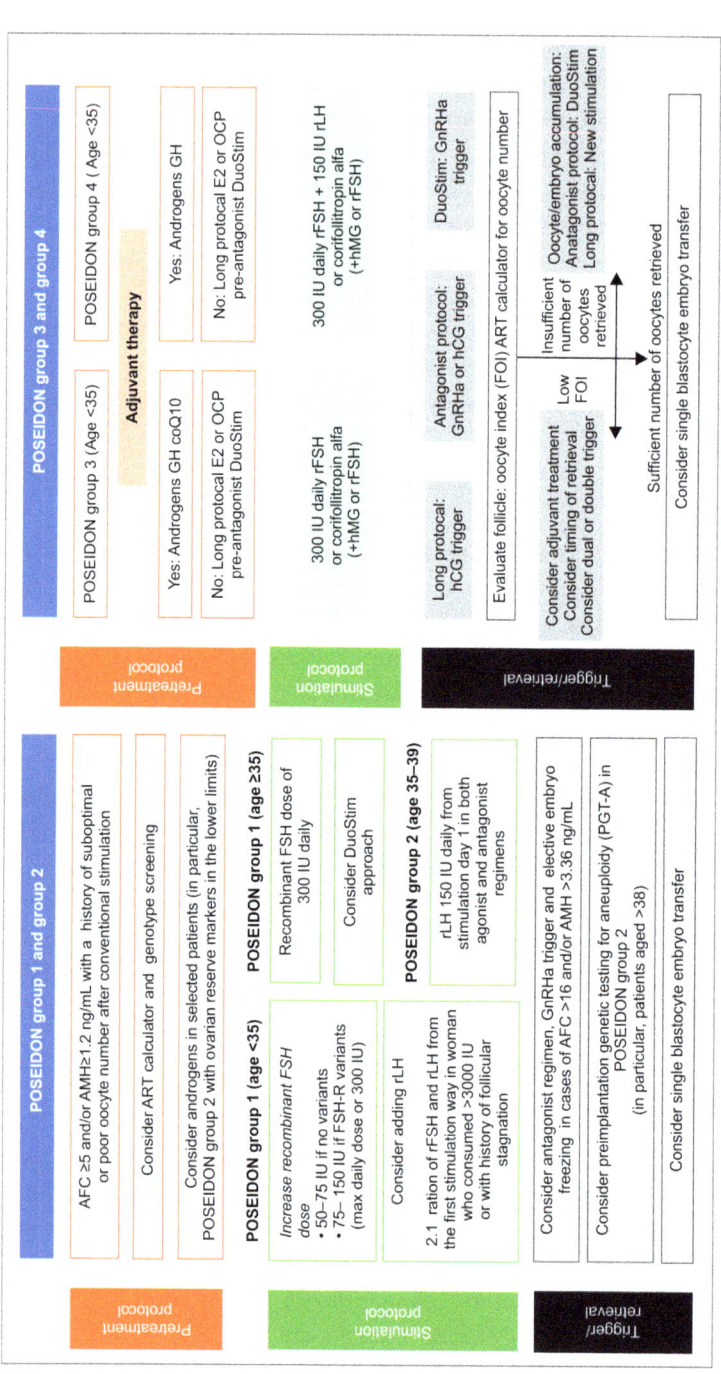

(AFC: antral follicle count; AMH: anti-Müllerian hormone; ART: assisted reproductive technology; FSH: follicle-stimulating hormone; GH: growth hormone; GnRHa: gonadotropin-releasing hormone agonist; hCG: human chorionic gonadotropin; hMG: human menopausal gonadotropin; OCP: oral contraceptive pill; rFSH: recombinant follicle-stimulating hormone; rLH: recombinant luteinizing hormone)

MANAGING DIMINISHED OVARIAN RESERVE PATIENTS BASED ON THE POSEIDON CRITERIA

The best practices according to the group are described in **Flowchart 2**; however there is a need of robust evidence to support the use of these in clinical practice.

CONCLUSION

Diminished ovarian reserve is one of the most common causes of infertility among the women, especially above 35 years of age. Prompt diagnosis of the underlying cause, if any, and individualized treatment may benefit the individuals and increase the rate of clinical pregnancy. Adjuvants such as DHEA or GH may have positive effect in women undergoing ART treatment for DOR. However, there is no conclusive evidence suggesting beneficial role of these treatments in IVF. Since most of these therapies are costly, it is important to ascertain the need of adjuvants on case-to-case basis and also prescribe them ethically to optimize their use.

REFERENCES

1. Dogan S, Cicek OSY, Demir M, Yalcinkaya L, Sertel E. The effect of growth hormone adjuvant therapy on assisted reproductive technologies outcomes in patients with diminished ovarian reserve or poor ovarian response. J Gynecol Obstet Hum Reprod. 2021;50(2):101982.
2. Kaur M, Arora M, Rao K. Diminished Ovarian Reserve, Causes, Assessment and Management. Int J Infertility Fetal Med. 2013;4:45-55.
3. Greene AD, Patounakis G, Segars JH. Genetic associations with diminished ovarian reserve: a systematic review of the literature. J Assist Reprod Genet. 2014;31(8):935-46.
4. Ata B, Seyhan A, Seli E. Diminished ovarian reserve versus ovarian aging: overlaps and differences. Curr Opin Obstet Gynecol. 2019;31(3):139-47.
5. Bunnewell SJ, Honess ER, Karia AM, Keay SD, Al Wattar BH, Quenby S. Diminished ovarian reserve in recurrent pregnancy loss: a systematic review and meta-analysis. Fertil Steril. 2020;113(4):818-27.e3.
6. Podfigurna A, Lukaszuk K, Czyzyk A, Kunicki M, Maciejewska-Jeske M, Jakiel G, et al. Testing ovarian reserve in pre-menopausal women: why, whom and how? Maturitas. 2018;109:112-7.
7. Pelosi E, Forabosco A, Schlessinger D. Genetics of the ovarian reserve. Front Genet. 2015;6:308.
8. Tal R, Seifer DB. Ovarian reserve testing: a user's guide. Am J Obstet Gynecol. 2017;217(2):129-40.
9. Practice Committee of the American Society for Reproductive Medicine. Testing and interpreting measures of ovarian reserve: a committee opinion. Fertil Steril. 2020;114(6):1151-7.
10. The Eshre Guideline Group On Ovarian Stimulation, Bosch E, Broer S, Griesinger G, Grynberg M, Humaidan P, et al. ESHRE guideline: ovarian stimulation for IVF/ICSI. Hum Reprod Open. 2020;2020(2):hoaa009.
11. Alborzi S, Madadi G, Samsami A, Soheil P, Azizi M, Alborzi M, et al. Decreased ovarian reserve: any new hope? Minerva Ginecol. 2015;67(2):149-67.
12. Esteves SC, Alviggi C, Humaidan P, Fischer R, Andersen CY, Conforti A, et al. The POSEIDON Criteria and Its Measure of Success Through the Eyes of Clinicians and Embryologists. Front Endocrinol (Lausanne). 2019;10:814.

13. Reed BG, Babayev SN, Bukulmez O. Shifting paradigms in diminished ovarian reserve and advanced reproductive age in assisted reproduction: customization instead of conformity. Semin Reprod Med. 2015;33(3):169-78.
14. Loutradis D, Drakakis P, Vomvolaki E, Antsaklis A. Different ovarian stimulation protocols for women with diminished ovarian reserve. J Assist Reprod Genet. 2007;24(12):597-611.
15. Nardo L, Chouliaras S. Adjuvants in IVF-evidence for what works and what does not work. Ups J Med Sci. 2020;125(2):144-51.
16. Segev Y, Carp H, Auslender R, Dirnfeld M. Is there a place for adjuvant therapy in IVF? Obstet Gynecol Surv. 2010;65(4):260-72.
17. Haahr T, Esteves SC, Humaidan P. Individualized controlled ovarian stimulation in expected poor-responders: an update. Reprod Biol Endocrinol. 2018;16(1):20.
18. Goyal R. Adjuvant therapy in poor ovarian response—Where do we stand? Fertil Sci Res. 2018;5:4-8.
19. Schwarze JE, Canales J, Crosby J, Ortega-Hrepich C, Villa S, Pommer R. DHEA use to improve likelihood of IVF/ICSI success in patients with diminished ovarian reserve: A systematic review and meta-analysis. JBRA Assist Reprod. 2018;22(4):369-74.
20. Gleicher N, Barad DH. Dehydroepiandrosterone (DHEA) supplementation in diminished ovarian reserve (DOR). Reprod Biol Endocrinol. 2011;9:67.
21. Zhang J, Qiu X, Gui Y, Xu Y, Li D, Wang L. Dehydroepiandrosterone improves the ovarian reserve of women with diminished ovarian reserve and is a potential regulator of the immune response in the ovaries. Biosci Trends. 2015;9(6):350-9.
22. Qin JC, Fan L, Qin AP. The effect of dehydroepiandrosterone (DHEA) supplementation on women with diminished ovarian reserve (DOR) in IVF cycle: Evidence from a meta-analysis. J Gynecol Obstet Hum Reprod. 2017;46(1):1-7.
23. Triantafyllidou O, Sigalos G, Vlahos N. Dehydroepiandrosterone (DHEA) supplementation and IVF outcome in poor responders. Hum Fertil (Camb). 2017;20(2):80-7.
24. Narkwichean A, Maalouf W, Campbell BK, Jayaprakasan K. Efficacy of dehydroepiandrosterone to improve ovarian response in women with diminished ovarian reserve: a meta-analysis. Reprod Biol Endocrinol. 2013;11:44.
25. Singh N, Zangmo R, Kumar S, Roy KK, Sharma JB, Malhotra N, et al. A prospective study on role of dehydroepiandrosterone (DHEA) on improving the ovarian reserve markers in infertile patients with poor ovarian reserve. Gynecol Endocrinol. 2013;29(11):989-92.
26. Fouany MR, Sharara FI. Is there a role for DHEA supplementation in women with diminished ovarian reserve? J Assist Reprod Genet. 2013;30(9):1239-44.
27. ScienceDirect. (2010). Androstenedione. [online] Available from https://www.sciencedirect.com/topics/medicine-and-dentistry/androstenedione. [Last accessed July, 2022].
28. Lu Q, Shen H, Li Y, Zhang C, Wang C, Chen X, et al. Low testosterone levels in women with diminished ovarian reserve impair embryo implantation rate: a retrospective case-control study. J Assist Reprod Genet. 2014;31(4):485-91.
29. Kim CH, Ahn JW, Moon JW, Kim SH, Chae HD, Kang BM. Ovarian Features after 2 Weeks, 3 Weeks and 4 Weeks Transdermal Testosterone Gel Treatment and Their Associated Effect on IVF Outcomes in Poor Responders. Dev Reprod. 2014;18(3):145-52.
30. Bosdou JK, Venetis CA, Dafopoulos K, Zepiridis L, Chatzimeletiou K, Anifandis G, et al. Transdermal testosterone pretreatment in poor responders undergoing ICSI: a randomized clinical trial. Hum Reprod. 2016;31(5):977-85.
31. Bosch E, Labarta E, Kolibianakis E, Rosen M, Meldrum D. Regimen of ovarian stimulation affects oocyte and therefore embryo quality. Fertil Steril. 2016;105(3):560-70.
32. Abir R, Garor R, Felz C, Nitke S, Krissi H, Fisch B. Growth hormone and its receptor in human ovaries from fetuses and adults. Fertil Steril. 2008;90(4 Suppl):1333-9.

33. Cai MH, Gao LZ, Liang XY, Fang C, Wu YQ, Yang X. The effect of growth hormone on the clinical outcomes of poor ovarian reserve patients undergoing in vitro fertilization/intracytoplasmic sperm injection treatment: a retrospective study based on POSEIDON criteria. Front Endocrinol (Lausanne). 2019;10:775.
34. Yang P, Wu R, Zhang H. The effect of growth hormone supplementation in poor ovarian responders undergoing IVF or ICSI: a meta-analysis of randomized controlled trials. Reprod Biol Endocrinol. 2020;18(1):76.
35. Alviggi C, Conforti A, Esteves SC, Andersen CY, Bosch E, Bühler K, et al. Recombinant luteinizing hormone supplementation in assisted reproductive technology: a systematic review. Fertil Steril. 2018;109(4):644-64.
36. Hill MJ, Levens ED, Levy G, Ryan ME, Csokmay JM, DeCherney AH, et al. The use of recombinant luteinizing hormone in patients undergoing assisted reproductive techniques with advanced reproductive age: a systematic review and meta-analysis. Fertil Steril. 2012;97(5):1108-14.e1.
37. Albu D, Albu A. The ratio of exogenous Luteinizing hormone to Follicle stimulating hormone administered for controlled ovarian stimulation is associated with oocytes' number and competence. Biosci Rep. 2020;40(1):BSR20190811.
38. Mignini Renzini M, Brigante C, Coticchio G, Canto MD, Caliari I, Comi R, et al. Retrospective analysis of treatments with recombinant FSH and recombinant LH versus human menopausal gonadotropin in women with reduced ovarian reserve. J Assist Reprod Genet. 2017;34(12):1645-51.
39. Dahan MH, Agdi M, Shehata F, Son W, Tan SL. A comparison of outcomes from in vitro fertilization cycles stimulated with either recombinant luteinizing hormone (LH) or human chorionic gonadotropin acting as an LH analogue delivered as human menopausal gonadotropins, in subjects with good or poor ovarian reserve: a retrospective analysis. Eur J Obstet Gynecol Reprod Biol. 2014;172:70-3.
40. Lee KH, Kim CH, Suk HJ, Lee YJ, Kwon SK, Kim SK, et al. The effect of aromatase inhibitor letrozole incorporated in gonadotrophin-releasing hormone antagonist multiple dose protocol in poor responders undergoing in vitro fertilization. Obstet Gynecol Sci. 2014;57(3):216-22.
41. Winer EP, Hudis C, Burstein HJ, Wolff AC, Pritchard KI, Ingle JN, et al. American Society of Clinical Oncology technology assessment on the use of aromatase inhibitors as adjuvant therapy for women with hormone receptor-positive breast cancer: status report 2002. J Clin Oncol. 2002;20(15):3317-27.
42. Elnashar A, Fouad H, Eldosoky M, Saeid N. Letrozole induction of ovulation in women with clomiphene citrate-resistant polycystic ovary syndrome may not depend on the period of infertility, the body mass index, or the luteinizing hormone/follicle-stimulating hormone ratio. Fertil Steril. 2006;85(2):511-3.
43. Goswami SK, Das T, Chattopadhyay R, Sawhney V, Kumar J, Chaudhury K, et al. A randomized single-blind controlled trial of letrozole as a low-cost IVF protocol in women with poor ovarian response: a preliminary report. Hum Reprod. 2004;19(9):2031-5.
44. Shapira M, Orvieto R, Lebovitz O, Nahum R, Aizer A, Segev-Zahav A, et al. Does daily co administration of gonadotropins and letrozole during the ovarian stimulation improve IVF outcome for poor and sub optimal responders? J Ovarian Res. 2020;13(1):66.
45. Moini A, Lavasani Z, Kashani L, Mojtahedi MF, Yamini N. Letrozole as co-treatment agent in ovarian stimulation antagonist protocol in poor responders: a double-blind randomized clinical trial. Int J Reprod Biomed. 2019;17(9):653-60.
46. Ebrahimi M, Akbari-Asbagh F, Ghalandar-Attar M. Letrozole+ GnRH antagonist stimulation protocol in poor ovarian responders undergoing intracytoplasmic sperm injection cycles: An RCT. Int J Reprod Biomed. 2017;15(2):101-8.
47. Conforti A, Esteves SC, Cimadomo D, Vaiarelli A, Di Rella F, Ubaldi FM, et al. Management of Women With an Unexpected Low Ovarian Response to Gonadotropin. Front Endocrinol (Lausanne). 2019;10:387.
48. Haahr T, Dosouto C, Alviggi C, Esteves SC, Humaidan P. Management strategies for POSEIDON groups 3 and 4. Front Endocrinol (Lausanne). 2019;10:614.

CHAPTER 22 | Diagnosis of Diminished Ovarian Reserve

Ameet Patki, Garima Sharma

INTRODUCTION

Ovarian reserve indicates the fertility potential of a woman at a particular age by defining the quantity and quality of primordial follicular pool.

The term "Diminished Ovarian Reserve (DOR)" has been used interchangeably with other terms like diminished ovarian response, poor ovarian reserve, poor ovarian response (POR).

Diminished ovarian reserve indicates a decline in the quantity and quality of oocytes in women of reproductive age group and is an important cause of infertility in many couples these days.[1]

Diminished ovarian reserve is a major challenge in assisted reproduction. It may occur due to either advanced female age or may also happen in young women due to diverse etiological factors.[1]

Early detection and individualization of treatment protocols is the only way of optimizing the success rate in these women.

DIAGNOSIS

Symptomatically, shortening of the menstrual cycles' secondary to early follicle selection and ovulation may indicate DOR. A lot of definitions have been formulated to define and diagnose DOR, taking into consideration several factors such as ovarian reserve markers, demographics, outcome of previous in vitro fertilization (IVF) cycles, age, and other etiological factors. However, these definitions show a lot of heterogeneity and none of them aids to optimize the IVF success rates in these women.

THE BOLOGNA CRITERIA

The European Society of Human Reproduction and Embryology (ESHRE) in 2011 made the first attempt to systematically define women with inadequate response to ovarian stimulation. This consensus definition was named as "Bologna criteria". This consensus was primarily made to standardize the definition of POR based on oocyte quantity.[2]

Flowchart 1: Bologna criteria for poor ovarian response (POR).

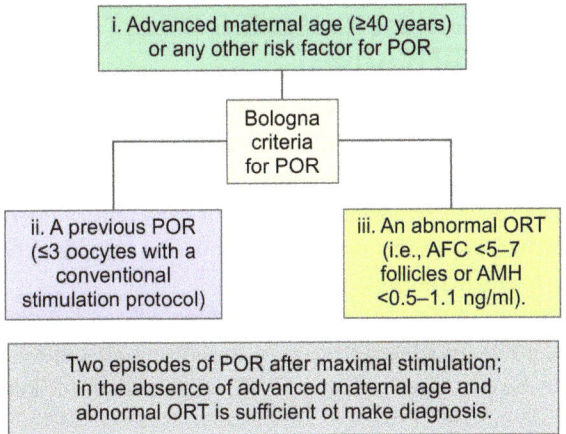

(AFC: antral follicle count; AMH: anti-Müllerian hormone; ORT: ovarian reserve test)

*Bologna criteria recommend the presence of at least two of the three features for diagnosis of POR (**Flowchart 1**):*[2]

By definition, the women may be classified as either the unexpected poor responder or expected poor responder.

LIMITATIONS OF THE EXISTING POR CRITERIA

- A 2016 review of interventional clinical trials in POR revealed that >90% trials were unable to detect meaningful differences in pregnancy rates.[3]
- Bologna criteria have received main criticism due to patient heterogeneity.[4]
- The risk factors defined for POR such as endometrioma, ovarian surgery, pelvic infection, and extensive periovarian adhesions have a variable impact on ovarian reserve. As a result, numerous patient categories with potentially different prognosis will be created with no focus on optimizing the assisted reproductive technology (ART) success rate.
- Biomarker's cut-off used to classify POR patients is another limitation of Bologna criteria. The antral follicle count (AFC) range of 5-7 and 0.5-1.1 ng/mL for anti-Müllerian hormone (AMH) appears quite wide. The authors did not provide much information on the accuracy of these ranges in predicting POR.
- Impact of oocyte quantity versus quality has not been discussed.
- Important factors which determine the ART success, like the embryo aneuploidy rates secondary to advancing age and the innate resistance of the ovaries to gonadotropin stimulation, are not taken into consideration.
- This criterion may lead to over diagnosis.[4]
- It does not give any clear-cut management strategies.

POSEIDON (PATIENT-ORIENTED STRATEGIES ENCOMPASSING INDIVIDUALIZED OOCYTE NUMBER) CLASSIFICATION

The limitations in earlier definitions lead to the development of new classification, the POSEIDON (patient-oriented strategies encompassing individualized oocyte number) classification. This was developed to provide a refined definition for POR, which can significantly reduce the heterogeneity involved in earlier definitions and at the same time provides counseling and management strategies in these patients.[5]

This criterion redefines patients as "expected" or "unexpected" poor ovarian responders to gonadotropin stimulation. This new classification challenges the current terminology of POR/DOR in favor of "low prognosis".[6]

Aims

- Early identification and classification of patients who can have low prognosis in ART.
- Individualize the treatment plan for these patients in order to optimize the success rates and reduce the time to pregnancy.
- Patient-oriented strategies to be used, considering the age parameter, in order to achieve the estimated individualized oocyte number required for attaining live birth.[7]

Classification (Figs. 1 and 2)

This classification system categorizes patient into one of the four groups based on:

1. Ovarian reserve markers (AFC and/or AMH)
2. Age of the female, and
3. The result of previous conventional ovarian stimulation in terms of number of oocytes retrieved (in cases where the information is available).

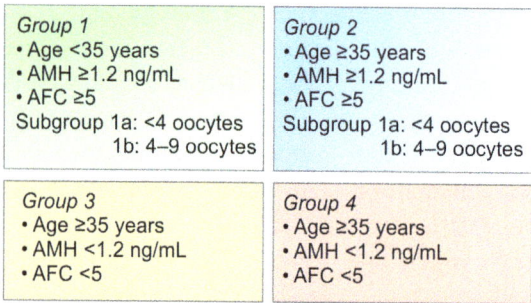

Fig. 1: Classification system of patients' categorization patient into four groups.

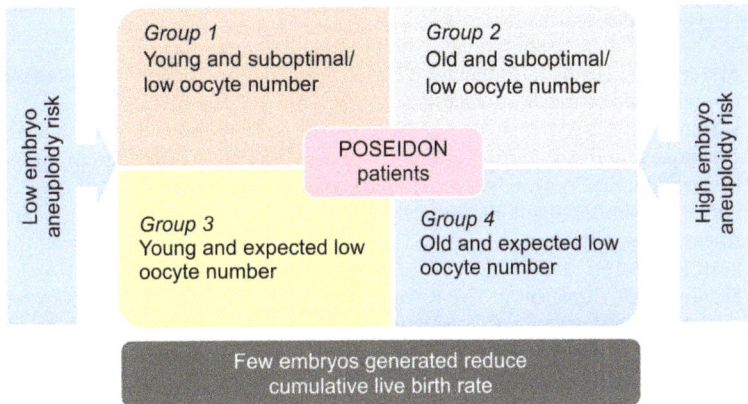

Fig. 2: POSEIDON (patient-oriented strategies encompassing individualized oocyte number) patients: Low and high embryo aneuploidy risk.

In addition to serving as a counseling tool, POSEIDON criteria should be used to optimize the follicle-to-oocyte index (FOI) for higher reproductive outcome.

- *Group 1 and 2* patients show an unexpected suboptimal/poor oocyte yield, probably due to a low FOI. These groups should individualize the ovarian stimulation along with higher gonadotropin doses in order to increase the number of oocytes retrieved.[8]
- *Group 3 and 4* patients with an expected low oocyte number also benefit from individualized regimens with focus on some pharmacological interventions along with oocyte/embryo accumulation.[9]

CONCLUSION

The recently established POSEIDON group is a new and more detailed stratification of low prognosis patients undergoing IVF. It aims to fine tune the management of POR for better outcomes.

"Low prognosis" seems to be an ideal terminology as it stratifies the patients into distinct categories based on quantitative and qualitative parameters and also prognosticates each group and helps in individualizing the treatment protocols per the patient group.[10]

This group also emphasizes the importance of oocyte quantity and age-related embryo euploidy in planning treatment protocols. Based on this, they introduced a new measure of clinical success, i.e., the ability to retrieve the number of oocytes which are required to obtain at least one euploid blastocyst for transfer.

In a nutshell, this new definition provides a more nuanced picture of DOR by using clinically relevant criteria in guiding the clinician for management of these patients.

Hopefully, this new classification system will help in improving pregnancy outcomes and reducing the time to pregnancy and live birth.

REFERENCES

1. Abu-Musa A, Haahr T, Humaidan P. Novel physiology and definition of poor ovarian response; clinical recommendations. Int J Mol Sci. 2020;21:2110.
2. Ferraretti AP, La Marca A, Fauser BC, Tarlatzis B, Nargund G, Gianaroli L. ESHRE consensus on the definition of 'poor response' to ovarian stimulation for in vitro fertilization: the Bologna criteria. Hum Reprod. 2011;26:1616-24.
3. Papathanasiou A, Searle BJ, King NM, Bhattacharya S. Trends in 'poor responder' research: lessons learned from RCTs in assisted conception. Hum Reprod Update. 2016;22:306-19.
4. Ferraretti AP, Gianaroli L. The Bologna criteria for the definition of poor ovarian responders: is there a need for revision? Hum Reprod. 2014;29(9):1842-5.
5. Esteves SC, Alviggi C, Humaidan P, Fischer R, Andersen CY, Conforti A, et al. The POSEIDON criteria and its measure of success through the eyes of clinicians and embryologists. Front Endocrinol; 2019.
6. Esteves SC, Roque M, Bedoschi GM, Conforti A, Humaidan P, Alviggi C. Defining low prognosis patients undergoing assisted reproductive technology: POSEIDON criteria—the why. Front Endocrinol. 2018;9:461.
7. Alviggi C, Andersen CY, Buehler K, Conforti A, De Placido G, Esteves SC, et al. POSEIDON group (patient-oriented strategies encompassing individualized Oocyte Number), A new more detailed stratification of low responders to ovarian stimulation: from a poor ovarian response to a low prognosis concept. Fertil Steril. 2016;105:1452-3.
8. Drakopoulos P, Blockeel C, Stoop D, Camus M, de Vos M, Tournaye H, et al. Conventional ovarian stimulation and single embryo transfer for IVF/ICSI. How many oocytes do we need to maximize cumulative live birth rates after utilization of all fresh and frozen embryos? Hum Reprod. 2016;31:370-6.
9. Vaiarelli A, Cimadomo D, Trabucco E, Vallefuoco R, Buffo L, Dusi L, et al. Double stimulation in the same ovarian cycle (DuoStim) to maximize the number of oocytes retrieved from poor prognosis patients: A multicenter experience and SWOT analysis. Front Endocrinol (Lausanne). 2018;9:317.
10. Cohen J, Chabbert-Buffet N, Darai E. Diminished ovarian reserve, premature ovarian failure, poor ovarian responder—aplea for universal definitions. J Assist Reprod Genet. 2015;32:1709-12.

CHAPTER 23

Pre-In Vitro Fertilization Evaluation

Sangeeta Tajpuriya, Umesh Sawarkar

INTRODUCTION

In vitro fertilization (IVF) a 4-decade old process, still has a success rate of 35–40% only.

Pre-IVF evaluation holds a very crucial step to increase the success rate and avoiding complications.

A checklist should be made available, so that entire team comprising nurse, counselor, physician (consultant), and embryologist can go through it before planning of the IVF cycle.

Evaluation would consist of two parts:
1. General evaluation
2. Reproductive system evaluation

GENERAL EVALUATION

Woman's general conditions, her basic investigations, and medical fitness for pregnancy and delivery are must before starting treatment for IVF.

General

Lifestyle factors play an important role in maximizing IVF outcome:
- Woman's body mass index (BMI) plays a very important role, as obesity is a state of oxidation stress and achieving ideal BMI by lifestyle modification will increase IVF results.
- General health of couple:
  - Blood group Rhesus (Rh) type
  - Hemoglobin (Hb) electrophoresis
  - Human immunodeficiency virus (HIV), hepatitis B surface antigen (HBsAg), hepatitis C, and venereal disease research laboratory (VDRL).
  - Thyroid-stimulating hormone (TSH) prolactin and related hormones

All these will help to identify the couple at risk and would help to prevent an offspring being born after so much efforts to be at risk for a serious and fatal disease:
- Woman should be screened for her rubella immunization status and vaccination can be advised if found nonimmune. General health

screening such as Pap smear and mammogram, electrocardiogram (ECG), and X-ray are advisable for woman aged 40 years and above.
- Stress, anxiety, and depression have been associated with IVF success rate. These mental states have to be dealt with counseling to overcome and improve the success rate.

Vitamin D level, thyroid, and prolactin hormones are essential hormones for the well being of woman at cellular level and hence required to be evaluated for increasing the IVF success rates.

REPRODUCTIVE SYSTEM EVALUATION

Assessment of Oocytes Quantity and Quality

Ovarian Reserve Test

Anti-Müllerian hormone (AMH) helps to predict the future status of woman, regarding ovarian response. It can be measured on any day of the menstrual cycle. It denotes primordial, primary follicle, secondary follicle, small antral follicle (AF), and large AF reserve of ovary.

Antral Follicle Count

Antral follicle count (AFC) denotes the present status of ovarian reserve. It is the AF which responds to ovarian stimulation. (Accordingly AFC count of 8–12 in each ovary is considered normal and anything below and above are considered low and high responder respectively.)

According to AFC, a woman is categorized into three groups:

1. Low responder   <10/ovary
2. Normal responder   10–12
3. Hyper responder   >12/ovary

Day 2 Follicle-stimulating Hormone and Estradiol
- Day 2 FSH level helps to formulate the ovarian stimulation protocol.
- Any level >10 mIU predicts poor response to stimulation.
- Day 2 FSH if coupled with serum E2 level will help to identify woman with accelerated follicular development and will help to predict poor responder to ovarian stimulation.

Tubal Abnormalities

Presence of hydrosalpinx, which is diagnosed by transvaginal sonography (TVS), should always be removed before IVF.

Studies have concluded a 50% reduction in live birth rate (LBR), in woman with hydrosalpinx as compared to woman with no hydrosalpinx.[1]

Salpingectomy or proximal occlusion has equal efficacy, either can be opted according to the patient profile.

Uterine Cavity

Transvaginal sonography and three-dimensional (3D) ultrasound have almost eliminated the need of routine endoscopy before IVF or ET. Color Doppler of the endometrium can evaluate spiral arterial blood flow which should be a low resistance flow. A thorough evaluation of uterine cavity is must. Direct visualization of uterine cavity by hysteroscopy enables one to diagnose endometritis and minute polyps as small as <1 cm, removal of such polyps has shown a higher pregnancy rate.[2] Uterine septum should be excised.

Semen Analysis

Semen analysis as per the World Health Organization (WHO) 2010 and WHO 2020 criteria is required to assess the semen quality.

There are three basic requirements:
1. Quantity
2. Morphology
3. Mortality

These are required to categorize into an IVF or intracytoplasmic sperm injection (ICSI) cycle.

Case of unexplained failure of fertilization may be due to unrecognized minute abnormalities of sperm morphology which can be subjected to ICSI in an otherwise normal semen count.

DNA Fragmentation Index

Although high DNA fragmentation index (DFI) is associated with abnormal sperm parameters, in unexplained infertility or infertility of long duration even with normal sperm parameters, a high level of DNA fragmentation may still persist **(Flowchart 1)**.

Treatment with antioxidant therapy for 3 months significantly reduces the DFI.[3]

Advising testicular sperm retrieval to a man with a very high DFI after all treatments also helps in choosing sperm with low DFI as level of fragmentation in testicular sperm averaged 5% compared to 24% in the ejaculate.

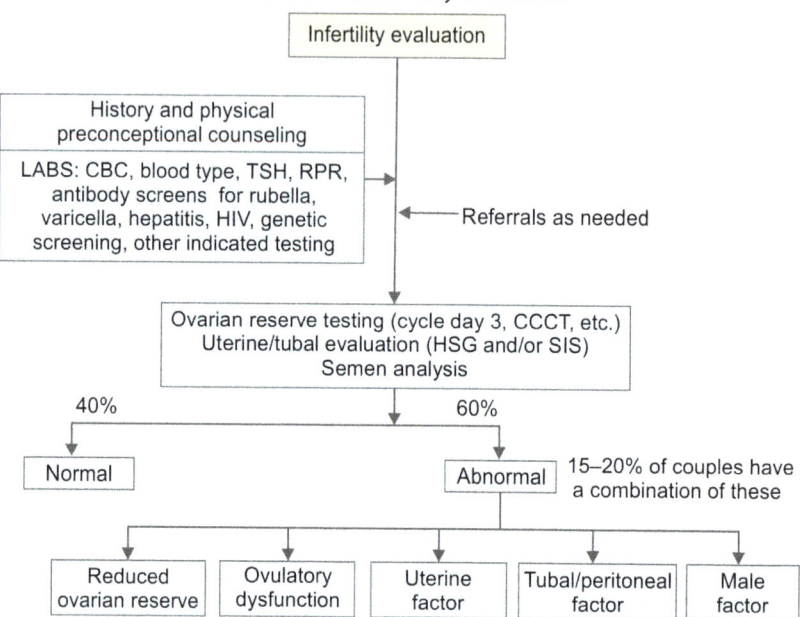

Flowchart 1: Infertility evaluation.

(CBC: complete blood count; CCCT: clomiphene citrate challenge test; HSG: hysterosalpingography; SIS: saline infusion sonohysterography; TSH: thyroid-stimulating hormone; RPR: rapid plasma regain)

REFERENCES

1. Camus E, Poncelet C, Goffinet F, Wainer B, Merlet F, Nisand I, et al. Pregnancy rates after in vitro fertilization in cases of tubal infertility with and without hydrosalpinx: a meta-analysis of published comparative studies. Hum Reprod. 1999;14(5):1243-9.
2. Perez-Medina T, Bajo-Arenas J, Salazar F, Redondo T, Sanfrutos L, Alvarez P, et al. Endometrial polyps and their implication in the pregnancy rates of patient undergoing intrauterine insemination: a prospective, randomized study. Hum Reprod. 2005;20(6):1632-5.
3. Greco E, Iacobelli M, Rienzi L, Ubaldi F, Ferrero S, Tesarik J. Reduction of the incidence of sperm DNA fragmentation by oral antioxidant treatment. J Androl. 2005;26(3):349-53.

CHAPTER 24: Ovarian Stimulation in Normal Responders

Sanjeev Madhav Khurd, Aditya Khurd, Sadhana Khurd

INTRODUCTION

Ovarian stimulation is at the top of the list of the various treatments that are offered to infertile couples, to increase their lowered chance at conception, and enable them to achieve their goal of having a baby. In women who have anovulatory infertility, any intervention that induces ovulation will help them to get pregnant, as an obvious problem gets corrected. But even women, who ovulate on regular basis, stand to benefit from ovarian stimulation and improve upon their chance of conception, as it enhances their ovulation, effects multiple follicular developments, and corrects subtle luteal phase defects, to favor implantation. Ovarian stimulation is often combined with timed intercourse, intrauterine insemination (IUI) or in vitro fertilization (IVF), as compelling evidence suggests that the combination of treatments increases the success rate even further. Since we deal with women of different ages, who are infertile due to a variety of different causes, their response to ovarian stimulation is bound to be highly variable. Also, there is cycle to cycle variation as well. In such a scenario, the anticipated response to ovarian stimulation is either normal, hyper or poor and study of patient's profile, sonographic and laboratory markers help clinicians to predict response and categorize women as normal, hyper and poor responders. Therefore, instead of having a standard "one-size-fits-all" line of treatment, the treating physician can design individualized ovarian stimulation protocols that are tailor made for that particular clinical situation, to effect the desired and optimum response which would then translate into better pregnancy outcomes, with minimization of risks.

DESIRED AND OPTIMUM RESPONSE TO OVARIAN STIMULATION

The desired response to ovarian stimulation will vary according to the clinical situation at hand and has to be planned with the selection of the appropriate drugs, planning and making adjustments in their doses and the duration they are given. Also, the desired response needs to be optimum, convenient and cost-effective as well. To achieve this desired and optimum response, the ovarian stimulation needs to be just appropriate to achieve the best results at pregnancy success and at the same time ensure safety, avoiding its possible complications.

In women who have chronic anovulation or oligo-ovulation, e.g., polycystic ovarian syndrome (PCOS), the aim is to produce just one mature oocyte every cycle, to achieve a pregnancy and at the same time avoiding chance of multiple pregnancy. However, in women who are undergoing IUI, the strategy is superovulation, with the plan to have two or three mature oocytes to ovulate. Superovulation therefore, does increase the chance of conception, as more than one oocyte are now available for fertilization. However, there is an increased risk of multiple pregnancy as well and the couple needs to be counselled appropriately regarding this important aspect.

In women who are on the IVF program, we aim to retrieve 10–15 mature oocytes which will optimize their cumulative pregnancy rate, by offering additional chances to conceive with fresh and/or frozen embryo transfer cycles as the need be. In this case we need to plan the ovarian stimulation which is not only optimum, but also a controlled one as well, so as to avoid the risk of potentially life-threatening ovarian hyperstimulation syndrome (OHSS). Limiting the number of embryos to be transferred will decrease the chance of multiple pregnancies and a single embryo transfer will prevent it all together.

FACTORS AFFECTING OVARIAN RESPONSE

While designing ovarian stimulation strategies we need to be aware of the factors affecting ovarian response. Following are the factors which affect the response to ovarian stimulation and have to be taken into account for planning and making adjustments in doses of the drugs and duration of stimulation.

Age and Ovarian Reserve

Woman's age is one of the most important determinants of the response to ovarian stimulation and success at achieving pregnancy, as it affects both, ovarian reserve and the quality of the oocytes.

Ovarian reserve is the number of oocytes in the residual pool in the ovaries. Anti-Müllerian hormone (AMH), antral follicle count (AFC) and follicle-stimulating hormone (FSH) give insights into the number of oocytes, while the woman's age largely determines their quality.

Women are born with a finite number of oocytes, 10–20 lakhs at birth, and as they advance in age, this number continuously declines, reducing to 2–5 lakhs at puberty to reaching as low as 8,000 by the time they reach the age of 40. Besides the reduction in number, more important is the fact that as their age advances, the residual pool of oocytes has an increasingly higher percentage of chromosomally abnormal oocytes. Till the age of 35 years, the chromosomally abnormal oocytes constitute about 25% of the oocyte pool and this dramatically increases to >90% when they cross 40 years of age. These chromosomally abnormal oocytes do not respond well to FSH and luteinizing hormone (LH), which is the cause of their declining fertility and increased miscarriage rates, thereby generally making women with advance age respond poorly to ovarian stimulation.

Younger women, due to their good ovarian reserve of chromosomally normal oocytes, are expected to respond well to FSH and LH and are therefore categorized as normal responders.

Sensitivity to FSH and LH

There is a subset of women who have increased sensitivity to FSH and LH and therefore respond excessively to ovarian stimulation and are categorized as hyper responders. Women who have PCOS belong to this subset and require lower doses of the drugs.

FSH Receptor Pleomorphism

Women with FSH receptor pleomorphism are less sensitive and require higher doses of FSH.

Body Mass Index

Women with higher body mass index (BMI) require higher doses of the drugs.

Previous Surgery on the Ovaries

For example, excision of ovarian cyst may negatively affect ovarian reserve.

Pelvic Infection and Oopheritis

For example, genital tuberculosis; higher doses of the drugs are required.

Previous Chemotherapy

Radiation negatively affects ovarian reserve.

GnRH Agonist and GnRH Antagonist Protocols in IVF

Gonadotropin-releasing hormone (GnRH) agonist protocol requires higher doses and longer duration of ovarian stimulation.

DRUGS FOR OVARIAN STIMULATION

Oral Ovulogens
- *Antiestrogens:* Clomiphene citrate, tamoxifen
- *Aromatase inhibitors:* Letrozole, anastrozole

Clomiphene citrate and letrozole are the most commonly used oral ovulogens. Both effect the release of FSH and LH from the pituitary gland, resulting in recruitment and growth of follicle/follicles. Letrozole (2.5-5 mg daily for 5 days) is the drug of first choice to induce ovulation in women with PCOS.[1] Letrozole usually results in mono-ovulation and gives superior pregnancy rate in comparison with clomiphene. Clomiphene (50-150 mg daily for 5 days) causes a higher incidence of multiple ovulations and therefore preferred for superovulation.[2] Combining clomiphene with gonadotropin, reduces the gonadotropin dose and the overall cost of stimulation.

Injectable Gonadotropins

- Follicle-stimulating hormone
- Human menopausal gonadotropin (hMG)
- Human chorionic gonadotropin (hCG)

All gonadotropins (urinary and recombinant) have the same live birth rates.[3] Choice of gonadotropin will depend on availability and cost of the drugs.

Gonadotropin (FSH, hMG) stimulation results in growth of multiple follicles. FSH recruits the follicles and keeping the FSH levels above the threshold ensures continued growth of the recruited follicles. With longer duration of FSH stimulation, more number of follicles are recruited and supported in their growth, causing multifollicular development, which is desired for superovulation and IVF cycles. hCG is a surrogate LH and causes final maturation of the oocytes and ruptures the follicles.

SUPEROVULATION FOR INTRAUTERINE INSEMINATION CYCLE

Menstrual Cycle

Day 2: Baseline sonography for AFC
- Rule out residual ovarian cysts from previous cycle, before starting ovarian stimulation.
- If residual cyst is present, do not give any ovarian stimulation. You may advice the couple to have coitus during the "fertile week"
  - Day 10 to day 17 and attempt natural conception.
- If pregnancy does not occur, then ask the patient to come for recheck sonography on day 2 of next menstrual cycle, to confirm that there is no cyst seen on scan, before proceeding for ovarian stimulation.
- Residual cyst/cysts from previous cycles usually regress in 2-3 months. Do not give oral contraceptive pill (OCP) with the aim to hasten regression of the cyst, as it will prevent a possible natural conception.

Days 2 to 6:
- *Tablet Clomiphene Citrate:* 50/100 mg—1 tablet daily × 5 days or
- *Tablet Letrozole:* 2.5/5 mg—1 tablet daily × 5 days

Days 2 to 6:
- Injection hMG 75 IU daily

Day 9 onwards:
- Monitor growth of the dominant follicle/follicles on sonography.
  - Follicles grow 1-2 mm/day. 2 or 3 follicles are expected to show dominance.
  - *Ovulation trigger:* When follicles reach a size of 18-23 mm and endometrial thickness 7 mm and above; injection hCG 5,000 IU given for final maturation of the oocytes and triggers ovulation.
  - *IUI:* Planned 36-44 hours after injection hCG trigger.
  - *Confirm:* Ovulation with rupture of follicle/follicles and fluid in the pelvis.
  - *Luteal phase support:* Progesterone is given for a period of 15 days, till the day of pregnancy test, when 2 or more follicles rupture. Luteal phase support is not required if only one follicle ovulates.

CONTROLLED OVARIAN STIMULATION FOR IVF/ICSI WITH GnRH ANTAGONIST PROTOCOL

Menstrual Cycle

Day 2:
- Baseline sonography for AFC
- Rule out residual ovarian cysts

Days 2 to 5:
- Injection FSH/hMG 225-300 IU daily

Day 6 onwards:
- Check follicular recruitment and growth
- Step up gonadotropin dose if required
- Monitor growth of follicles and when follicles reach size of 13-14 mm, start injection GnRH antagonist (cetrorelix 0.25 mg) daily, along with gonadotropins

Days 9 to 11:
- Monitor growth of follicles and when they reach a size of 17-23 mm and endometrial thickness of 7 mm and above
- Injection hCG 5,000-10,000 IU or recombinant hCG 250 µg trigger is given for final maturation of oocytes *or*
- Injection GnRH agonist trigger (leuprolide acetate 2 mg or treptorelin 0.2 mg) is given if a hyper-response is observed
- Usually 10 days of ovarian stimulation suffices for GnRH antagonist protocol

Day 13/14:
- Oocyte retrieval is timed 34-36 hours after hCG/GnRH agonist trigger followed by IVF/ICSI.

Day 16/17:
- Embryo transfer of day 3 embryos

Day 18/19:
- Embryo transfer of day 5 embryos
- *Luteal phase support* with progesterone started from the day of oocyte retrieval and continued for 15 days after embryo transfer, till day of pregnancy test.

CONTROLLED OVARIAN STIMULATION FOR IVF/ICSI WITH LONG GnRH AGONIST PROTOCOL

Pre-IVF Cycle

Menstrual Cycle

Day 10:
- Oral contraceptive pill (OCP) daily for 21 days.

Day 21:
- Injection GnRH agonist (leuprolide acetate: 0.5 mg) daily
- Menses start after stopping OCP

IVF cycle

Down regulation is confirmed by the following criteria:
- Endometrial thickness <5 mm
- Estradiol <50 pg/mL
- Injection GnRH agonist is continued at half dose (leuprolide acetate 0.25 mg) daily, till the day of injection hCG trigger.

Ovarian Stimulation

Day 1:
- Baseline sonography for AFC
- Start injection FSH/hMG 225–300 IU daily

Day 5/6:
- Check follicular recruitment and growth
- Step up gonadotropin dose if required

Day 11/12:
- Monitor growth of follicles and when they reach a size of 17–23 mm and endometrial thickness of 7 mm and above
- Injection hCG 10,000 IU or recombinant hCG 250 µg trigger is given for final maturation of oocytes
- Usually 12 days of ovarian stimulation is necessary for GnRH agonist cycle

Day 13/14:
- Oocyte retrieval is timed 34–36 hours after hCG trigger followed by IVF/ICSI

Day 16/17:
- Embryo transfer of day 3 embryos

Day 18/19:
- Embryo transfer of day 5 embryos
- *Luteal phase support* with progesterone started from the day of oocyte retrieval and continued for 15 days after embryo transfer, till the day of pregnancy test.

REFERENCES

1. Franik S, Kremer JAM, Nelen WLDM, Farquhar C. Aromatase inhibitor for subfertility treatment in women with polycystic ovary syndrome: Summary of a Cochrane review. Fertil Steril. 2015;103(2):1-9.
2. Cantineau AE, Cohlen BJ. Ovarian stimulation protocols (anti-estrogens, gonadotrophins with and without GnRH agonists/antagonists) for intrauterine insemination in women with subfertility. Cochrane Database Syst Rev. 2007:CD005356.
3. van Wely M, Kwan I, Burt AL, Thomas J, Vail A, Van der Veen F, et al. Recombinant versus urinary gonadotrophins for ovarian hyperstimulation in IVF or ICSI cycles. Cochrane Database Syst Rev. 2011(2):CD00534.

25 | Preinduction Adjuvants

Paresh Gandecha, Shalaka Mamidwar

INTRODUCTION

The term "adjuvant therapy" is used for the agents, tools or procedures that can be implemented alongside the core assisted reproductive techniques. For usages convenience, we have divided these adjuvants in following four groups:

1. *For hyper-responders:* Metformin and myoinositol (MI)
2. *For poor responders:* Dehydroepiandrosterone (DHEA), testosterone and growth hormones (GH)
3. *For normal responders:* Antioxidants, folic acid
4. *For all:* Corticosteroids, estrogen, aspirin, low-molecular-weight heparin (LMWH)

METFORMIN

- *Use:* Polycystic ovary syndrome (PCOS—obese/insulin resistant)
- *Mode of action:* It is insulin-sensitizing agent. It increases the sensitivity of peripheral tissues to insulin. It inhibits gluconeogenesis and increases glucose uptake by peripheral tissues and reduces fatty acid oxidation. It has positive effect on endometrium. It restores ovulation, reduces weight, reduces circulating androgen levels, reduces risk of miscarriage, and reduces risk of gestational diabetes mellitus (GDM). The available evidence also suggests that metformin may have some beneficial effect in women with PCOS by reducing risk of ovarian hyperstimulation syndrome (OHSS) and increasing pregnancy rates.
- *Doses:* Starting dose 500 mg/day *increase to:* 1,500 mg/day.
- *Benefits:*
  - Reduction in risk of OHSS
  - Metformin may improve endometrial receptivity (ER) in PCOS patients by increasing endometrial thickness (EMT) and reducing endometrial artery resistance index (RI).[1]

Recommendations (PCOS Evidence-based Guidelines 2018)[2]

1. *Evidence-based recommendation (EBR):* Metformin, in addition to lifestyle, could be recommended in adult women with PCOS, for the treatment of weight, hormonal, and metabolic outcomes.
2. *EBR:* Metformin, in addition to lifestyle, should be considered in adult women with PCOS with body mass index (BMI) ≥ 25 kg/m^2 for management of weight and metabolic outcomes.
3. *EBR:* Metformin, in addition to lifestyle, could be considered in adolescents with a clear diagnosis of PCOS or with symptoms of PCOS before the diagnosis is made.
4. *Clinical practice point (CPP):* Metformin may offer greater benefit in high metabolic risk groups including those with diabetes risk factors, impaired glucose tolerance or high-risk ethnic groups.

Cochrane Database 2020[3]

1. No conclusive evidence that metformin improves live birth rates.
2. In a long gonadotropin-releasing hormone (GnRH)-agonist cycles, metformin may increase the clinical pregnancy rate.
3. Metformin may reduce the incidence of OHSS but may result in a higher incidence of side effects.
4. Uncertain of the effect of metformin on miscarriage rate per woman.

MYOINOSITOL

- *Uses:* Used for metabolic syndrome and PCOS. It lowers triglyceride and testosterone levels, improves insulin resistance and helps in ovulation.
- *Mode of action:* It mediates all signal transduction in response to various hormones, neurotransmitters, growth factors and helps these factors in binding their receptors.
- *Doses:* Used as dietary supplementation in management of PCOS. 4 g per day (2 g twice per day).
- *Evidence:* Minimal evidence suggesting its efficiency in increasing fertility in women with PCOS.

Myoinositol 3 months prior to ovarian stimulation, is effective in normalizing ovarian function, improving oocyte and embryo quality in PCOS.[4]

Recommendations (PCOS Evidence-based Guidelines 2018)[2]

1. *EBR:* Inositol (in any form) should currently be considered an experimental therapy in PCOS, with emerging evidence on efficacy highlighting the need for further research.
2. *CPP:* Women taking inositol and other complementary therapies are encouraged to advise their health professional.

Cochrane Database 2018[5]

1. Uncertain whether MI improves live birth rate or clinical pregnancy rate in subfertile women with PCOS undergoing IVF pretreatment taking MI compared to standard treatment.
2. It is also uncertain whether MI decreases miscarriage rates or multiple pregnancy rates for these same women taking MI compared to standard treatment.

DEHYDROEPIANDROSTERONE

- *Uses:* In poor ovarian reserve and poor responders.
- *Mode of action:* It enhances follicular function by increasing the production of insulin-like growth factor-1 (IGF-1) and augmenting estradiol production ion granulose cells acting as precursor of androstenedione and testosterone in theca cells. It improves the number of antral follicles available for stimulation.
- *Dose:* 75 mg/day for 2–3 months prior to planned conception.

ESHRE Guidelines 2019[6]

Recommendations: Use of DHEA before and/or during ovarian stimulation is probably not recommended for poor responders (Conditional).

This is due to inconsistent evidence that adjuvant DHEA use before and during ovarian stimulation improves ovarian response in terms of live birth/ongoing pregnancy rate in poor responders undergoing IVF treatment. The studies varied in duration of DHEA treatment, possibly contributing toward the inconsistence in observed results.

Recent Randomized Clinical Trial: Listed in Cochrane 2020[7]

Ovarian stimulation after DHEA supplementation in poor ovarian reserve: A randomized clinical trial was conducted by Elprince et al.

It concluded that DHEA may help many poor responders, so better considered for poor responder patients.

TESTOSTERONE

- *Use:* Poor responders
- *Doses:* Transdermally—Testosterone Gel or patches
  - 10 mg/day or 12.5 mg/day of testosterone gel for 15–21 days during pituitary downregulation Or
  - 2.5 mg testosterone patches for 5 days during pituitary downregulation preceding gonadotropin stimulation.

ESHRE Guidelines 2019[6]

Recommendations: Use of testosterone before ovarian stimulation is probably not recommended for poor responders. Conditional ⊕⊕⊕☐

Cochrane Database 2015[8]

A Cochrane meta-analysis investigated the effect of testosterone pretreatment before ovarian stimulation in poor responder women and reported improved live birth rate with testosterone pretreatment (4 RCT, OR 2.60, 95% CI 1.30–5.20, 345 women) (Nagels et al., 2015). However, in a sensitivity analysis, removing all studies at high risk of performance bias as there was no evidence of an association between pretreatment with testosterone and improved live birth rates in the remaining study.

GROWTH HORMONES

- *Use:* Poor responders.
- *Mode of action:* Regulate the effect of FSH on granulosa cells by increasing IGF-1 and have a role in ovarian function including follicle development, estrogen synthesis and oocyte maturation.
- *Doses:* Started on first day of ovulation induction, given daily or on alternate days. 8–24 IU/day. Doses as low as 0.5 IU/day are also seen to be effective.
- *Evidence:* Clinical pregnancy rates are better than live birth rates only in poor responders.

ESHRE Guidelines 2019[6]

Use of adjuvant growth hormone before and/or during ovarian stimulation is probably not recommended for poor responders. Conditional ⊕⊕☐☐

Cochrane Database 2010[9]

A Cochrane meta-analysis including 80 women considered as normal responder undergoing IVF treatment reported no significant difference in live birth rate (2 RCT, OR 1.32, 95% CI 0.40–4.43) with routine use of GH in women undergoing IVF treatment compared to placebo (Duffy et al., 2010).

ANTIOXIDANTS

- *Use:* Prevention of negative effect due to oxidative stress, which can lead to cell membrane damage, lipid peroxidation, cellular protein oxidation and DNA damage.
- *Mode of action:* They counteract the negative impact of oxygen free radicals by acting as free radical scavengers.
- *Evidence:* A very low quality evidence of increased pregnancy rates and increased live birth rates.

FOLIC ACID

- *Use:* It is used not exactly to increase pregnancy rates or implantation rate, but used to prevent neural tube defects (NTD) in baby to be born.
- *Mode of action:* It is involved the regulation of homocysteine metabolism.
- *Dose:* 5 mg/day is standard recommended dose.

Note: Newer drugs like L-Methylfolate claim to more effective in patients with MTHFR mutation.

ASPIRIN

- *Use:* Thought to improve ovarian flow and stimulation outcome. It improves implantation rate.
- *Mode of action:* It inhibits cyclooxygenase enzyme in platelets and reduction of prostaglandin synthesis. It may enhance endometrial receptivity and improve implantation rates.
- *Doses:* Daily administration in doses of 150 mg/day causes a shift from thromboxane A2 to prostacyclin leading to vasodilatation and increased peripheral blood flow.
- *Evidence:* There is lack of proven efficiency for routine use of aspirin as adjuvant.

ESHRE Guidelines 2019[6]

Use of aspirin before and/or during ovarian stimulation is not recommended in the general in vitro fertilization (IVF)/intracytoplasmic sperm injection (ICSI) population and for poor responders. Strong ⊕⊕⊕☐

The existing evidence suggests that adjuvant aspirin before and/or during ovarian stimulation does not improve ovarian response in terms of number of oocytes retrieved and clinical outcomes of clinical or ongoing pregnancy, or live birth rates following IVF treatment.

Cochrane Database 2016[10]

A Cochrane meta-analysis combining three RCTs with 1,053 women reported no significant difference in the live birth rate (3 RCT, RR 0.91, 95% CI 0.72–1.15) or ongoing pregnancy rate (2 RCT, RR 0.94, 95% CI 0.69–1.27) between the aspirin and the control group.

LOW-MOLECULAR-WEIGHT HEPARIN

- *Use:* It is to be used in recurrent implantation failure and thrombophilia cases.
- *Mode of action:* LMWH may facilitate implantation process by downregulating the E-cadherin expression in the decidua.
- *Dose:* Enoxaparin 40 mg/day.

CORTICOSTEROIDS

- *Use:* In PCOS cases during simulation, especially cases of hyperandrogenism (clinical and biochemical). Also, in cases of repeated IVF failures and recurrent miscarriages.
- *Mode of action:* Anti-inflammatory and immune modulator.
- *Dose:* Methylprednisolone 10–60 mg/day.

ESTROGEN

- *Use:* Pretreatment to ovulation induction to synchronize follicular growth. Also, to increase endometrial thickness.
- *Mode of action:* Reduces endogenous FSH rise and follicular recruitment till stimulation is started.
- *Dose:* Estradiol valerate 4–6 mg/day.
- *Limitation:* No evidence of a beneficial effect on live birth rate/ongoing pregnancy rate using estrogen as pretreatment in GnRH antagonist protocol.

ESHRE Guidelines 2019[6]

Pretreatment with estrogen before ovarian stimulation using the GnRH antagonist protocol is probably not recommended for improving efficacy and safety. Conditional ⊕☐☐☐

There is no evidence of a beneficial effect on live birth rate/ongoing pregnancy rate using estrogen as pretreatment in GnRH antagonist protocol, compared to no pretreatment. The evidence regarding the effect of estradiol pretreatment on the number of oocytes retrieved is conflicting.

CONCLUSION

We need to use specific adjuvant in specific patients, some have strong evidence in support to its use in specific situation and some have weak to poor evidence in support to their use. We need to rationalize and individualize our approach while treating our infertility patients with adjuvant as we do for our stimulation protocol.

REFERENCES

1. Yuan L, Wu H, Huang W, Bi Y, Qin A, Yang Y. The function of metformin in endometrial receptivity (ER) of patients with polycyclic ovary syndrome (PCOS): a systematic review and meta-analysis. Reprod Biol Endocrinol. 2021;19(1):89.
2. Teede HJ, Misso ML, Costello MF, Dokras A, Laven J, Moran L, et al. Recommendations from the international evidence-based guideline for the assessment and management of polycystic ovary syndrome. Hum Reprod. 2018;33(9):1602-18.
3. Tso LO, Costello MF, Albuquerque LET, Andriolo RB, Macedo CR. Metformin treatment before and during IVF or ICSI in women with polycystic ovary syndrome. Cochrane Database Syst Rev. 2020;12: CD006105.

4. Merviel P, James P, Bouée S, Le Guillou M, Rince C, Nachtergaele C, et al. Impact of myoinositol treatment in women with polycystic ovary syndrome in assisted reproductive technologies. Reprod Health. 2021;18:13.
5. Showell MG, Mackenzie-Proctor R, Jordan V, Hodgson R, Farquhar C. Inositol for subfertile women with polycystic ovary syndrome. Cochrane Database Syst Rev. 2018;12:CD012378.
6. ESHRE. (2019). Ovarian stimulation for IVF/ICSI. [online] Available from: https://www.eshre.eu/-/media/sitecore-files/Guidelines/COS/ESHRE-COS-guideline_for-stakeholder-review_versie-2.pdf?la=en&hash=461B6F7899B5D272FB7AC8AD98892E82777A3461. [Last Accessed May, 2022].
7. Elprince M, Kishk EA, Metawie OM, Albiely MM. Ovarian stimulation after dehydroepiandrosterone supplementation in poor ovarian reserve: a randomized clinical trial. Arch Gynecol Obstet. 2020;302(2):529-34
8. Nagels HE, Rishworth JR, Siristatidis CS, Kroon B. Androgens (dehydroepiandrosterone or testosterone) for women undergoing assisted reproduction. Cochrane Database Syst Rev. 2015:Cd009749.
9. Duffy JM, Ahmad G, Mohiyiddeen L, Nardo LG, Watson A. Growth hormone for in vitro fertilization. Cochrane Database Syst Rev. 2010:Cd000099.
10. Siristatidis CS, Basios G, Pergialiotis V, Vogiatzi P. Aspirin for in vitro fertilisation. Cochrane Database Syst Rev. 2016;11:Cd004832.

CHAPTER 26

Various Ovarian Stimulation Protocols and their Clinical Significance

Sanjay Gupte, Sachin Jadhav

INTRODUCTION

The goals of protocols have changed from "one size fits all" to tailor-made plans nuanced to patient's needs.

Optimal ovarian stimulation protocol should:
- Synchronize growth maximizing oocyte yield: A Dutch Group (van der Gaast MH, et al.) proved that the average number of oocytes required to achieve highest number of pregnancy/embryo transfer (ET) was 13.1 and no improvement beyond this.[1]

    Another study by Datta AK and Law YJ et al., observed that the retrieval of 12–18 oocytes is associated with maximal fresh live birth rate (LBR), and a strong positive association was noted between number of oocytes retrieved and CBR.[2,3]

    Recent studies positively correlated between the number of oocytes retrieved and the number of euploid embryos, therefore affirming no detrimental effect of hyper ovarian response on embryo euploidy rates.[4]

- Prevent ovarian hyperstimulation syndrome: Ovarian hyperstimulation syndrome (OHSS) though it is uncommon, but is a serious complication associated with assisted reproductive technology.

    1–5% of assisted reproductive technology (ART) cycles are affected with moderate to severe OHSS.[5]

- *Prevent premature luteinizing hormone (LH) surge and premature elevation of progesterone:* Incidence of premature LH surge is high with short or ultrashort protocol—almost 12% and is Reduced to <1–2% in long agonist or multidose antagonist protocol.

    Premature elevation of progesterone is associated with lower clinical pregnancy rates in fresh cycles and was detrimental to LBRs. A high serum estradiol concentration on the day of human chorionic gonadotropin (hCG) administration did not affect the in vitro fertilization (IVF) pregnancy outcome.[6]

- *Patient friendly*

OVARIAN STIMULATION PROTOCOLS

The different types of ovarian stimulation protocols are enlisted here.

Conventional

Involve use of high dose gonadotropins >150 IU: The commonly used protocols are the long agonist protocol and the antagonist protocols. The other protocols such as ultralong down regulation, short, and ultrashort flare up protocols are sparingly used in special scenarios.[6,7]

Mild Stimulation In Vitro Fertilization

Encompasses use of lower dose of follicle-stimulating hormone (FSH) or menopausal gonadotropins in antagonist cycles with or without adjuvant role of oral ovulogens in patients with expected poor ovarian response, with the aim of collecting fewer oocytes **(Table 1)**.[7,8]

Standard Agonist Protocols

These involve inhibition of premature LH rise by downregulating the pituitary that requires at least 8 days of administration.[9] Initial FSH flare starts at 4–12 hours and remains elevated for 24–34 hours before downregulation happens and is maintained **(Fig. 1)**.[10]

GnRH Antagonist Protocols

Antagonists competitively block the gonadotropin hormone-releasing hormone (GnRH) at the pituitary and stop release of gonadotropins.

TABLE 1: The comparison of conventional and mild stimulation protocols.[19,32,36]

Conventional stimulation	Mild stimulation
Advantages: • It maximizes the number of oocytes retrieved • The greater number of embryos for cryopreservation • It may help patients complete their family in fewer stimulated cycles • It has higher pregnancy rates per cycle	*Advantages:* • It minimizes the treatment burden and reduces the risk of complications • It has lower doses of gonadotropins and fewer injections • It has possible association with better embryo quality • It has lower per-cycle drop-out rates
Disadvantages: • It has greater patient discomfort and increased risk of complications, including OHSS • It has increased per-cycle costs associated with higher gonadotropin dosage	*Disadvantages:* • It has higher per-cycle cancellation rate; may require multiple stimulated cycles to achieve a pregnancy • It has few embryos available for cryopreservation • It has increased cumulative costs associated with multiple fresh cycles

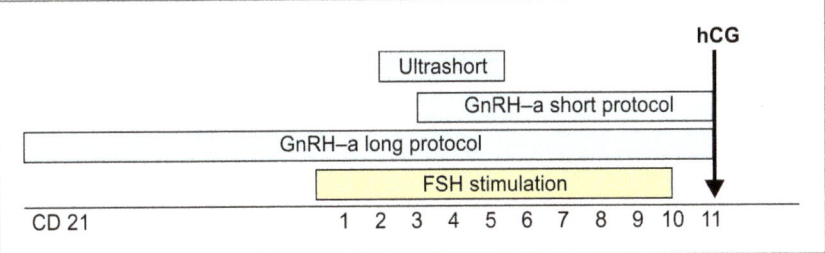

Fig. 1: GnRH agonist protocols.

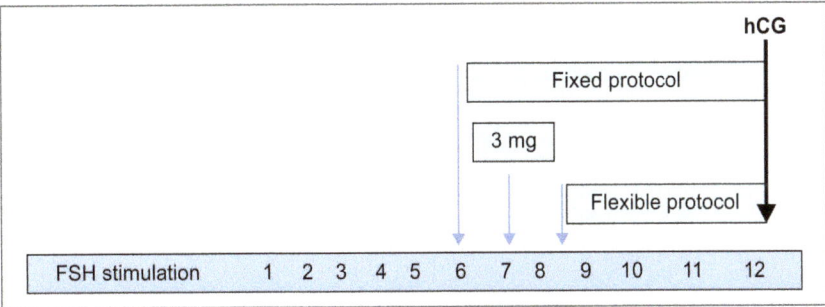

Fig. 2: GnRH antagonist protocols.

A single dose of 0.25 mg acts within 2-4 hours and lasts for 20-22 hours.[12] Usually suppress LH by 75% and FSH by 25% with 6 hours (**Fig. 2**).[11]

Multiple Dose Protocol

Infixed protocol antagonist is started on day 5 or 6 irrespective of the follicular size. In flexible dose it is started when the follicles reach 13-14 mm size.

In good responders, fixed dose protocol produced better clinical pregnancy rates. While flexible dose protocol is used in expected poor responder for better follicular growth.[12]

Single Dose Antagonist

It uses 3 mg of cetrorelix on day 6 commonly. Its action lasts for 4 days. It may cause profound LH suppression. Statistically, it is not different compared with daily dosing.[12]

Follicular cohort synchronization can be done with GnRH antagonists prior to the start of gonadotropins—a new modification protocol for IVF for better recruitment has been recommended with similar results as in agonist downregulation protocol.[13,14]

Cetrorelix versus Ganirelix

With similar pharmacokinetics and dynamics they are equally good in preventing LH surge. Ganirelix was less likely to prevent or reduce the incidence of OHSS.[13] Also, cetrorelix has better pregnancy rates.

Flowchart 1: Different modulations of these phases constitute an individualized COH strategy.

OC pills, estrogen alone, antagonist, and no medicines	Pre-IVF priming
rFSH or hMG, or rFSH + rLH	Gonadotropin stimulation
Agonist protocol of antagonist single of multidose	Control of LH surge with agonist/antagonist
hCG trigger hCG or urinary of GnRH analog	Final oocyte maturation trigger

(COH: controlled ovarian hyperstimulation; hCG: human chorionic gonadotropin; hMG: human menopausal gonadotropin; IVF: in vitro fertilization; LH: luteinizing hormone; OC: oral contraceptive; rFSH: recombinant follicle-stimulating hormone; rLH: recombinant luteinizing hormone)

Agonist Protocol versus Multidose Antagonist

- The clinical outcomes are fare equally well between the two protocols.[15,16]
- The total gonadotropin dose is reduced, and safety is improved.
- In particular, the antagonist protocols have paved a way for OHSS free clinics.
- Also, patient surveys have inclined a preference for antagonist over agonist treatment cycles.
- These benefits made GnRH antagonist-based protocols popular and thus have replaced the agonist treatment protocols in current clinical practice-assisted reproductive techniques.[14]

An ovarian stimulation protocol has four components (our suggested analysis) (in our unique perspective) (**Flowchart 1**).

PRE-IN VITRO FERTILIZATION PRIMING

- *Short priming of OC pills* as compared with direct stimulation on day 2 of the cycle in patients treated with GnRH antagonist and recombinant FSH, appears to be associated with *slightly low* but insignificant difference in ongoing pregnancy rates per started cycle. Secondly it resulted in, a *significant higher early pregnancy loss.*[17]

It was also associated with higher gonadotropin dose requirement.[17,18]

- *Prolonged combined oral contraceptive pill (COCP) pretreatment (>12 days) is not recommended in the GnRH antagonist protocol.* The adverse outcomes in the form of lower live birth/ongoing pregnancy rate have been noted. The Guideline Development Group (GDG) recommends against (12-28 days) COCP pretreatment in GnRH antagonist protocol.[19] Estrogen alone or progestins alone can be used in antagonist cycles without any detrimental effects. It helps in serving the purpose of scheduling cycles, especially in batch IVF. This is probably acceptable by the given data on efficacy and safety. No benefit on live birth rates.
- *In poor responders:* In previous failed cycles, estrogen priming through luteal phase and stimulation phase improved the follicular cohort recruitment and with every additional egg retrieved, the pregnancy rates got improved.[20]

WHICH GONADOTROPIN?

According to MENOPUR® in GnRH Antagonist Cycles with Single Embryo Transfer (MEGASET) trial, highly purified human menopausal gonadotropin (hp-hMG) is as effective in achieving pregnancy as treatment with recombinant follicle-stimulating hormone (rFSH) in GnRH antagonist protocols. Even cumulative pregnancy rates over a period of one 1 year were similar.[21]

In oocyte donation the cycles in luteal phase down regulation protocols human menopausal gonadotropin (hMG) compared with rFSH, recombinant luteinizing hormone (rLH) have provided similar serum and follicular fluid hormonal profiles. Comparable cycle outcome is observed in terms of follicle oocyte index, embryo grading, and clinical pregnancy rates.[22]

The use of hMG in long GnRH agonist cycles was associated with a 3-4% increase in LBRs. There was insufficient evidence to make definitive conclusions on the need for exogenous LH activity in GnRH antagonist cycles or the benefit of recombinant LH and hCG protocols. Poor responders and patients of 35 years of age and older may benefit from exogenous LH.[23,24]

Addition of Luteinizing Hormone

The addition of LH is required in:
- Hypogonadotropic hypogonadism
- Poor responders
- The known poor response with previous FSH cycles
- Patients with FSH and LH receptor polymorphism.

Gonadotropin Dosage

Currently there is no established consensus on how to determine the optimal recombinant human FSH (r-FSH) starting dose for ovarian stimulation and often the choice of initial dose is based on the clinical experience and judgment.

The Consolidated Standards of Reporting Trials (CONSORT) calculator has been proposed. It uses four baseline factors [patient age, body mass index (BMI), early follicular phase serum FSH level and antral follicle count (AFC)].[25] Its role in clinical practice is limited, in our understanding due to the diverse influence of ethnicity and hormonal and receptor polymorphism.

Total gonadotropin dose was inversely associated with LBRs irrespective of the number oocytes retrieved. Even in good prognosis patients this decline was evident, regardless of the female age. Except in poor responders aged >35 years with 1–5 oocytes retrieved there was no negative impact.[26-31]

For every 500-unit increase in FSH dose, there was a 3% reduction in the odds of a live birth and an equal reduction in the odds of a clinical pregnancy. Duration of COH and average daily dose were not significantly associated with the live birth or clinical pregnancy. No significant association was found between miscarriage rates and total FSH dose, days of stimulation, or average daily dose.[26]

DECISION MAKING ON TYPE OF PROTOCOL TO USE

Assisted reproductive technologies clinicians should individualize taking into view patient clinical characteristics, medical history, and IVF goals when determining the best treatment options.

In good and hyper responders mild protocols may have a draw back by limiting the cumulative pregnancy rates.

In poor responders, adequate evidence to suggest that clinical pregnancy rates after IVF are not substantially different when comparing mild ovarian stimulation protocols to conventional-gonadotropin protocols.[32]

In our experience this fact can be utilized in clinical practice judiciously to provide cost benefits to the patients.

NEWER PROTOCOLS

Dual Stimulation Protocol[33,34]

Poor responders and emergency fertility preservation in cancer **(Fig. 3)**.

Controlled ovarian hyperstimulation with same gonadotropin dosage in the follicular phase and luteal phase of the same menstrual cycle resulted in a similar number of oocytes in patients with reduced ovarian response. The luteal phase stimulation statistically significantly contributed to the final transferable blastocyst yield, thus increasing the number of patients undergoing transfer per menstrual cycle and reducing cancellation rates.

Poor Responder

Agonist Microdose Flare Protocol with Antagonist added as in flexible protocol **(Fig. 4)**

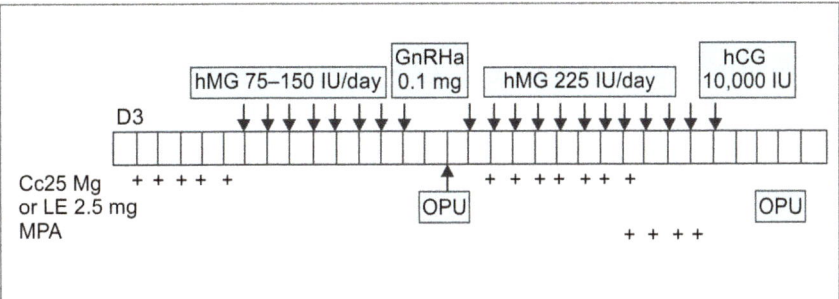

Fig. 3: Dual stimulation protocol. (GnRHa: gonadotropin-releasing hormone agonist; hMG: human menopausal gonadotropin; OPU: ovum pick-up; IU: international unit; LE: letrozole; MPA: medroxyprogesterone acetate)

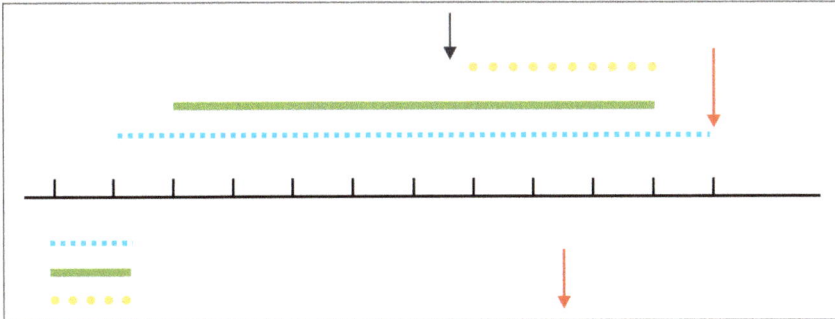

Fig. 4: Poor responder. [Blue: agonist 40–60 μg/day (microdose); green: gonadotropins; yellow: antagonist; red arrow 1st hCG trigger; 2nd oocyte pickup (OPU)]

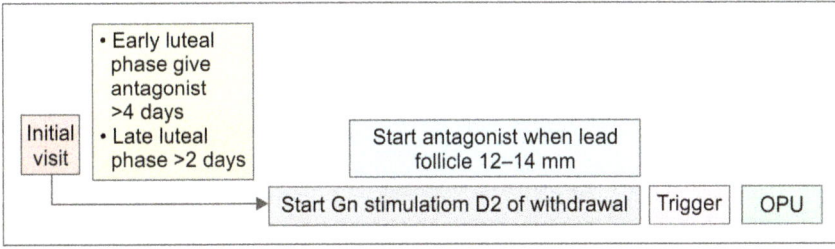

Fig. 5: Conventional multidose antagonist protocol.

Random Stimulation Protocol

Multiple follicular waves form the basis on which dual or random stimulations are based **(Fig. 5)**.[35-38]

It involves initial luteolysis with antagonist for 3 days for conventional multidose antagonist protocol.

In estrogen-dependent cancer, letrozole is added daily.

OUR EXPERIENCE AND CLINICAL EVIDENCE

- Individualization of protocol is must. Optimization of oocyte yields the most important factor to improve live birth rates in all age groups.
- OHSS is a completely preventable condition, and every ART clinic should strive to become an OHSS free clinic.
- High dose gonadotropins (doses >300 IU) does not offer additional advantage.

REFERENCES

1. van der Gaast MH, Eijkemans MJ, van der Net JB, de Boer EJ, Burger CW, van Leeuwen FE, et al. Optimum number of oocytes for a successful first IVF treatment cycle. Reprod Biomed Online. 2006;13(4):476-80.
2. Datta AK, Campbell SJ, Felix N, Singh JSH, Nargund G. How many oocytes or embryos are required to optimise live birth rate and cumulative live birth rate in mild stimulation In vitro fertilisation cycles? Reprod Biomed Online. 2021;43(10).
3. Law YJ, Zhang N, Kolibianakis EM, Costello MF, Keller K, Chanmber GM, et al. Is there an optimal number of oocytes retrieved at which live birth rates or cumulative live birth rates per aspiration are maximized after ART? A systematic review. Reprod Biomed Online. 2021;42(1)83-104.
4. Vermey BG, Chua SJ, Zafarmand MH, Wang R, Longobardi S, Cottell E, et al. Is there an association between oocyte number and embryo quality? A systematic review and meta-analysis. Reprod Biomed Online. 2019;39(5):751-63.
5. Practice Committee of the American Society for Reproductive Medicine, Practice Committee of the American Society for Reproductive Medicine. Prevention and treatment of moderate and severe ovarian hyperstimulation syndrome: a guideline. Fertil Steril. 2016;106(7)1634-47.
6. Wu Ze, Li R, Ma Y, Deng Bo, Zhang X, Meng Y, et al. Effect of HCG-day serum progesterone and oestradiol concentrations on pregnancy outcomes in GnRH agonist cycles. Reprod Biomed Online. 2012;24(5)511-20.
7. Nargund G, Fauser BCJM, Macklon NS, Ombelet W, Nygren K, Frydman R, et al. The ISMAAR proposal on terminology for ovarian stimulation for IVF. *Hum Reprod.* 2007;22(11):2801-4.
8. Nargund G, Datta AK, Fauser BCJ. Mild stimulation for in vitro fertilization. Fertil Steril. 2017;108(4):558-67.
9. Tarlatzis BC, Fauser BC, Kolibianakis EM, Diedrich K, Rombauts L, Devroy P, et al. GnRH antagonists in ovarian stimulation for IVF. Hum Reprod Update. 2006;12:333-40.
10. Gardner DK, Weissman A, Howles CM, Shoham Z. Textbook of Assisted Reproduction Techniques, 4th edition. CRC Press: Boca Raton; 2012.
11. Check ML, Check JH, Choel JK, Davies E, Kiefer D. Effect of antagonists vs agonists on in vitro fertilization outcome. Clin Exp Obstet Gynecol. 2004;31(4):257-9.
12. Duijikers IJ, Klipping C, Willemsen WN, Krone D, Schneider E, Niebch G, et al. Single and multiple dose pharmacokinetics and pharmacodynamics of the gonadotrophin-releasing hormone antagonist cetrorelix in healthy female volunteers. Hum Reprod. 1998;13(9):2392-8.
13. Papier S, Lipowicz R, Miranda ME, Sueldo C, Fiszbajn G, Olmedo SB. A Prospective Randomized Clinical Study Comparing a Single vs. Multiple Doses of GnRH Antagonists in ART. Fertil Steril. 2005;84(Suppl 1):S429.
14. Maletteri N, Dietterich C, Check JH, Dix E, Brasile D. The Adverse Effect of Ganirelix Versus Cetrorelix on Pregnancy Rates (PRs) and Implantation Rates Is Not Associated With Midluteal Phase Echo Patterns. Fertil Steril. 2008;89(4)S24.

15. Doody K, Langley M, Marek DE, Nackley AC, Doody KM. Synchronization of the follicle cohort with GnRH antagonist prior to the start of gonadotropins, a novel stimulation protocol for IVF. Fertil Steril. 2003;80(3):105-6.
16. Barri PN, Martinez F, Coroleu B, Tur R. The role of GnRH antagonists in assisted reproduction. Reprod Biomed Online. 2002;5(Suppl 1):14-9.
17. Al-Inany H, Aboulghar M. GnRH antagonist in assisted reproduction: a Cochrane review. Hum Reprod. 2002;17(4):874-85.
18. Griesinger G, Venetis CA, Marx T, Diedrich K, Tarlatzis BC, Kolibianakis EM. Oral contraceptive pill pretreatment in ovarian stimulation with GnRH antagonists for IVF: a systematic review and meta-analysis. Fertil Steril. 2008;90(4):1055-63.
19. Kolibianakis EM, Papanikolaou EG, Camus M, Tournaye H, Van Steirteghem AC, Devroey P. Effect of oral contraceptive pill pretreatment on ongoing pregnancy rates in patients stimulated with GnRH antagonists and recombinant FSH for IVF. A randomized controlled trial. Hum Reprod. 2006;21(2):352-7.
20. European Society of Human Reproduction and Embryology. (2019). Ovarian Stimulation for IVF/ICSI. [online] Available from https://www.eshre.eu/Guidelines-and-Legal/Guidelines/Ovarian-Stimulation-in-IVF-ICSI [Last accessed July, 2022].
21. Chang EM, Han JE, Won HJ, Kim YS, Yoon TK, Lee WS. Effect of estrogen priming through luteal phase and stimulation phase in poor responders in in-vitro fertilization. J Assist Reprod Genet. 2012;29(3):225-30.
22. Westergaard LG, Erb K, Laursen SB, Rex S, Rasmussen PE. Human menopausal gonadotropin versus recombinant follicle-stimulating hormone in normogonadotropic women down-regulated with a gonadotropin-releasing hormone agonist who were undergoing in vitro fertilization and intracytoplasmic sperm injection: a prospective randomized study. Fertil Steril. 2001;76(3):543-9.
23. Bosch E, Pellicer A, Pau E, Zuzuarregui J, Albert C, Remohí J. HMG vs. rFSH + rLH: Analysis of Hormonal Serum and Follicular Profiles, and Cycle Outcome in Oocyte Donation. Fertil Steril. 2005;84(Suppl 1):S257-8.
24. Fertilization, Implantation, and Pregnancy Rates With Recombinant Follicle Stimulating Hormone (rFSH) Versus rFSH Combined With Human Menopausal Gonadotropins (HMG) in Women Over Forty Undergoing In-Vitro Fertilization (IVF). Fertil Steril. 2000;74(3):S231.
25. Hill MJ, Levy G, Levens ED. Does exogenous LH in ovarian stimulation improve assisted reproduction success? An appraisal of the literature. Reprod Biomed Online. 2012;24(3):261-71.
26. Pouly JL, Olivennes F, Massin N, Celle M, Caizergues N, Contard F, et al. Usability and utility of the CONSORT calculator for FSH starting doses: a prospective observational study. Reprod Biomed Online. 2015;31(3):347-55.
27. Baker VL, Brown MB, Luke B, Smith GW, Ireland JJ. Gonadotropin dose is negatively correlated with live birth rate: analysis of more than 650,000 assisted reproductive technology cycles. Fertil Steril. 2015;104(5):1145-52.e1-5.
28. Shaia KL, Acharya KS, Harris BS, Webber JM, Truong T, Muasher SJ. Total follicle stimulating hormone dose is negatively correlated with live births in a donor/recipient model with fresh transfer: an analysis of 8,627 cycles from the Society for Assisted Reproductive Technology Registry. Fertil Steril. 2020;114(3):545-51.
29. Lin MH, Wu FS, Lee RK, Li SH, Lin SY, Hwu YM. Dual trigger with combination of gonadotropin-releasing hormone agonist and human chorionic gonadotropin significantly improves the live-birth rate for normal responders in GnRH-antagonist cycles. Fertil Steril. 2013;100(5):1296-302.
30. Castillo JC, Haahr T, Martínez-Moya M, Humaidan P. Gonadotropin-releasing hormone agonist for ovulation trigger—OHSS prevention and use of modified luteal phase support for fresh embryo transfer. Ups J Med Sci. 12(2).131-7.
31. Haas J, Bassil R, Cadesky K, Casper R. Dual trigger vs. HCG for final oocyte maturation. A prospective randomized controlled, double blinded study: preliminary results. Fertil Steril. 2017;108(3):e229.

32. Papanikolaou EG, Fatemi H, Camus M, Kyrou D, Polyzos NP, Humaidan P, et al. Higher birth rate after recombinant hCG triggering compared with urinary-derived hCG in single-blastocyst IVF antagonist cycles: a randomized controlled trial. Fertil Steril. 2010;94(7):2902-4.
33. American Society for Reproductive Medicine. (2022). Practice Committee of the American Society for Reproductive Medicine American Society for Reproductive Medicine. [online] Available from https://www.asrm.org/news-and-publications/practice-committee-documents/ [Last accessed July, 2022].
34. Ubaldi FM, Capalbo A, Vaiarelli A, Cimadomo D, Colamaria S, Alviggi C, et al. Follicular versus luteal phase ovarian stimulation during the same menstrual cycle (DuoStim) in a reduced ovarian reserve population results in a similar euploid blastocyst formation rate: new insight in ovarian reserve exploitation. Fertil Steril. 2016;105(6):1488-95.e1.
35. Kuang Y, Chen Q, Hong Q, Lyu Q, Ai A, Fu Y, et al. Double stimulations during the follicular and luteal phases of poor responders in IVF/ICSI programmes (Shanghai protocol). Reprod Biomed Online. 2014;29(6):684-91.
36. Effective method for emergency fertility preservation: random-start controlled ovarian stimulation. Cakmak H, Kartz A, Cedars MI, Rosen MP. Fertil Steril. 2013;100(6):1673-80.
37. Benadiva CA, Ben-Rafael Z, Strauss JF 3rd, Mastroianni L Jr, Flickinger GL. Ovarian response of individuals to different doses of human menopausal gonadotropin. Fertil Steril. 1988;49(6):997-1001.
38. Franco JG Jr, Baruffi RL, Mauri AL, Petersen CG, Felipe V, Cornicelli J, et al. GnRH agonist versus GnRH antagonist in poor ovarian responders: a meta-analysis. Reprod Biomed Online. 2006;13(5):618-27.

CHAPTER 27

Complications of Ovarian Stimulation

Kedar N Ganla, Priyanka Harshavardhan Vora, Rana Choudhary

INTRODUCTION

With the advent of rise in use of ovarian stimulating drugs even by the general gynecologists in assisted reproduction technology (ART), it is not only important to achieve results but also to plan patient management wisely so as to avoid the complications associated with the same. In this chapter, we will discuss the iatrogenic complications with use of ovulation induction agents such as ovarian hyperstimulation syndrome (OHSS), multiple pregnancies, ectopic gestations, adnexal torsion and cancer risks.

OVARIAN HYPERSTIMULATION SYNDROME (TABLE 1)[1-5]

- Incidence: 0.1–2% of all ART cycles

TABLE 1: RCOG classification of severity of ovarian hyperstimulation syndrome (OHSS).

Category	Features
Mild OHSS	Abdominal bloating
	Mild abdominal pain
	Ovarian size usually <8 cm
Moderate OHSS	Moderate abdominal pain
	Nausea ± vomiting
	Ultrasound evidence of ascites
	Ovarian size usually 8–12 cm
Severe OHSS	Clinical ascites (±hydrothorax)
	Oliguria (<300 mL/day or <30 mL/h)
	Hematocrit >0.45
	Hypernatremia (sodium <135 mmol/L)
	Hypo-osmolality (osmolality <282 mOsm/kg)
	Hyperkalemia (potassium >5 mmol/L)
	Hypoproteinemia (serum albumin <35 g/L)
	Ovarian size usually >12 cm

(RCOG: Royal College of Obstetricians and Gynaecologists)

- It is associated with increased capillary permeability and ovarian neoangiogenesis. This in turn causes fluid accumulation in the third space from intravascular spaces along with cystic enlargement of the ovaries.
- *Increased risk:* Younger women with polycystic ovary syndrome (PCOS), high anti-Müllerian hormone (AMH) >3.4 ng/dL, antral follicle count (AFC) >24, estradiol (E2)> 4,000 pg/dL, >24 oocytes retrieved and in women with gonadotropins.
- Risk is higher in women who achieve pregnancy—secondary OHSS.
- Recommendations for strategies to prevent OHSS are described in **Table 2**.

Management of Ovarian Hyperstimulation Syndrome

The management of OHSS is given in **Table 3**.

Practical Pointers

- Use metformin 2 g for 3 months prior
- Watch for previous history of OHSS, start with lesser dose
- Look for recruitment of smaller follicles (Cohort)
- Use the step-down protocol and do serial E2 for slope of rise
- Use antagonist protocol with agonist trigger
- Avoid hCG trigger (If dual trigger, use lowest possible dose of Injection hCG 1,500 IU)
- If agonist trigger is given, do LH levels 12 hours later
- Do not give hCG in the luteal phase
- Give progesterone as luteal phase support
- Avoid isotonic solutions such as Ringer's lactate (RL), normal saline (NS), as they will increase the fluid in the third space
- *Postretrieval:* Cabergoline, steroids, aromatase inhibitors and gonadotropin-releasing hormone (GnRH) antagonist till menses.

MULTIPLE GESTATION (TABLE 4)[6,7]

- *Incidence:* 30% of twin gestation, 5% are triplets.
- Total motile sperm count (TMSC) has a correlation with it.
- Increase in monozygotic twinning attributed to the in vitro culture environment and to extended duration of culture (i.e., day 5 to 6 embryos).
- This in turn leads to an increase in the risk of miscarriage, first trimester bleeding, abnormalities in the infant, preterm delivery sometimes resulting in handicap, increased blood pressure in pregnancy, thromboembolic other maternal complications along with burden socially and financially.
- Strategies to reduce iatrogenic epidemic of pregnancy must include begin with a lower gonadotropin dose at recruitment, conversion to IVF, cryopreservation, elective single embryo transfer, cycle cancellation and multifetal pregnancy reduction (MFPR).

TABLE 2: Recommendations for strategies to prevent ovarian hyperstimulation syndrome (OHSS).

S. No	Intervention	Recommendation	Effect of intervention	Level of evidence*
1.	Reducing gonadotropin dose	Recommended	"Step-up regimen" has a lower risk of OHSS, cycle cancellation from hyperstimulation, and higher rate of monofollicular ovulation in contrast to other protocols	1b, 4
2.	Reducing gonadotropin duration	Utilized as clinically appropriate	"Mild" stimulation protocol with gonadotropin-releasing hormone (GnRH) antagonist for late suppression has a lower risk of OHSS and multiple pregnancies and is cost effective	1b
			It also is less effective in terms of pregnancy rates than "long" protocols	1a
3.	Individualized controlled ovarian stimulation (iCOS)	Further research required	iCOS can reduce OHSS rates and associated cycle cancellations. It also produces a significant oocyte yield and good pregnancy rates	1b, 2a
4.	GnRH agonist (GnRHa) as an ovulation trigger	Recommended	GnRHa use virtually eliminates OHSS rates	1b
5.	Human chorionic gonadotropin (hCG) as an ovulation trigger	Further research required	Lowest dose of hCG does not seem to reduce OHSS rates	2a, 2b, 4
6.	Adjuvant metformin therapy	Recommended	Metformin is associated with a lower risk of OHSS and increased clinical pregnancy rate	1a, 4
7.	Cabergoline	Recommended	Cabergoline reduces the incidence of OHSS without an effect on pregnancy rates	1a
8.	Hydroxyethyl starch (HES)	Utilized as clinically appropriate	HES causes a decrease in OHSS without an effect on pregnancy rates	1a

Contd...

Contd...

S. No	Intervention	Recommendation	Effect of intervention	Level of evidence*
9.	Coasting	Further research required	Coasting does not completely prevent OHSS, is associated with a lower oocyte yield, and has no benefit in contrast to other interventions. The protocols are also very diverse	1a, 4
10.	Cryopreservation	Utilized as clinically appropriate	Cryopreservation alone does not reduce rates of OHSS	1a
			GnRHa followed by cryopreservation virtually eliminates OHSS	1b
11.	Cycle cancellation	Utilized as clinically appropriate	Cancellation completely eliminates risk of OHSS but has a high financial and emotional burden	4
12.	Adjunct GnRHa use	Not recommended	GnRHa use increases the associated costs and rate of OHSS while lowering the pregnancy rates	1a
13.	Aromatase inhibitors (AIs) for ovulation induction (OI)	Not recommended	AIs have shown no reduction in rates of OHSS in contrast to other methods of OI	1a
14.	Human recombinant luteinizing hormone (rhLH)	Not recommended	rhLH use does not reduce the risk of OHSS and has higher costs and lower pregnancy rates	1a, 1b
15.	hCG for luteal phase support	Not recommended	Progesterone significantly reduces the risk of OHSS with improved clinical pregnancy rates and live birth rates in comparison to hCG for luteal-phase support (LPS)	1a
16.	Albumin infusion	Not recommended	Albumin does not reduce OHSS rates and may cause lower pregnancy rates. There are also associated risks with anaphylaxis and disease transmission	1a
17.	Vasopressin V1a receptor antagonist	Further research required	It appears to reduce the ovarian weight gain and multiple corpus luteum development in OHSS	2b

*Note—Glossary for levels of evidence:
1a: Systematic review and/or meta-analysis; 1b: ≥1 RCT; 2a: ≥1 well-designed controlled study without randomization; 2b: ≥1 well-designed quasi experimental study; 3: ≥1 well-designed descriptive study; 4: Committee or expert opinions

TABLE 3: Management of ovarian hyperstimulation syndrome (OHSS).

Mild and moderate	Severe and critical
Outpatient	Inpatient and ICU management
<ul><li>Reassurance</li><li>Self-limiting condition</li><li>Resolves within 7–10 days</li><li>Easy recovery in the absence of pregnancy</li><li>If pregnancy occurs, OHSS worsens</li></ul>	<ul><li>Fluid management<ul><li>IV colloids</li><li>HES</li></ul></li><li>Renal protection<ul><li>Catheter to monitor I/O Chart</li><li>Furosemide 10–20 mg IV SOS</li></ul></li><li>Paracentesis<ul><li>Ascitic fluid aspiration</li><li>Peritoneal venous shunting</li></ul></li><li>Thromboprophylaxis:<ul><li>LMWH (40 mg/day)</li><li>Therapeutic heparin in case of DVT/PE</li><li>LMWH: 1.5 mg/kg/day</li></ul></li></ul>

(DVT: deep vein thrombosis; HES: hydroxyethyl starch; I/O: intake/output; LMWH: low-molecular-weight heparins; PE: pulmonary embolism)

TABLE 4: Problems related to multiple gestations.

Characteristics	Twins	Triplets	Quadruplets
Average birth weight	2,347 g	1,687 g	1,309 g
Average gestational age at delivery	35.3 weeks	32.2 weeks	29.9 weeks
Percentage with growth restriction	14–25	50–60	50–60
Percentage requiring admission to neonatal intensive care unit	25	75	100
Average length of stay in neonatal intensive care unit	18 days	30 days	58 days
Percentage with major handicap	-	20	50
Risk of cerebral palsy	Five times more than singletons	17 times more than singletons	-
Risk of death by age 1 year	Seven times higher than singletons	20 times higher than singletons	-

ECTOPIC (TUBAL) PREGNANCIES[8]

- *Incidence:* 2.1%, and in patients with tubal damage it is 11%.
- Common causes leading to the same are PID, prior ectopic pregnancy, tubal surgery, pelvic adhesions, endometriosis, high estrogenic or a high

progestogenic environment, partial or complete blockage of the fallopian tube due to either infection or inflammation, implantation occurs in the tubal mucosa itself if the transport of the fertilized ovum is delayed in the tube.
- Heterotopic pregnancy is far more common in pregnancies conceived by ART than spontaneous conceptions (1/100 vs. 1/30,000). This increase mirrors the dramatic increase in multiple gestations after IVF due to the transfer of multiple embryos.
- *In early assisted reproductive pregnancies:* Think ectopic to not miss one!

ADNEXAL TORSION (OVARIAN TWISTING)[9]

- *Incidence:* 2% of gonadotropin cycles
- Ovarian torsion results from twisting of the ovary around its own axis, resulting in occlusion of the artery and vein **(Figs. 1A and B)**.

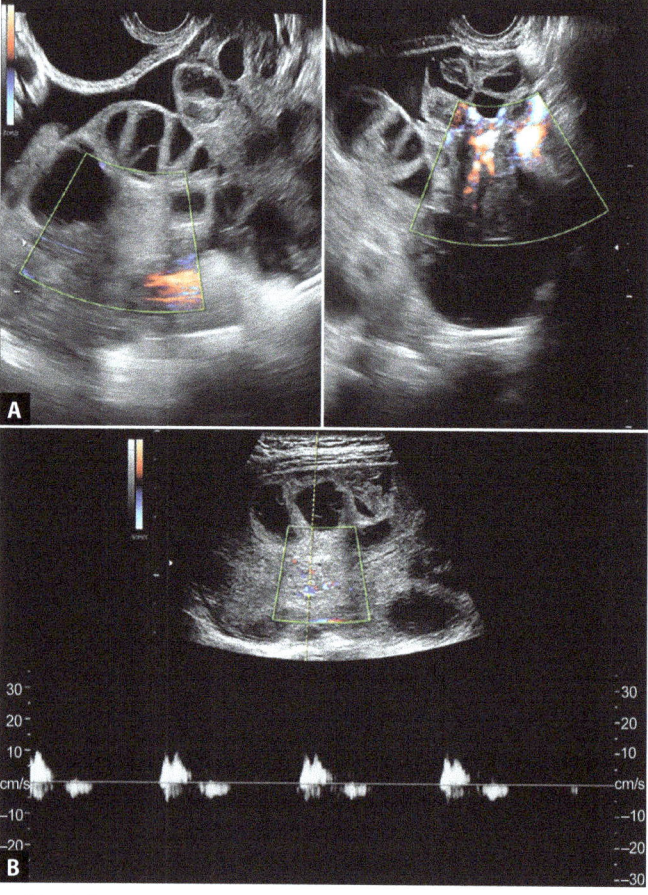

Figs. 1A and B: Color Doppler demonstrating (A) Postpickup enlarged right ovary with less blood flow; (B) Ultrasonography suggestive of right ovarian torsion.

- The use of gonadotropins for ovarian stimulation, ovarian cysts, and pregnancy causes ovarian enlargement, which predisposes such ovaries to torsion.
- The risk of torsion increases when OHSS develops, especially when the patient is pregnant.
- A suspicion of torsion should be raised in any woman undergoing stimulation of the ovaries and presenting with acute sharp abdominal pain and nausea. Associated important findings are leukocytosis and anemia.
- A study conducted by Murat Berkkanoglu and associates in 15,577 subjects in 2018 stated that use of GnRH agonist trigger in an antagonist cycle significantly reduced incidence of OHSS and further ovarian torsion than use of hCG trigger.

CANCER[10]

- Polyfollicular growth and high levels of gonadotropins due to repeated high doses of injectable gonadotropins causes malignant changes in the ovaries due to stimulation of the ovarian epithelium.
- Risk of ovarian cancer in *BRCA* mutation carriers undergoing fertility treatment, as this high-risk group may also be more likely to undergo fertility treatment for fertility preservation or diminished ovarian reserve.
- A Cochrane-based systematic review concluded that some studies suggested an increased risk of ovarian and borderline ovarian tumors (of serous type) in subfertile women treated with infertility drugs when compared to general population or subfertile women not being treated. However, the number of cancers and the number of studies are still very small.
- Increasing age, obesity, strong family history, PCOS, anovulation and tamoxifen use, excess estrogen use are all predisposing factors for endometrial cancer. Progesterone, however, has a protective effect.
- No increased risk of corpus uteri or invasive breast cancer was detected in women who had assisted reproduction, but increased risks of in situ breast cancer and invasive and borderline ovarian tumors were found in a large cohort study performed in Great Britain including 2.2 million person years of observation.
- A cohort study of 12,193 infertile women followed for 30 years found no increased risk of breast cancer after clomiphene citrate (hazard ratio: 1.05, 95% CI 0.9–1.22) or gonadotropin (hazard ratio: 1.14, 95% CI 0.89–1.44) exposure compared to infertile controls.
- Cervical cancer risk is not shown to have an increased risk in either the general population or infertile patients.
- Clomiphene citrate or gonadotropins or GnRH may lead to an increased risk of melanoma.

LIMITED OR OVERALL BODY REACTIONS

- Sometimes the injections may lead to local skin irritation
- Allergy to the gonadotropins is a rarity. However, breast tenderness, headaches, or mood swings are seen in a few women.

CONCLUSION

It is of utmost importance to first think of any likelihood of complications. If one is present, correct insight into the problem, helps in adequate counseling, diagnosing and treating these patients correctly on an individual basis.

REFERENCES

1. Joint SOGC-CFAS Clinical Practice Guideline. The diagnosis and management of ovarian hyperstimulation syndrome. JOGC. 2011;2068:1156-62.
2. RCOG. The Management of Ovarian Hyperstimulation Syndrome. Green-top Guideline No. 5. London: RCOG; 2016.
3. Choudhary RA, Vora PH, Darade KK, Pandey S, Ganla KN. A prospective comparative study of luteal phase letrozole versus ganirelix acetate administration to prevent severity of early onset OHSS in ARTs. Int J Fertil Steril. 2021;15(4):263-8.
4. D'Angelo A, Amso N. Embryo freezing for preventing ovarian hyperstimulation syndrome. Cochrane Database Syst Rev. 2007;(3):CD002806.
5. Klemetti R, Sevón T, Gissler M, Hemminki E. Complications of IVF and ovulation induction. Hum Reprod. 2005;20(12):3293-300.
6. Veleva Z, Karinen P, Tomás C, Tapanainen JS, Martikainen H. Elective single embryo transfer with cryopreservation improves the outcome and diminishes the costs of IVF/ICSI. Hum Reprod. 2009;24(7):1632-9.
7. American College of Obstetricians and Gynecologists' Committee on Obstetric Practice; Committee on Genetics; US Food and Drug Administration. Committee Opinion No 671: Perinatal risks associated with assisted reproductive technology. Obstet Gynecol. 2016;128(3):e61-8.
8. Fonslick JA, Seifer DB. Complications of ovulation induction. In: Seifer DB, Collins RL (Eds). Office-Based Infertility Practice. Berlin, Heidelberg: Springer; 2002.
9. Ganla KN, Choudhary RA, Vora PH, Athavale UV. Sildenafil Citrate: Novel therapy in the management of ovarian torsion. J Hum Reprod Sci. 2019;12(4):351-4.
10. Kroener L, Dumesic D, Al-Safi Z. Use of fertility medications and cancer risk: a review and update. Curr Opin Obstet Gynecol. 2017;29(4):195-201.

28 | Controlled Ovarian Hyperstimulation and Management of Polycystic Ovaries in In Vitro Fertilization

Nagadeepti Naik, Duru Shah

INTRODUCTION

Polycystic ovarian syndrome (PCOS) is a multifaceted, complex, heterogeneous endocrine disorder with variable endocrine, genetic, metabolic and environmental etiology. Prevalence of PCOS is around 8-13%.[1] Various diagnostic criteria are used for the diagnosis of PCOS, but the most commonly followed criteria are the Rotterdam criteria. The Rotterdam criteria include (any 2 out of 3):
1. Oligo/anovulation
2. Clinical/biochemical signs of hyperandrogenism (raised free androgen index or testosterone)
3. Ultrasound diagnosis of polycystic ovaries (12 or more follicles measuring 2-9 mm in diameter or increased ovarian volume, >10 cm^3 in any one of the ovary.)

Other etiologies such as androgen secreting tumors, thyroid dysfunction, congenital adrenal hyperplasia, hyperprolactinemia need to be excluded.[2]

Women having polycystic ovarian syndrome are mainly manifest with:
- Menstrual irregularities
- Features of hyperandrogenism (acne, hirsutism)
- Altered metabolic profile leading to metabolic syndrome
- Infertility

The prevalence of infertility is 70-80% in PCOS women.[1]

PATHOGENESIS (FIG. 1)

It is a vicious cycle with complex interaction between hyperinsulinemia, insulin resistance, and hyperandrogenemia leading to anovulation, infertility and decreased oocyte quality.[3]

Management

Lifestyle modifications such as exercise, and calorie restriction leading to weight loss have been strongly recommended in the management of PCOS. Studies have shown that a minimal weight loss of 5% has helps to restore ovulation, improve the menstrual cycle in women and is also associated with

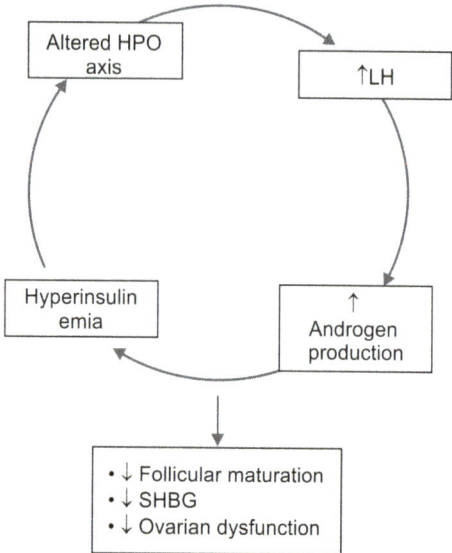

Fig. 1: Pathogenesis. (HPO: hypothalamic-pituitary-ovarian; LH: luteinizing hormone; SHBG: sex hormone binding globulin)

improved response to ovarian stimulation. Exercise is seen to be associated with a decrease in visceral fat, thus improving insulin sensitivity and decreasing resistance, decrease in the free testosterone levels, modulating the hypothalamopitutary axis and thus improving ovarian follicular response.[4]

Metformin: It is an oral biguanide, insulin sensitizer with a theoretically promising effect on the follicular growth. It acts by:[5]
- ↓ Peripheral glucose levels
- ↓ Systemic insulin levels
- Ovaries acts by decreasing the activity of cytochrome P450c 17a → androgen production
- ↓ VEGF → Indirectly decrease the incidence of OHSS.

As per the Cochrane review, metformin use alone or along with ovulation induction drugs or in IVF/ICSI has shown to be effective.[6]

Use of *ovulation induction drugs* such as selective estrogen receptor modulator (Clomiphene citrate), aromatase inhibitors (letrozole) are considered as the first line of management in PCOS.

Clomiphene citrate:

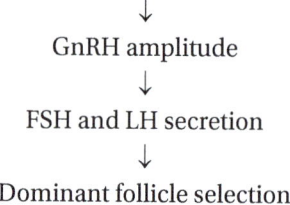

It is given in a dose of 50 mg/day for 5 days starting between day 2 and 5 of the menstrual cycle. It can be increased up to 250 mg/day. No additional benefits have been seen with dose >100 mg/day.[7]

Aromatase inhibitors (Letrozole):

Blocks aromatase enzyme responsible for conversion of androgen to estrogen
↓
FSH and follicular sensitivity to FSH
↓
Improved follicular response

It is given in a dose of 2.5–5 mg/day for 5 days starting from day 2 to 5 of the menstrual cycle. It does not have any negative effect on the endometrial thickness. US Food and Drug Administration (FDA) has not approved the use of letrozole but evidence-based guidelines strongly recommend use of letrozole.[8]

Gonadotropins (Gn): Gonadotropins along with/without intrauterine insemination are considered as the second line of management in anovulatory PCOS. It is associated with multifollicular growth, ovarian hyperstimulation and multiple pregnancies. Studies have shown no significant difference in the type of gonadotropin used [FSH or human menopausal gonadotropin (hMG)] for ovarian stimulation.

Low dose step-up or step-down protocol are mainly used to have a unifollicular growth and avoid hyperstimulation.

Tubal evaluation to establish tubal patency prior to start of gonadotropins is mandatory. Increased cost, duration, regular ultrasound monitoring and conversion to IVF in case of multifollicular growth (>2 follicles above 16 mm or >3 intermediate follicles) are the drawbacks of gonadotropin usage.[9]

Laparoscopic ovarian drilling (LOD): It is the second line of management mainly indicated in clomiphene resistant women who would require laparoscopy for other indications. It is an invasive procedure requiring general anesthesia with increased cost. Side effects such as adhesion formation and decrease reserve have been seen in few cases postoperatively.[10]

It acts by decreasing the ovarian androgen levels
↓
Release of negative feedback of estrogen on the hypothalamus
↓
↓ LH and ↑ FSH
↓
Dominant follicle recruitment

Farquhar et al., in his Cochrane review has shown no significant difference between laparoscopic ovarian drilling and medical management of PCOS.[11]

In vitro fertilization: IVF/ICSI has been considered as the third line of management in PCOS patients.

INDICATIONS

Previous failed ovulation induction with oral induction agents/gonadotropins. Other confounding factors such as bilateral blocked tubes, altered semen parameters, endometriosis altering the success rates.

Women undergoing IVF/ICSI have to be clearly explained/counselled regarding the risk of multifollicular growth, ovarian hyperstimulation and multiple gestation.

Points to be considered before ovarian stimulation in PCOS women are:
- Treatment protocol to be used
- Type and dose of gonadotropin used
- Trigger used for final oocyte maturation.

Aim of these protocols is controlled ovarian stimulation leading to good cohort of follicles **(Fig. 2)**.

The two commonly used protocols are the gonadotropin-releasing hormone (*GnRH*) agonist or the GnRH antagonist protocol.[9]

1. *GnRH agonist protocol:* They are of two types (long luteal and short luteal phase protocol). They mainly act by suppressing the hypothalamopituitary axis to avoid premature luteinization.[12]
   a. *Long luteal phase protocol:* In this protocol GnRH agonist is started on day 21 of the previous cycle and gonadotropins are started from day 2, after complete downregulation, i.e., (E2 <50 pg/mL and serum progesterone <0.5).
   b. *Short GnRH agonist protocol:* It is started from day 1 of the menstrual cycle followed by gonadotropins till the final trigger injection. It initially leads to a flare effect followed by pituitary desensitization. Increased risk of OHSS is associated with short agonist protocol. This protocol has found to be helpful mainly in cases with decreased ovarian reserve.

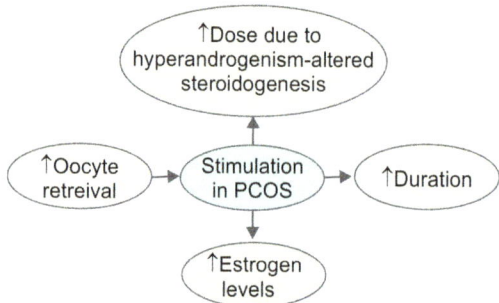

Fig. 2: Stimulation in polycystic ovarian syndrome (PCOS).

Gonadotropin-releasing hormone agonist protocol is associated with complete depletion of LH, so human chorionic gonadotropin (hCG) is considered for the final trigger, due to its structural similarities to LH.[12] This protocol is associated with increased risk of ovarian hyperstimulation. Cryopreservation of the embryos with single embryo transfer is considered in these cases.

2. *GnRH antagonist protocol (Friendly IVF protocol)*: Gonadotropins are started from day 2 of the menstrual cycle, GnRH antagonist is added daily when the follicle reaches 12 or 13 mm in case of flexible protocol or on day 5 in case of fixed protocol. A single dose of 3 mg GnRH antagonist can also be considered.

In these cases GnRH agonist or hCG can be considered for the trigger injection.[13] hCG has a long half-life (24 hours) as compared to GnRH agonist (60 minutes). It stimulates the corpus lutea leading to ↑VEGF and thus increase risk of OHSS. Therefore GnRH agonist trigger with freeze-all strategy has shown to have a favorable outcome in IVF in PCOS women.

Several studies have shown that GnRH antagonist protocol should be preferred over an agonist protocol in view of decrease dose of gonadotropins, duration of stimulation and decreased incidence of OHSS.[14]

Administration of oral contraceptive pills before ICSI has shown no beneficial effect.

CRYOPRESERVATION OF EMBRYOS (FREEZE-ALL STRATEGY)[15,16] (FIG. 3)

Many studies have shown increased risk of aneuploidy in PCOS women undergoing IVF/ICSI. The exact mechanism is unknown. It has been hypothesized that altered steroidogenesis and impaired oocyte metabolism is associated with DNA instability. But, more research is still needed.

COMPLICATIONS

- Ovarian hyperstimulation syndrome (OHSS)
- Multiple gestation
  - *Ovarian hyperstimulation syndrome:* It is an iatrogenic condition caused due to ovarian stimulation.

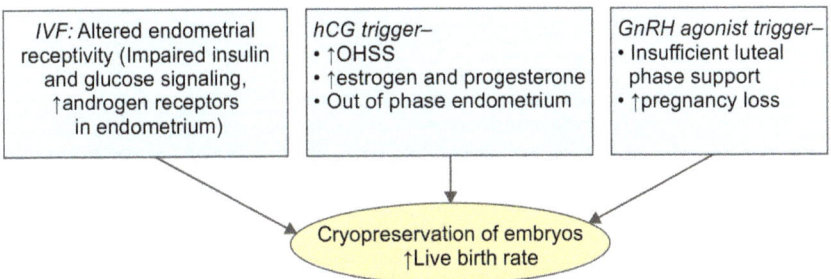

Fig. 3: Cryopreservation of embryos.

Pathophysiology[17,18] **(Fig. 4):**

Young women, low BMI, polycystic ovaries on ultrasound, serum AMH >3.36 ng/mL, antral follicle count >24 and previous history of OHSS are all considered as high risk factors in the development of OHSS.

Treatment of OHSS includes, identification of high-risk factors and its management.

Prevention of OHSS:[19]
- Individualizing the treatment protocol and decreasing the gonadotropin use on the basis of age, AFC, AMH and BMI to be considered.
- Use of GnRH antagonist protocol as an alternative has proven to minimize the risk of OHSS.
- Studies have shown that use of Metformin prior and during the ovarian stimulation has led to 63% decrease in incidence of OHSS.
- hCG
  - Decreasing the dose of hCG trigger as compared to 10,000 IU. But studies have shown not much difference in the clinical impact on OHSS
  - Use of GnRH agonist trigger-freeze all embryos.
  - *Recombinant LH:* As compared to hCG it has a short half-life of 10 hours but no significant difference has been documented. Further studies are recommended.
- In GnRH agonist cycles with increased estradiol levels, withholding the hCG trigger and cancellation of the cycle was been considered.
- *Coasting:* It is a condition in which hCG trigger is delayed till the serum estradiol levels plateau. On with holding gonadotropins the follicles continue to grow for 4 days and serum estradiol levels increase in 1–2 days. With holding the hCG trigger for more than 4 days is associated with decreased outcome.
- Use of volume expanders:
  - *Albumin:* Prevents the release of vasoactive substances and oncotic effect maintains the intravascular compartment. Dose: 20–50 g of 25% albumin on the day of oocyte retrieval.

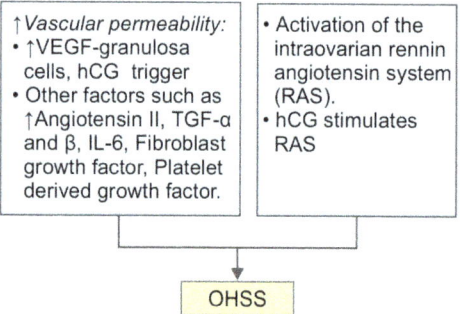

Fig. 4: Pathophysiology.

- *Hydroxyethyl starch:* Studies have shown beneficial effect when 1,000 mL of 6% HESS was used on the day of oocyte retrieval.
- *Calcium:* Naredi N, in his study has shown that 10% of 10 mL calcium gluconate in 200 mL of normal saline has shown decreased incidence of OHSS.
- *Low dose aspirin:* Supraphysiological estradiol levels has been associated with platelet aggregation. Studies have shown that low dose aspirin during ovarian stimulation has beneficial effects in decreasing the risk of OHSS.
- *Dopamine agonist (Cabergoline):* As per the Cochrane review, administration of cabergoline 0.5 mg for 8 days starting from the day of oocyte retrieval has shown comparable decrease in the incidence of mild to moderate OHSS.
- Cryopreservation of embryos
- *In vitro maturation (IVM):* Women with estrogen sensitive cancers, high risk of OHSS are ideal candidates for IVM. In this condition the immature oocytes are retrieved at an earlier stage when the follicle is around 14 mm, thus decreasing the incidence of OHSS. They are then cultured in IVM media which contains mainly a combination of FSH, growth hormone and hCG. Some studies have considered IVM to be a good alternative. But further randomized controlled trials are needed as the level of evidence is low.[20]
- *Multiple gestation:* Multiple gestation is one of the major complications of IVF in PCOS women to avoid the risks of prematurity, IUGR and other maternal effects due to multiple pregnancy and with the advances in reproductive medicine transfer of single embryo with pregenetic analysis has shown to have higher success rate and live birth rates.[21]

In PCOS, use of GnRH antagonist protocol with GnRH agonist trigger followed by adoption of freeze-all strategy should be the treatment of choice. Preparation of endometrium using artificial hormonal replacement therapy with/without prior downregulation using GnRH analogs in a thaw transfer cycle combined with pregenetic analysis has shown to considerable success rates.

Luteal support in the form of vaginal progesterone till 12 weeks of gestation has demonstrated higher pregnancy rates and live birth rates. Various studies have shown improved results in cases of cotreatment with GnRH agonist along with vaginal progesterone as it extends the LH production thus preventing premature luteolysis and direct effect on the endometrium and early embryo cannot be excluded.[22,23]

REFERENCES

1. Maqbool M, Gani I, Geer MI. Polycystic ovarian syndrome-a multifaceted disease. Int J Pharmaceut Sci Res. 2018;10(3):1072-9.
2. Rotterdam ESHRE/ASRM-Sponsored PCOS consensus workshop group. Revised 2003 consensus on diagnostic criteria and long-term health risks related to polycystic ovary syndrome (PCOS). Hum Reprod. 2004;19:41-7.

3. Strauss JF. Some new thoughts on the pathophysiology and genetics of polycystic ovary syndrome. Ann N Y Acad Sci. 2003;997:42-8.
4. Giallauria F, Palomba S, Vigorito C, Tafuri MG, Colao A, Lombardi G, et al. Androgens in polycystic ovary syndrome: the role of exercise and diet. Semin Reprod Med. 2009;27:306-15.
5. Diamanti-Kandarakis E, Christakou CD, Kandaraki E, Economou FN. Metformin: an old medication of new fashion: evolving new molecular mechanisms and clinical implications in polycystic ovary syndrome. Eur J Endocrinol. 2010;162:193-212.
6. Tso LO, Costello MF, Albuquerque LE, Andriolo RB, Macedo CR. Metformin treatment before and during IVF or ICSI in women with polycystic ovary syndrome. Cochrane Database Syst Rev. 2014:CD006105.
7. Perales-Puchalt A, Legro RS. Ovulation induction in women with polycystic ovary syndrome. Steroids. 2013;78(8):767-72.
8. Kar S. Current evidence supporting "letrozole" for ovulation induction. J Hum Reprod Sci. 2013;6:93-8.
9. Melo AS, Ferriani RA, Navarro PA. Treatment of infertility in women with polycystic ovary syndrome: approach to clinical practice. Clinics. 2015;70(11):765-9.
10. Amer SA, Li TC, Metwally M, Emarh M, Ledger WL. Randomized controlled trial comparing laparoscopic ovarian diathermy with clomiphene citrate as a first-line method of ovulation induction in women with polycystic ovary syndrome. Hum Reprod. 2009;24:219-25.
11. Farquhar C, Brown J, Marjoribanks J. Laparoscopic drilling by diathermy or laser for ovulation induction in anovulatory polycystic ovary syndrome. Cochrane Database Syst Rev. 2012;13(6):CD001122.
12. Shrestha D, La X, Feng HL. Comparison of different stimulation protocols used in in vitro fertilization: a review. Ann Transl Med. 2015;3:137.
13. Van Loenen AC, Huirne JA, Schats R, Hompes PG, Lambalk CB. GnRH agonists, antagonists, and assisted conception. Semin Reprod Med. 2002;20:349-64.
14. Lin H, Li Y, Li L, Wang W, Yang D, Zhang Q. Is a GnRH antagonist protocol better in PCOS patients? A meta-analysis of RCTs. PLoS One. 2014;9:e91796.
15. D'Angelo A. Ovarian hyperstimulation syndrome prevention strategies: cryopreservation of all embryos. Semin Reprod Med. 2010;28:513-8.
16. D'Angelo A, Amso N. Embryo freezing for preventing ovarian hyperstimulation syndrome. Cochrane Database Syst Rev. 2007:CD002806.
17. Naredi N, Talwar P, Sandeep K. VEGF antagonist for the prevention of ovarian hyperstimulation syndrome: Current status. Med J Armed Forces India. 2014;70:58-63.
18. Pellicer A, Albert C, Mercader A, Bonilla-Musoles F, Remohi J, Simon C. The pathogenesis of ovarian hyperstimulation syndrome: In vivo studies investigating the role of interleukin-1beta, interleukin-6, and vascular endothelial growth factor. Fertil Steril. 1999;71:482-9.
19. Jahromi BN, Parsanezhad ME, Shomali Z, Bakhshai P, Alborzi M, Vaziri NM. Ovarian hyperstimulation syndrome: a narrative review of its pathophysiology, risk factors, prevention, classification, and management. Iranian J Med Sci. 2018;43(3):248-60.
20. Fadini R, Dal Canto M, Mignini Renzini M, Milani R, Fruscio R, Cantù MG, et al. Embryo transfer following in vitro maturation and cryopreservation of oocytes recovered from antral follicles during conservative surgery for ovarian cancer. J Assist Reprod Genet. 2012;29:779-81.
21. Tandulwadkar SR, Lodha PA, Mangeshikar NT. Obstetric complications in women with IVF conceived pregnancies and polycystic ovarian syndrome. J Hum Reprod Sci. 2014;7(1):13-8.
22. Boutzios G, Karalaki M, Zapanti E. Common pathophysiological mechanisms involved in luteal phase deficiency and polycystic ovary syndrome. Impact on fertility. Endocrine. 2013;43:314-7.
23. Yazici G, Savas A, Tasdelen B, Dilek S. Role of luteal phase support on gonadotropin ovulation induction cycles in patients with polycystic ovary syndrome. J Reprod Med. 2014;59:25-30.

CHAPTER 29: Management in Diminished Ovarian Reserve and Controlled Ovarian Hyperstimulation

Jatin Shah, Amiti Agrawal

INTRODUCTION

Poor ovarian reserve (POR) is the most challenging area of reproductive medicine. There is no uniform definition and there is a lot of low quality or empirical data **(Box 1)**.[1]

BOX 1: Bologna criteria for poor responders.[2]

At least two of the following:
1. *Advanced maternal age:* ≥30 years or risk factor for poor ovarian reserve
2. *Previous poor ovarian reserve:* ≤3 oocytes with conventional stimulation
3. *Abnormal ovarian reserve biomarker:* AFC <5–7; AMH <0.5–1.1 ng/mL

Or, two episodes of poor ovarian reserve after maximal stimulation

POSEIDON Group 1	POSEIDON Group 2
• Young patients <35 years with adequate ovarian reserve parameters (AFC ≥5; AMH ≥1.2 ng/mL) and with an unexpected poor or suboptimal ovarian response • Subgroup 1a: <4 oocytes* • Subgroups 1b: 4–9 oocytes retrieved*	• Older patients ≥35 years with adequate ovarian reserve parameters (AFC ≥1.2 ng/mL) and with an unexpected poor or suboptimal ovarian response • Subgroup 1a: <4 oocytes* • Subgroups 1b: 4–9 oocytes retrieved*
POSEIDON Group 3	**POSEIDON Group 4**
Young patients (<35 years) with poor ovarian reserve prestimulation parameters (AFC <5; AMH <1.2 ng/mL)	Young patients (≥35 years) with poor ovarian reserve prestimulation parameters (AFC <5; AMH <1.2 ng/mL)

*After standard stimulation
(AFC: antral follicle count; AMH: anti-Müllerian hormone)

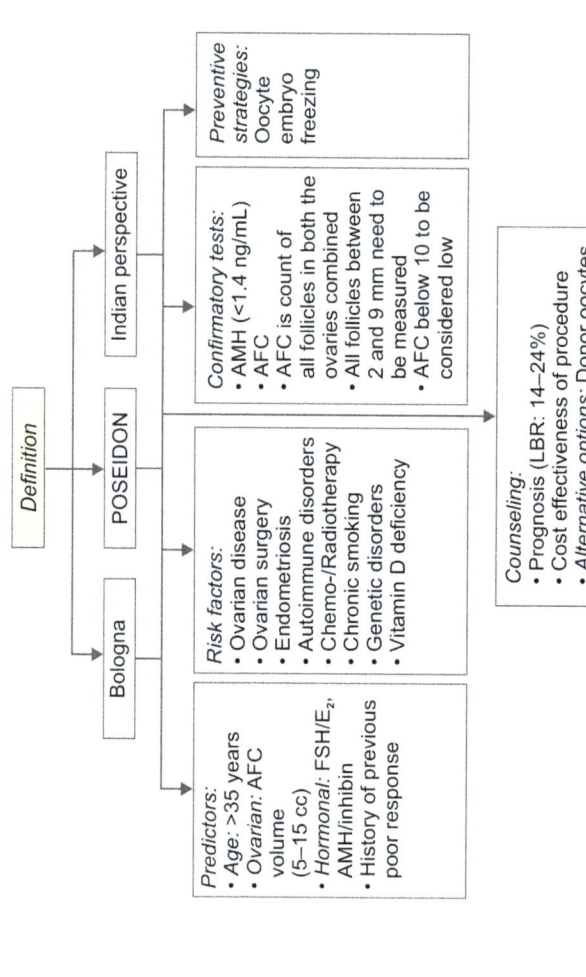

(AFC: antral follicle count; AMH: anti-Müllerian hormone; E2: estradiol; FSH: follicle-stimulating hormone; LBR: live birth rates)

Management in Diminished Ovarian Reserve and Controlled Ovarian...

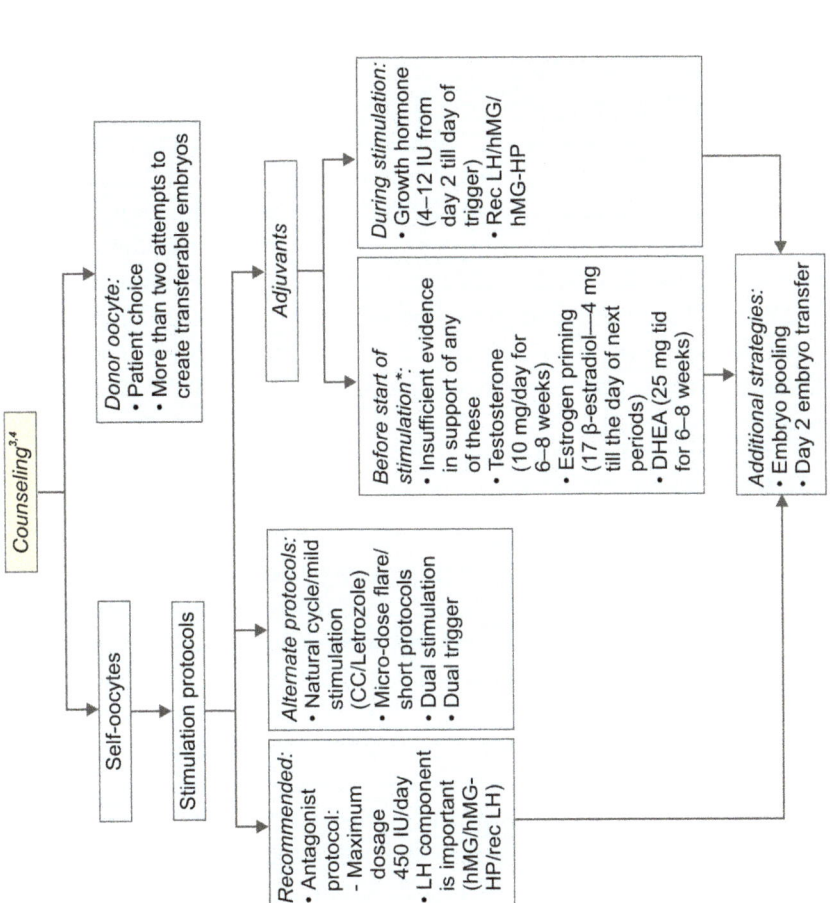

*Enumerated in the order of proven benefit
(CC: clomiphene citrate; DHEA: dehydroepiandrosterone; hMG: human menopausal gonadotropin; HP: highly purified; LH: luteinizing hormone; rec: recombinant)

NEWER ADVANCES

Intraovarian Autologous Platelet-rich Plasma Therapy

Platelet-rich plasma (PRP) is separated after centrifugation for preparing PRP. Initially, 20 mL of blood sample is collected. This is done under sterile conditions. PRP is prepared using T-lab autologous platelet rich plasma kit. The tubes are centrifuged at 830 g for 8 minutes, briefly after blood collection. 16 G needle connected to a 5-mL syringe and is inserted into the tube and advanced to the buffy coat layer. Needle tip is rotated to collect the PRP. Once collected, approximately 2–4 cc PRP from the first tube, the second tube is processed similarly (a total 4–8 cc PRP was collected). Then collected solution was transferred to the re-suspension tube. This is then shaken gently for 30 s–1 min. Within 2 hours of sample preparation, PRP injection is performed. This is done transvaginally and under ultrasound guidance. Sedation anesthesia is preferred. Injection carried out into at least one ovary. This is done using a 35-cm 17 G single lumen needle. Baseline antral follicle count (AFC) and anti-Müllerian hormone (AMH) are checked before the procedure and response is seen after 6 weeks. This approach is still under experimental stage and still needs further studies to prove its efficacy for poor responders.

Oocyte Cryopreservation

Oocyte cryopreservation has opened a new era in the field of assisted reproductive technology (ART). This is possible because of vitrification process. In the past the only indication was for women, suffering with various premalignant or malignant conditions. This was to prevent them infertility after cancer therapy. However, it has expanded its role in several nonmedical indications as well. This includes the women at risk of reduced reproductive capacity due to age-related fertility decline and as a part of oocyte donation programs. Vitrification techniques have proven results in terms of post-thaw survival and pregnancy rates. Thus, oocyte freezing has gained popularity in egg donation services. It is also a viable alternative to embryo cryopreservation because this does not carry the same ethical and legal issues. Oocyte cryopreservation will soon play an integral role in infertility treatments.

CONCLUSION

Treatment of diminished ovarian reserve is a challenge. Evaluating ovarian reserve and individualizing the therapeutic strategies are important. They optimize the success rate. Bologna criteria offer right direction and are useful to identify homogenous groups for evaluating efficacy of various therapies. The therapeutic interventions in this situation includes—avoiding prolonged pituitary suppression, prevention of premature luteinizing hormone (LH) surge, and controlled ovarian stimulation (COS) to maximize oocyte yield and achieve embryos with good implantation potential.

REFERENCES

1. Cohen J, Chabbert-Buffet N, Darai E. Diminished ovarian reserve, premature ovarian failure, poor ovarian responder—a plea for universal definitions. J Assist Reprod Genet. 2015;32(12):1709-12.
2. Ferraretti AP, La Marca A, Fauser BC, Tarlatzis B, Nargund G, Gianaroli L; ESHRE working group on Poor Ovarian Response Definition. ESHRE consensus on the definition of "poor response" to ovarian stimulation for in vitro fertilization: the Bologna criteria. Hum Reprod. 2011;26(7):1616-24.
3. Jeve YB, Bhandari HM. Effective treatment protocol for poor ovarian response: A systematic review and meta-analysis. J Hum Reprod Sci. 2016;9(2):70-81.
4. Pandian Z, McTavish AR, Aucott L, Hamilton MP, Bhattacharya S. Interventions for "poor responders" to controlled ovarian hyperstimulation (COH) in in-vitro fertilisation (IVF). Cochrane Database Syst Rev. 2010;(1):CD004379.

CHAPTER 30

Trigger in In Vitro Fertilization

Sonali Tawde, Revati Rane, Milind Patil

PHYSIOLOGY OF TRIGGER

Introduction

In natural menstrual cycle, follicle-stimulating hormone (FSH) levels start to rise gradually from the mid luteal phase of the preceding cycle. Selection of dominant follicle is established during cycle days 5-7. With the growth of the dominant follicle, estradiol levels start rising. Once it crosses the threshold, negative feedback switches to positive feedback effect, causing mid-cycle surge of gonadotropins from the pituitary. Luteinizing hormone (LH) and FSH surge leads to sequence of events causing final oocyte maturation and ovulation.

During controlled ovarian stimulation, endogenous LH surge is prevented by agonist or antagonist preparations. For final oocyte maturation, timely trigger needs to be given which aims at oocyte maturation and ovulation **(Fig. 1)**. For many years, human chorionic gonadotropin (hCG) was the only trigger available. Ever since antagonist cycles gained popularity, agonist trigger is being used more commonly by assisted reproductive technology (ART) clinicians, especially in high responders.

Types of triggers and their pharmacodynamics are shown in **Table 1 and Figure 2**.

LH plays an important role in:
- Maturation of oocyte from arrested prophase 1 stage by reduction in cAMP and activation of CDK kinase enzymes which causes resumption of meiosis and brings about cytoplasmic changes.
- Luteinization of granulosa cells
- Cumulus expansion.

FSH surge in the mid-cycle:
- Leads to nuclear maturation of oocyte
- Resumption of meiosis and further expansion of cumulus cells
- Release of proteolytic enzymes necessary in the process of ovulation
- Induction of LH receptors on granulosa cells to promote corpus luteum.
- Similar alpha subunit and 85% similar beta subunit as that of LH.

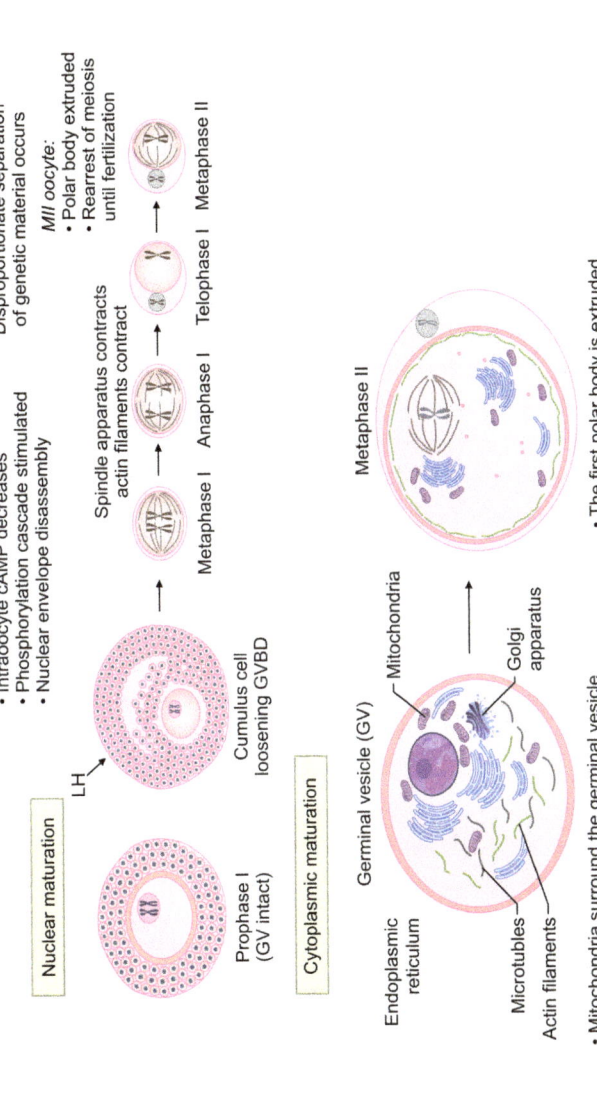

Fig. 1: Physiology of oocyte maturation.

TABLE 1: Types of triggers.

	hCG	GnRH agonist	Recombinant LH	Kisspeptins
Site of action	Ovary	Pituitary	Ovary	Hypothalamus
Receptors	LH	GnRH	LH	Kisspeptin receptors
Action	LH	LH + FSH	LH	LH + FSH
Peak of action (hours)	18–22	4	Variable (Depending on dose)	4–6
Duration of action	5–7 days	20–24 hours	5–7 days	12–24 hours
Use in protocols	• Short • Long	• Short • Antagonist	• Short • Long	• Short • Antagonist
Luteal phase defect	✗	✓	✗	✓
Risk of OHSS	✓	✗	✓	✗

(FSH: follicle-stimulating hormone; GnRH: gonadotropin-releasing hormone; LH: luteinizing hormone; OHSS: ovarian hyperstimulation syndrome)

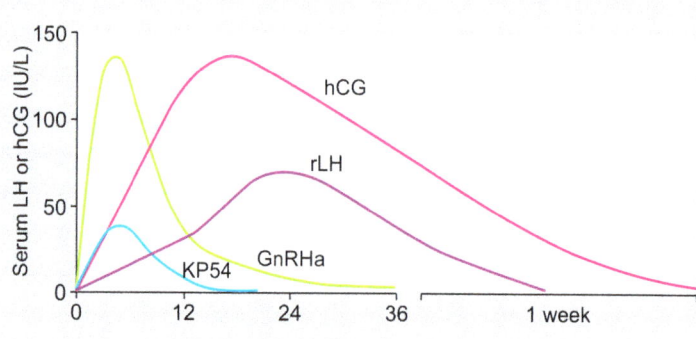

Fig. 2: Pharmacodynamics of various triggers.

- The major difference being, LH has a circulating half-life of 25–30 minutes, while hCG, has a circulating half-life of approximately 37 hours **(Table 2)**.
- Available in two forms—urinary and recombinant as shown in **Table 3**.

Choice of hCG Trigger

- The use of recombinant hCG and urinary hCG is equally recommended for triggering final oocyte maturation during ovarian stimulation protocols.[1]
- A reduced dose of 5,000 IU urinary hCG for final oocyte maturation is probably recommended over a 10,000 IU dose in GnRH agonist protocols, as it may improve safety.

TABLE 2: Luteinizing hormone (LH) versus human chorionic gonadotropin (hCG) trigger.

	LH	hCG
Glycosylation	Less	More
Affinity to LH receptors	Less	More
Potency	Less	5 times more
Effect on cAMP	Less	More
Action	Through extracellular signaling effective in oocyte maturation and ovulation	Steroidogenic and maintenance of corpus luteum

TABLE 3: Urinary versus recombinant trigger.

	Urinary	Recombinant
Obtained from	Urine of pregnant woman	Chinese Hamster ovary cell
Standard dose	5,000–10,000 IU	250 (equivalent to 6,500 IU uhCG)/500 μg depending on BMI
Route	Intramuscular/subcutaneous	Subcutaneous
Batch to batch variability	✓	✗
Epidermal growth factors[1]	Present and causes negative influence on trophoblast	Absent so does not affect implantation

- Similarly, low dose (250 μg) of recombinant hCG does not appear to influence the probability of pregnancy as compared to a higher dose (500 μg).
- Higher dose is recommended in cases with body mass index (BMI) >30
- Lower doses of hCG could be considered when an unpredicted high response has occurred, and GnRH long agonist protocol is applied.[2]

GnRH Agonist

GnRH agonist trigger has revolutionized IVF treatment in terms of safety and OHSS prevention **(Figs. 3 and 4)**.

No significant dose-dependent difference in oocyte retrieval or fertilization or pregnancy rate.[3]

Has greater affinity for the GnRH receptor than GnRH antagonists. It will displace the GnRH antagonist from the GnRH receptor in the pituitary, eliciting an endogenous surge of FSH, as well as LH, that is similar, although not identical, to the natural midcycle surge of gonadotropins (**Table 4**). This is known as "Flare effect" of GnRH analogue trigger.

Triggering of final oocyte maturation with a bolus of GnRH-a could be considered more physiological than the use of hCG for trigger because GnRH-a trigger also introduces a surge of FSH.

Fig. 3: Advantages of agonist trigger.

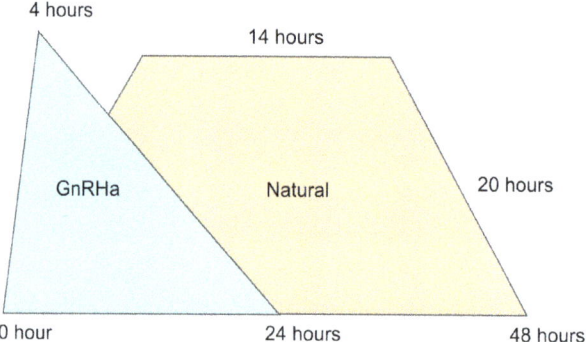

Fig. 4: Pharmacodynamics of agonist trigger versus luteinizing hormone (LH).

TABLE 4: Action of endogenous LH versus agonist trigger.

	Endogenous LH	**GnRH (a)**
Phases	Three phases 1. Ascending 14 hours 2. Plateau 14 hours 3. Descending 20 hours	Two phases 1. Ascending 4 hours 2. Descending 20 hours
Peak	14 hours	4 hours
Total duration	48 hours	24 hours
Risk of OHSS	More	Less
Action	Only LH	LH + FSH

(FSH: follicle-stimulating hormone; GnRH: gonadotropin-releasing hormone; LH: luteinizing hormone; OHSS: ovarian hyperstimulation syndrome)

Dual Trigger

- GnRH agonist + concomitant uhCG 1,500/2,500/5,000 IU or 250 μg rhCG (**Table 5**)
- Preferred in normoresponders/hyporesponders POSIEDON Group 4/ history of immature oocytes in previous cycle[4,5]

GnRHa trigger advantages and disadvantages are described in **Table 6**.

TABLE 5: Gonadotropin-releasing hormone (GnRH) preparations and dose.

Name	Dose	Route
Leuprolide	1–4 mg	Subcutaneous
Buserelin	0.5 mg	Subcutaneous
Triptorelin	0.2 mg	Subcutaneous
Nafarelin	100 µg	Nasal

TABLE 6: GnRHa trigger advantages and disadvantages.

Advantages	Disadvantages
1. Simultaneous induction of an FSH surge comparable to the surge of the natural cycle **(Fig. 4)** 2. Retrieval of more mature oocytes (Oktay et al., 2010) 3. Prevents OHSS due to shorter half-life (Hernandez et al., 2009) 4. Ideal trigger for oocyte donors, high responders, PCOS, fertility preservation cycles, follicular stimulation in dual stimulation cycles, due to rapid luteolytic action	1. Luteal phase insufficiency despite standard LPS with progesterone and estradiol 2. Poor clinical outcome with an extremely high early pregnancy loss rate in fresh ET cycles (Kolibianakis et al., 2005)

(ET: embryo transfer; FSH: follicle-stimulating hormone; GnRHa: gonadotropin-releasing hormone agonist; OHSS: ovarian hyperstimulation syndrome; PCOS: polycystic ovary syndrome; LPS: luteal phase support)

Advantages

- Increased number of mature oocytes (MII)
- Better fertilization rates
- Increased implantation rates
- Increased clinical pregnancy rates.

Disadvantages

OHSS not eliminated but reduced to 0.5%.

Double Trigger

- GnRH agonist trigger 40 hours before OPU + hCG 34–36 hours prior to OPU
- Causes prolongation of time interval between trigger and pickup with added advantage of FSH.

Advantages

- More useful in cases of empty follicle syndrome (EFS)[6]
- The GnRH agonist trigger should be followed by luteal phase support with LH-activity. The use of GnRH agonist for final oocyte maturation with

conventional luteal phase support and fresh transfer is not recommended in the general IVF/ICSI population **(Table 5)**.[2]
- The addition of a GnRH agonist to hCG as a dual trigger for final oocyte maturation is probably not recommended for predicted normal responders.
- In patients at risk of OHSS, the use of a GnRH agonist for final oocyte maturation is probably recommended over hCG in cases where no fresh transfer is performed.[2]

Recombinant LH Trigger

- Shorter half-life than hCG, more physiological
- Variable dose used in studies
- 15,000–30,000 IU has similar efficacy as 5,000 IU uhCG
- Not used in practice, commercially unavailable.

Kisspeptins

- Acts on hypothalamus to release GnRH
- KP10, KP54 have been extensively studied
- Results in 3-4 fold rise in LH levels if given in preovulatory phase
- Better safety profile, no risk of OHSS
- More research is needed.

PREREQUISITES OF TRIGGER

Ultrasound Criteria

- Majority cohort of follicles between 16 and 22 mm is considered optimum before giving trigger[7]
- Size of follicles can be 1-2 mm bigger in agonist cycles than antagonist at the time of trigger
- >22 mm size may give less favorable yield
- Subendometrial vascularity reaching zone 3 or 4 is desirable for fresh ET cycles.

Hormonal Evaluation at the Time of Trigger

- E2 if there is a high risk of OHSS (approximately 200 pg/mL per mature follicle)
- P4 on the day of trigger, should be <1.5 ng/mL if fresh ET is planned. If >1.5 ng/mL, freeze-all policy should be implemented.

The decision on timing of triggering in relation to follicle size is multifactorial, considering the size of the growing follicle cohort, the hormonal data on day of pursued trigger, duration of stimulation, patient burden, financial costs, experience of previous cycles and organizational factors for the center. The Guideline Development Group (GDG) does not recommend to base timing of final oocyte maturation triggering on estradiol levels alone, or estradiol/follicle ratio alone.[2]

Interval between Trigger and Ovum Pickup

Optimum interval to:
- Get mature oocytes
- Prevent spontaneous ovulation.

CHOICE OF TRIGGER

It depends upon:
- Type of ET planned
- Risk of OHSS
- Previous h/o stimulation outcome in terms of mature oocytes, fertilization rate, pregnancy outcome.

Agonist Protocol (Long/Short) (Table 7)

Only hCG trigger can be used.

Antagonist Protocol (Table 7)

- Either hCG alone/GnRH agonist alone/dual trigger/double trigger option available
- Those with very low levels of LH on day 2, due to prolonged suppression, may fail to respond to only agonist trigger, e.g., oocyte donors on prolonged OCPs.

Hypogonadotropic Hypogonadism

Only hCG trigger should be used.

Post-trigger Check Points (12 Hours Post-trigger)

- *hCG trigger:* Sr. hCG > 50 mIU/mL, Sr. progesterone >2.3 ng/mL
- *Agonist only trigger:* Serum LH >15 IU/L, serum progesterone >9 ng/mL[8]
- *Dual trigger:* hCG >50 mIU/mL, LH >15 IU/L
- LH and hCG levels may vary according to BMI, dose of trigger
- If less values of hCG/LH at 12 hours, retrigger with hCG and schedule OPU at 34–36 hours from hCG.

TABLE 7: Timing the trigger.

Time	Stimulation protocol
34–36 hours	Agonist
35 hours	Antagonist

Luteal Phase Support Recommendation for Fresh ET Cycles

After hCG trigger: Vaginal micronized progesterone ± Oral dydrogesterone.

After dual trigger:
- Estradiol tablets/transdermal preparations/Patch
- Vaginal micronized progesterone ± Oral dydrogesterone
- Injection hCG 1,500 IU on day 5 post-trigger, thereafter every 5 days

or

Inj. progesterone 50–100 mg daily/25–50 mg aqueous progesterone daily depending upon weight and BMI of patient.

After agonist only trigger:
Ideally "Freeze-all policy" should be implemented.

If at all fresh ET is planned:
- 1,500 IU hCG on day of OPU and every 5 days thereafter,

or

GnRh agonist (0.1 mg Triptorelin) on D6 of OPU

or

Inj. Progesterone to rescue luteal phase.
- Carries mild risk of OHSS.
- Recommended cut off of <25 follicles of ≥11 mm, when considering fresh ET.

EMPTY FOLLICLE SYNDROME

It is characterized by lack of retrieval of oocytes from apparently normal growing ovarian follicles with normal estradiol levels after ovarian stimulation **(Table 8)**.

TABLE 8: Empty follicle syndrome (EFS).

	False	Genuine
Incidence	0.04–3.4 %	0–1%
Cause	Inadequate trigger, low baseline luteinizing hormone (LH) level due to prolonged suppression, variable threshold for follicular response to trigger	LH receptor defect, defective granulosa cell function
LH levels	<15 IU/L	>15 IU/L
Human chorionic gonadotropin (hCG) levels	<50 mIU/mL	>50 mIU/mL
Management	1. hCG rescue dose followed OPU at 34–36 hours 2. GnRH/dual trigger in next cycle	Dual/double trigger might help

According to recent large database, incidence of false EFS is similar with GnRH agonist and hCG trigger (3.5 vs. 3.1%).[9]

CONCLUSION

- In controlled ovarian stimulation, trigger plays very crucial role in oocyte maturation and ovulation
- In natural cycle, both LH and FSH surge occurs
- Agonist cycle—only hCG trigger works
- Antagonist cycle—hCG or agonist trigger can be given, dual trigger is the best for poor responders and normoresponders
- Only agonist trigger prevents OHSS in PCOS, hyper-responders, oocyte donors and dual stimulation. To be used in *freeze-all cycles*
- Only agonist trigger leads to luteal phase insufficiency, hence needs robust luteal support.

REFERENCES

1. Youssef M, Al-Inany H, Aboulghar M, Mansour R, Abou-Setta A. Recombinant versus urinary human chorionic gonadotrophin for final oocyte maturation triggering in IVF and ICSI cycles. Cochrane Database Syst Rev. 2016;4:CD003719.
2. Youssef M, Al-Inany H, Aboulghar M, Mansour R. Recombinant versus urinary human chorionic gonadotropin for final oocyte maturation triggering in IVF/ICSI cycles. Cochrane systematic review and meta-analysis. Fertil Steril. 2011; 94(4 Suppl 1):S141.
3. Reproductive Endocrinology Guideline Group. Ovarian Stimulation for IVF-ICSI. Belgium: ESHRE; 2019.
4. Pabuccu EG, Pabuccu R, Caglar GS, Yilmaz B, Yarci A. Different gonadotropin releasing hormone agonist doses for the final oocyte maturation in high-responder patients undergoing in vitro fertilization/intra-cytoplasmic sperm injection. J Hum Reprod Sci. 2015;8(1):25-9.
5. Lin MH, Wu FS, Lee RK, Li SH, Lin SY, Hwu YM. Dual trigger with combination of gonadotropin-releasing hormone agonist and human chorionic gonadotropin significantly improves the live-birth rate for normal responders in GnRH-antagonist cycles. Fertil Steril. 2013;100:1296-302.
6. Shapiro BS, Daneshmand ST, Garner FC, Aguirr M, Thomas S. Gonadotropin-releasing hormone agonist combined with a reduced dose of human chorionic gonadotropin for final oocyte maturation in fresh autologous cycles of in vitro fertilization. Fertil Steril. 2008;90:231-3.
7. Beck-Fruchter R, Weiss A, Lavee M, Geslevich Y, Shalev E. Empty follicle syndrome: successful treatment in a recurrent case and review of the literature. Hum Reprod. 2012;27:1357-67.
8. Revelli A, Martiny G, Delle Piane L, Benedetto C, Rinaudo P, Tur-Kaspa I. A critical review of bidimensional and three-dimensional ultrasound techniques to monitor follicle growth: do they help improving IVF outcome? Reprod Biol Endocrinol. 2014;12(1):107.
9. Gupta M, Ghumman S, Khanna SC, Patel S. Variation of post trigger LH, progesterone and HCG levels with BMI and its impact on recovery rates of oocytes during IVF/ICSI cycles. Fertil Sci Res. 2020;7(1):92.
10. Castillo JC, Juan G, Humaidan P. Empty follicle syndrome after GnRHa triggering versus hCG triggering in COS. J Assist Reprod Genet. 2012;29(3):249-53.

31 | Luteal Phase Support

Nisha Nikheel Pansare, Chaitanya Shembekar

INTRODUCTION

Luteal phase extends from ovulation to the establishment of pregnancy or beginning of menses. In the luteal phase of menstrual cycle, human chorionic gonadotropin (hCG) (secreted by corpus luteum) and progesterone hormone prepares the endometrium for pregnancy. This progesterone and hCG levels are insufficient in assisted reproductive technique (ART) cycles and may lead to poor implantation rate or pregnancy loss. In ART, there is a supra-physiological concentrations of steroids secreted by high number of corpora lutea during early luteal phase, which directly inhibits luteinizing hormone (LH) release via negative feedback actions at hypothalamopituitary axis level.[1,2] Multiple follicles of different sizes ovulate at different time which expands the fertilization window. In gonadotropin-releasing hormone (GnRH) agonist protocol, there is prolonged suppression of pituitary LH after 3 weeks of downregulation.[3,4] In GnRH antagonist protocol, there is direct effect on LH receptors hence less LH secretions.[5]

Human chorionic gonadotropin trigger for ovulation in ART cycle, leads to inhibition of endogenous LH secretion. All of this affects receptivity of endometrium, luteal insufficiency, insufficient progesterone secretion and early luteolysis.[6]

LUTEAL PHASE DEFECT MECHANISM

Luteal phase support (LPS) in the form of medications in ART improves implantation rates and pregnancy rates significantly **(Flowchart 1)**.

Luteal phase defect in ART can occur due to:
- Continuation of pituitary downregulation effect
- Shortened duration of luteal phase
- Formation of multiple corpus lutea leading to inhibition of pulsatile LH release
- Loss of granulosa cells during oocyte retrieval **(Flowchart 1)**.

DURATION OF LUTEAL PHASE SUPPORT

There is still no definitive consensus about the progesterone initiation, dose and duration of the treatment. This is because of the duration and timing

Flowchart 1: Luteal defect mechanism.

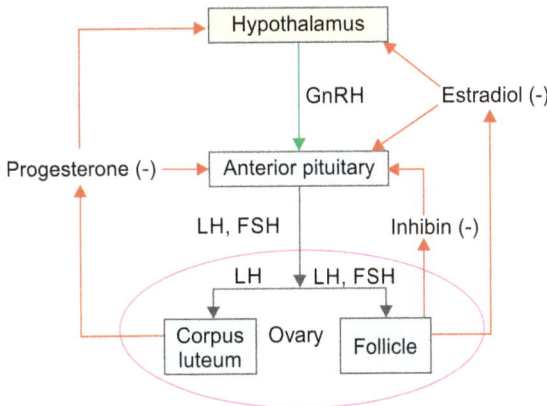

of implantation is not precisely known. Some studies have recommended starting the progesterone from the day of ovum pick-up (OPU).
- In most of the cases progesterone is started after OPU and it is continued until 8–10 weeks of gestation in fresh embryo transfer cycles[7,8]
- In donor oocyte cycle LPS is continued till 10–12 weeks of gestation
- In frozen embryo transfer cycle, LPS is continued till placental takeover (around 10–12 weeks).

DRUGS USED IN LUTEAL PHASE SUPPORT (FLOWCHART 2)

Progesterone

Progesterone supplementation is available in the form of intramuscular, vaginal, rectal, oral and subcutaneous preparation.
- Two preparations are available as dydrogesterone (synthetic progesterone) and natural micronized progesterone. These preparations are known to undergo first pass prehepatic and hepatic metabolisms which reduce their bioavailability. So there is more drug requirement and more dosages.[9]
  - Dydrogesterone is the biologically active metabolite of progesterone, thereby having a good oral bioavailability. It induces the secretory transformation of the endometrium through its antiestrogenic effect. Many studies have shown that dydrogesterone has immunological effects which are associated with higher rates of pregnancy **(Fig. 1)**. Dydrogesterone in 10 mg thrice daily dose is recommended.[10]
  - Natural micronized progesterone has high protein binding with long half-life (18 hours) giving once a dosage benefit. Micronized progesterone, if used orally, has poor absorption <10%. So oral use is to be avoided ideally. Vaginal or rectal route is preferred 600–800 per day in divided doses. Progesterone gel 8%, 90 mg per day is also available.[11]

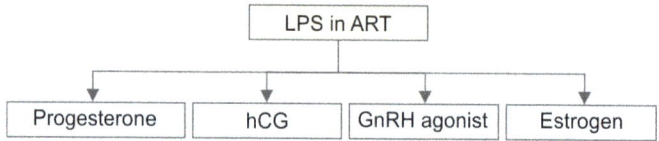

Flowchart 2: Drugs used in luteal phase support (LPS).

(ART: assisted reproductive technique; hCG: human chorionic gonadotropin; GnRH: gonadotropin-releasing hormone)

Year	Review	Conclusion
2011	Cochrane review	Oral synthetic progesterone is more efficacious
2015	Cochrane review	No longer concludes that oral synthetic progesterone is more efficacious
2016	Barbosa meta-analysis	Oral dydrogesterone seems to be as effective as vaginal progesterone for LPS in ART cycles and is better tolerated
2018	LOTUS I / LOTUS II	Dydrogesterone 30 mg vs. 8% micronized vaginal progesterone gel 90 mg daily to be started from OPU until 12 weeks of gestation

Fig. 1: Review or study review for luteal phase support (LPS).
(ART: assisted reproductive technique; OPU: ovum pick-up)

TABLE 1: Various progesterone preparations.

Drug	Route	Dose	Remark
Micronized progesterone	Vaginal/Rectal/Oral	600–800 mg/day in divided doses	*Oral use:* Not reliable because of poor absorption (<10%)
Dydrogesterone	Oral	10 mg thrice a day	Well tolerated
Progesterone gel	Vaginal	8%, 90 mg/day	*Side effects:* Vaginal discharge, gel accumulation
Progesterone injection (Oil base)	Intramuscular	50–100 mg/day	*Side effect:* Pain at injection site, sterile abscess
Progesterone injection (Aqueous)	Subcutaneous	25 mg/day	*Side effect:* Local irritation

- Injectable progesterone comes in the form of oil base intramuscular and aqueous solution of subcutaneous preparations. Subcutaneous injections are well-tolerated as compared to intramuscular injections. Dosage of injectable progesterone may vary from 25 to 100 mg/day. Side effects of injectable progesterone are pain and rashes at injection site, more commonly with intramuscular preparation **(Table 1)**.

Progesterone Plus Estrogen

Corpus luteum secretes progesterone, estrogen and other steroid hormones. So, it was suggested that to improve implantation rate estrogen can be added to progesterone for luteal phase defect (LPD).[12]

But in a meta-analysis, it has been shown that routine use of estrogen is not justified in progesterone supported luteal phase in IVF cycle.[13]

Human Chorionic Gonadotropin

Dose of hCG for LPS (only in fresh cycles) is 1,500 IU every 3rd day for 3-4 doses. Luteal support with hCG should be avoided if estradiol (E2) concentrations are above 2,500-2,700 pg/mL on the day of hCG trigger in IVF cycle or if there are more than 10 follicles.[14,15] Cochrane review (2015) states that hCG with or without progesterone is associated with high live birth rates but with higher risk of ovarian hyperstimulation syndrome, so it should be avoided.[16]

Few prefer daily micro dose hCG (100-150 IU) throughout the luteal phase without exogenous progesterone in GnRH agonist triggered IVF cycle.

Gonadotropin-releasing Hormone Agonist

Gonadotropin-releasing hormone agonist acts at three levels—(1) pituitary, (2) endometrium, and (3) embryo.[17] It also supports the corpus luteum by stimulating the secretion of LH at pituitary or at endometrial level directly through the locally expressed GnRH receptors.[18] Single dose 0.1 mg of Triptorelin acetate after 5-6 days of oocyte retrieval was suggested earlier. Many trials have shown opposing effects of GnRH agonist with low quality of evidence.[19] Recent Cochrane review showed increased pregnancy, ongoing pregnancy and live birth rates in subjects receiving luteal GnRH agonist.

Adjuvants

- *Heparin:* Low-molecular-weight heparin is used in cases of recurrent implantation failure and recurrent pregnancy loss. It has an anticoagulant and immunomodulatory action which helps in adhesion of blastocyst to endometrial epithelium and subsequent invasion. Few studies have shown improved implantation rate[20] while other studies do not find any role of low molecular weight heparin.[17,18] Recommended daily dose is 20-40 mg subcutaneously.[21]
- *Aspirin:* Aspirin inhibits enzyme cyclooxygenase in platelets which increases uterine and ovarian blood flow and tissue perfusion. Low dose aspirin (75 mg) is preferred in tablet form. Although there is no substantial evidence supporting role of aspirin in pregnancy and delivery rates.[22,23]

- *Sildenafil:* Sildenafil citrate increases endometrial vascularity and thickness by inhibiting 5-phosphodiesterase leading to vasodilatation. Luteal supplementation of vaginal Sildenafil is beneficial in improving endometrial receptivity.[24] It is administered vaginally in a dosage of 25–50 mg started from the day of OPU or embryo transfer.

LUTEAL PHASE SUPPORT IN INTRAUTERINE INSEMINATION AND OVULATION INDUCTION CYCLE

Luteal phase support in the form of progesterone may be useful in ovulation induction with Gonadotropins as there is basic difference in endogenous luteal phase function depending on method of ovulation induction.[25] LPS is not useful in clomiphene citrate-induced intrauterine insemination (IUI) cycle. There was a study where 400 women were analyzed and found no difference in ongoing pregnancy with progesterone support (8.8%, 17/196) and without progesterone support (9.3%, 19/204).[26] Luteal phase is shortened in IUI cycle when induced with FSH. In a meta-analysis of five trials involving 1,938 cycles in 1,298 patients, LPS with progesterone improves success rate.[25] In one of the RCTs it was studied that 300 mg of intravaginal micronized progesterone found to be beneficial for LPS in gonadotropin induced IUI cycles.[27]

CONCLUSION

- LPS in ART is essential in frozen embryo transfer cycle and donor cycle.
- Cochrane 2015 supports LPS in ART to improve implantation and pregnancy rate
- The European Society of Human Reproduction and Embryology (ESHRE) 2019 strongly recommends progesterone use for LPS in ART cycle commenced at the day of OPU till the day of pregnancy test at least.
- As per American Society for Reproductive Medicine (ASRM), LPS is not essential once the pregnancy is established.
- Though optimum duration of LPS is not yet formalized, common practice is to continue LPS till luteoplacental shift is achieved (10–11 weeks).
- LPS is not beneficial in natural or unstimulated cycles. LPS (Progesterone) is useful in ovulation induction with gonadotropins in IUI cycles.

REFERENCES

1. Fauser BCJM, Devroey P. Reproductive Biology and IVF: ovarian stimulation and luteal phase consequences. Trends Endocrinol Metab. 2003;14(5):236-42.
2. Fatemi HM. The luteal phase after 3 decades of IVF: what do we know? Reprod Biomed Online. 2009;19:4331.
3. Pritts EA, Atwood AK. Luteal phase support in infertility treatment: a meta-analysis of the randomized trials. Hum reprod. 2002;17(9):2287-99.
4. Daya S, Gunby J. Luteal phase support in assisted reproduction cycles. Cochrane Database Syst Rev. 2004;3:CD004830.

5. Beckers NGM, Macklon NS, Eijkemans MJ, Ludwig M, Felberbaum RE, Diedrich K, et al. Nonsupplemented luteal phase characteristics after the administration of recombinant human chorionic gonadotropin, recombinant luteinizing hormone, or gonadotropin releasing hormone (GnRH) agonist to induce final oocyte maturation in in vitro fertilization patients after ovarian stimulation with recombinant follicle stimulating hormone and GnRH antagonist cotreatment. J Clin Endocrinol Metab. 2003;88:4186-92.
6. Tavaniotou A, Albano C, Smitz J, Devroey P. Impact of ovarian stimulation on corpus luteum function and embryonic implantation. J Reprod Immunol. 2002;55:123-30.
7. Sohn SH, Penzias AS, Emmi AM, Dubey AK, Layman LC, Reindollar RH, et al. Administration of progesterone before oocyte retrieval negatively affect the implantation rate. Fertil Steril.1999;71:11-4.
8. Mochtar MH, Van Wely M, Van der Veen F. Timing luteal phase support in GnRH agonist downregulated IVF/Embryo transfer cycles. Hum Reprod. 2006;21:905-8.
9. Kleinstein J, Luteal Phase Study Group. Efficacy and tolerability of vaginal progesterone capsules (Utrogest 200+) compared with progesterone gel (Crinone 8%) for luteal phase support during assisted reproduction. Fertil Steril. 2005;83:1641-9.
10. Griesinger G, Blockeel C, Sukhikh GT, Patki A, Dhorepatil B, Yang DZ, et al. Oral dydrogesterone versus intravaginal micronized progesterone gel for luteal phase support in IVF: a randomized clinical trial. Hum Reprod. 2018;33:2212-21.
11. ESHRE Reproductive Endocrinology Guideline Group. Controlled ovarian stimulation for IVF/ICSI. Belgium: ESHRE Reproductive Endocrinology Guideline Group; 2019. pp.106-12.
12. Fatemi HM, Popvic-Todorovic B, Papanikolaou E, Donoso P, Devroey P. An update of luteal phase support in stimulated IVF cycles. Hum Reprod Update. 2007;13:581-90.
13. Kolibianakis EM, Griesinger G, Venetis CA, Papanikolaou EG, Diedrich K, Tarlatzis BC. Estrogen addition to progesterone for luteal phase support in cycles stimulated with GnRH analogues and gonadotrophins for IVF: a systemic review and meta-analysis. Hum Reprod. 2008;23(6):1346-54.
14. Araujo Jr E, Bernardini L, Frederick JL, Asch RH, Balmacedaet JP. Prospective randomized comparison of human chorionic gonadotropin versus intramuscular progesterone for luteal phase support in assisted reproduction. J Assist Reprod Genet. 1994;11(2):74-8.
15. Farhi J, Weissman A, Steinfeld Z, Shorer M, Nahum H, Levran D. Estradiol supplementation during the luteal phase may improve the pregnancy rate in patients undergoing in vitro fertilization-embryo transfer cycles. Fertil Steril. 2000;73(4):761-6.
16. Van der Linden M, Buckingham K, Farquhar C, Kremer JAM, Metwally M. Luteal phase support for assisted reproduction cycles. Cochrane Database Syst Rev. 2015;2015(7):CD009154.
17. Tesarik J, Hazout A, Mendoza-Tesarik R, Mendoza N, Mendoza C. Beneficial effect of luteal phase GnRH agonist administration on embryo implantation after ICSI in both GnRH agonist and antagonist treated ovarian stimulation cycles. Hum Reprod. 2006;21:2572-9.
18. Pirard C, Donnez J, Loumaye E. GnRH agonist as novel luteal support: results of randomized, parallel group, feasibility study using intranasal administration of buserelin. Hum Reprod. 2005;20:1798-804.
19. de Ziegler D, Pirtea P, Anderson CY, Ayoubi JM. Role of gonadotropin releasing hormone agonist, human chorionic gonadotropin, progesterone and estrogen in luteal phase support after hCG triggering and when in pregnancy hormonal support can be stopped Fertil Steril. 2018;109(5):749-55.
20. Tesarik J, Hazout A, Mendoza C. Enhancement of embryo developmental potential by a single administration of GnRH agonist at the time of implantation. Hum Reprod. 2004;19:1176-80.

21. Casanova P, Szilt Feldman, Blanco LA. The addition of GnRH agonist for luteal phase support in ovum donation cycles. Fertil Steril. 2015;104(3):e346.
22. Pakkila M, Rasanen J, Heinonen S, Tinkanen H, Tuomivaara L, Mäkikallio K. Low dose aspirin does not improve ovarian responsiveness for pregnancy rate in IVF and ICSI patients: a randomized, placebo controlled double blind study. Hum Reprod. 2005;20:2211-4.
23. Hurst BS, Bhojwani JT, Marshburn PB, Papadakis MA, Loeb TA, Matthews ML. Low dose aspirin does not improve ovarian stimulation, endometrial response or pregnancy rate for in vitro fertilisation. J Exp Clin Assist Reprod. 2005;2:8-12.
24. Kim KR, Lee HS, Ryu HE, Park CY, Min SH, Park C, et al. Efficacy of luteal supplementation of vaginal sildenafil and oral estrogen on pregnancy rate following IVF ET in women with a history of thin endometria: a pilot study. J Wowens Med. 2010;3:155-8.
25. Hill MJ, Whitcomb BW, Lewis TD, Wu M, Terry N, DeCherney AH, et al. Progesterone luteal support after ovulation induction and intrauterine insemination: a systematic review and meta-analysis. Fertil Steril. 2013;100(5):1373-80.
26. Devroey P, Kyrou D, Fatemi HM, Tournaye H. Luteal phase support in normo-ovulatory women stimulated with clomiphene citrate for intrauterine insemination: need or habit? Hum Reprod. 2010;25(10):2501-6.
27. Biberoglu EH, Tanrikulu F, Erdem M, Erdem A, Biberoglu KO. Luteal phase support in intrauterine insemination cycles: a prospective randomized study of 300 mg versus 600 mg intravaginal progesterone tablet. Gynecol Endocrinol. 2016;32:55-7.

CHAPTER 32: Managing Quality Control and Quality Management of IVF Laboratory

Kalyan Baramade, Manisha Barmade

INTRODUCTION

"Quality of the IVF laboratory is invisible when it is good but impossible to ignore when it is bad".

The in vitro fertilization (IVF) is the heart of assisted reproductive technology (ART), which is explicitly designed for the development of 3–5 initial days of the imminent child's life **(Fig. 1)**. The quality management (QM) is a program that pinpoints and rectifies issues or defects in the overall laboratory system in order to ensure the whole process. The two considerations of quality management are—(1) quality assurance (QA) and (2) quality control (QC) **(Fig. 2)**.

In any laboratory, generating high-quality work does not occur by accident; it necessitates the acquisition of skills as well as ongoing performance evaluation. Each process in your laboratory should have its own set of standard operating procedures (SOPs), which each professional in your laboratory, including yourself, should follow.

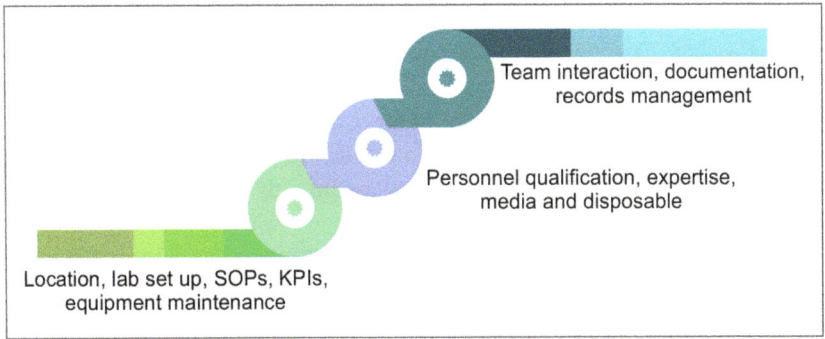

Fig. 1: ART quality management principle protocols. *(SOPs for the specific laboratory, KPIs, equipment maintenance, laboratory set-up, personnel qualification, and expertise, records management and documentation, all forms of media and disposable vendors, and effective team interaction play a vital role in quality management to maximize laboratory outputs)* **(Fig. 3)**
(ART: assisted reproductive technology; KPIs: key performance indicators; SOPs: standard operating procedures)

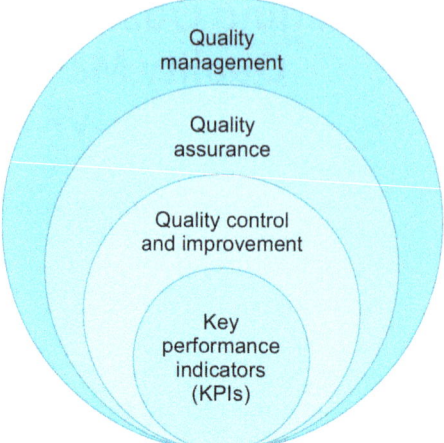

Fig. 2: Relationship between quality management, quality assurance, quality control, and key performance indicators (KPIs).
Source: Fabozzi G, Cimadomo D, Maggiulli R, Vaiarelli A, Ubaldi FM, Rienzi L. Which key performance indicators are most effective in evaluating and managing an in vitro fertilization laboratory? Fertil Steril. 2020;114(1):9-15.

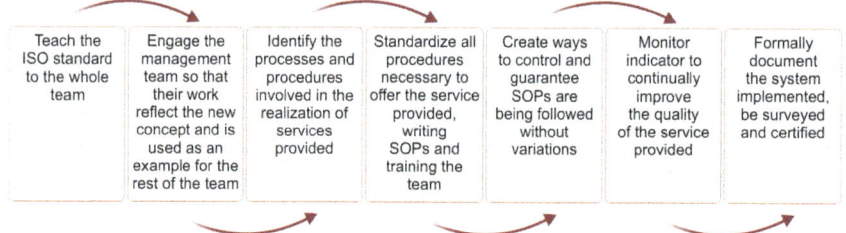

Fig. 3: Regulation of SOPs and their implementation in the ART laboratory. (ART: assisted reproductive technology; ISO: International Organization for Standardization; SOPs: standard operating procedures)

Quality of care is a multifaceted phenomenon that includes the effectiveness of the treatment as well as the effects on the well-being of each patient and their descendants, and it should not be jeopardized. Furthermore, quality embraces the economic and human value of acquiring the desired goal. However, the "process" is the only fundamental objective and observable aspect of quality.

Every IVF laboratory must be certified and accredited by a reputable organization. Contrariwise, take cognizance that proper QA and QC are not only necessary for the accreditation of a human IVF laboratory, but they are also vital for sustainability.

WHAT ARE THE STANDARD QUALITY INDICATORS? (FIG. 4)

Only those metrics whose significance is solely determined by laboratory procedures and protocols should be embodied in an IVF laboratory's PIs.

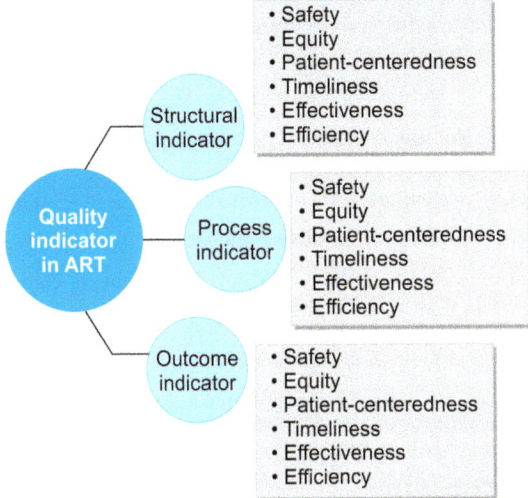

Fig. 4: Quality indicators in assisted reproductive technology (ART). [Security, equality, patient-centeredness, punctuality, efficacy, and quality are the six areas of health care that should often be considered when choosing KPIs **(Fig. 4)**. PIs should, in principle, encompass all of them. The most critical and commonly used metrics for monitoring ART are safety and effectiveness].
Source: Fabozzi G, Cimadomo D, Maggiulli R, Vaiarelli A, Ubaldi FM, Rienzi L. Which key performance indicators are most effective in evaluating and managing an in vitro fertilization laboratory? Fertil Steril. 2020;114(1):9-15.

(e.g., Pregnancy rate, its prominence is determined by clinical practices and patient behaviors).

Structural Indicators

It assesses the consistency of the following:
- Facilities, machinery, and finances are examples of physical aspects.
- Human resources (e.g., operators count, and their qualifications and abilities).

Process Indicators

It evaluates the laboratory's performance in terms of safety, quality, and promptness.

Outcome Indicators

It estimates the efficiency. of an IVF laboratory performance indicators for ART laboratories, i.e., reference indicators to assess performance **(Table 1)**, PIs, and KPIs **(Tables 2 and 3)**, are as follows, as per the Vienna consensus report.

TABLE 1: Reference indicators (RIs) for evaluating the ART laboratory's efficiency.

RI	Calculation	Benchmark value
The proportion of oocytes recovered (stimulated cycles)	$\dfrac{\text{Number of oocytes retrieved}}{\text{Number of follicles on day of trigger}} \times 100$	80–95% of follicles measured
Proportion of MII oocytes at ICSI	$\dfrac{\text{Number of MII oocytes at ICSI}}{\text{Number of COCs retrieved}} \times 100$	75–90%

(ART: assisted reproductive technology; COC: cumulus-oocyte complex; ICSI: intracytoplasmic sperm injection; MII: metaphase II)

TABLE 2: Performance indicators (PIs) for the ART laboratory.

PI	Calculation	Competency value (%)	Benchmark value (%)
Sperm motility postpreparation (for IVF and IUI)	$\dfrac{\text{Progressively motile sperm}}{\text{All sperm counted}} \times 100$	90	≥95
IVF polyspermy rate	$\dfrac{\text{Number of fertilized oocytes with >2PN}}{\text{Number of COCs inseminated}} \times 100$	<6	
1 PN rate (IVF)	$\dfrac{\text{Number of 1PN oocytes}}{\text{Number of COCs inseminated}} \times 100$	<5	
1 PN rate (ICSI)	$\dfrac{\text{Number of 1PN oocytes}}{\text{Number of MII oocytes injected}} \times 100$	<3	
Good blastocyst development rate	$\dfrac{\text{Number of good quality blastocysts on day 5}}{\text{Number of 2PN/2PB oocytes on day 1}} \times 100$	≥30	≥40

(COCs: cumulus-oocyte complexes; ICSI: intracytoplasmic sperm injection; IUI: intrauterine insemination; IVF: in vitro fertilization; MII: metaphase II; PB: polar body; PN: pronucleus)

To optimize the exploitation of the entire quality management approach, the emphasis should be on the **Figure 5 and Flowchart 1**.

QUALITY MANAGEMENT IN ART LABORATORY

The general ambience of the IVF laboratory, and the expertise of the working clinician and embryologists have a noteworthy impact on the progress rate of IVF. Couples receiving IVF treatment should bear the responsibility for

TABLE 3: KPIs for the ART laboratory.

KPI	Calculation	Competency value (%)	Benchmark value (%)
ICSI damage rate	$\dfrac{\text{Number of damaged or degenerated}}{\text{All oocytes injected}} \times 100$	≤10	≤5
ICSI normal fertilization rate	$\dfrac{\text{Number of oocytes with 2PN and 2P}}{\text{Number of MII oocytes injected}} \times 100$	≥65	≥80
IVF normal fertilization rate	$\dfrac{\text{Number of oocytes with 2PN and 2PB}}{\text{Number of COCs inseminated}} \times 100$	≥60	≥75
Failed fertilization rate (IVF)	$\dfrac{\text{Number of cycles with no evidence of fertilization}}{\text{Number of stimulated IVF cycles}} \times 100$	<5	
Cleavage rate	$\dfrac{\text{Number of cleaved embryos on day 2}}{\text{Number of 2PN/2PB oocytes on day 1}} \times 100$	≥95	≥99
Day 2 embryo development rate	$\dfrac{\text{Number of 4-cell embryos on day 2}}{\text{Number of normally fertilized oocytes}^a} \times 100$	≥50	≥80
Day 3 embryo development rate	$\dfrac{\text{Number of 8-cell embryos on day 3}}{\text{Number of normally fertilized oocytes}^a} \times 100$	≥45	≥70
Blastocyst development rate	$\dfrac{\text{Number of blastocysts on day 5}}{\text{Number of normally fertilized oocytes}^a} \times 100$	≥40	≥60
Successful biopsy rate	$\dfrac{\text{Number of biopsies with DNA detected}}{\text{Number of biopsies performed}} \times 100$	≥90	≥95
Blastocyst cryo-survival rate	$\dfrac{\text{Number of blastocysts appearing intact}}{\text{Number of blastocysts warmed}} \times 100$	≥90	≥99
Implantation rate (cleavage-stage)[b]	$\dfrac{\text{Number of sacs seen on ultrasound}^c}{\text{Number of embryos transferred}} \times 100$	≥25	≥35
Implantation rate (blastocyst-stage)[b]	$\dfrac{\text{Number of sacs seen on ultrasound}^c}{\text{Number of blastocysts transferred}} \times 100$	≥35	≥60

[a]Defined as oocytes with 2PN and 2PB on day 1.
[b]Based on the overall number of embryos delivered to all of the patients in the reference group, not just those who had successful insertion.
[c]After some debate, it was decided that the number of fetal hearts/number of embryos implanted was a more reliable marker.
(COCs: cumulus-oocyte complexes; DNA: deoxyribonucleic acid; ICSI: intracytoplasmic sperm injection; IVF: in vitro fertilization; KPI: key performance indicator; MII: metaphase II)

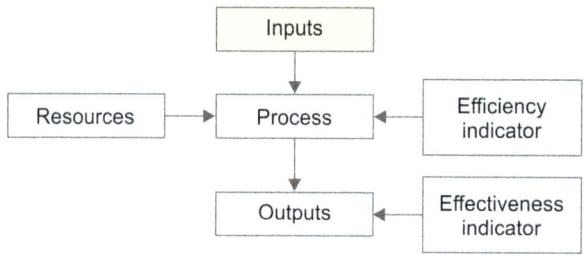

Fig. 5: Process mapping.

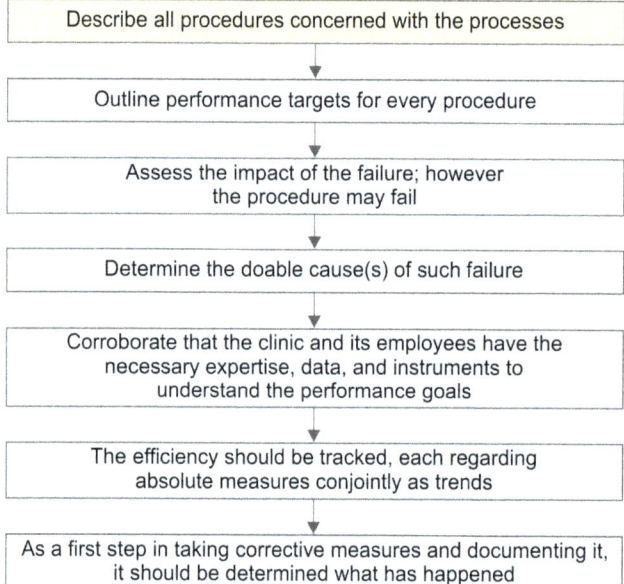

Flowchart 1: Protocol for quality management.

concerns such as when to go to the clinics, when to take medicines and doses, abstinence, and when and where to collect the semen, among other things **(Flowchart 1)**.

Both of the above aspects promote the high quality and acceptable results of an IVF laboratory to an ART clinic **(Fig. 6)**. Consequently, effective coordination among all parties (the IVF staff, team members, and patients) is critical to maintaining the IVF laboratory's performance.

Many countries have developed ART regulatory bodies and associations in response to the requirements of ART treatment, which are detailed in **Table 4**.

Indian Council of Medical Research (ICMR) has authorized ART clinic specifications in India. The quality standard that assures patient safety, care quality, and the desire for success and progress. Total quality management (TQM) is both a philosophy and a way of life. The sterile zone of an ART

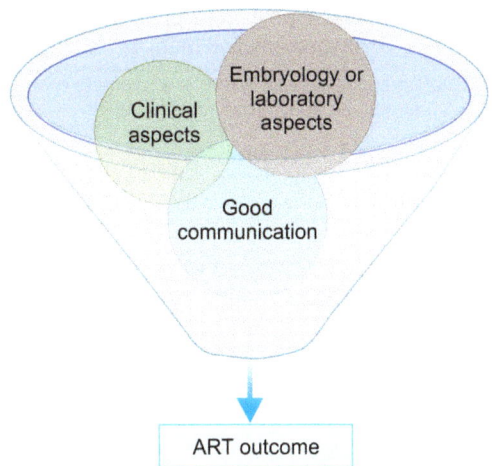

Fig. 6: The essential aspects affecting the ART outcome.

TABLE 4: Various ART regulatory organizations and their provisions.	
Organizations	**Functions**
Clinical Laboratory Improvement Amendments of 1988 (CLIA'88)	It establishes laboratory protocol guiding principles and technical standards
The Society for Assisted Reproductive Technologies (SART) and the European Society of Human Reproduction and Embryology (ESHRE)	It introduces and implements ART standards. It offers recommendations on how to manage clinical and laboratory operations safety and quality assurance
Canadian Fertility and Andrology Society (CFAS) and American Society for Reproductive Medicine (ASRM)	They fulfill their mission by achieving excellence in evidence, lifelong learning, promoting and supporting ground-breaking research, developing and promoting the highest safety and technical standards in patient care, and advocating on behalf of physicians and healthcare affiliates and their patients

clinic is determined chiefly by where and how it is designed, so a good IVF laboratory QC is nothing more than a sterile QC area.

STERILITY AND INFECTION CONTROL IN THE STERILE ZONE

Infection management is pivotal for quality control and progress in the IVF laboratory. The key vectors of contamination are the outside world, sperm, and people permissible to enter the laboratory. Into the bargain, the growth culpable for infection dissemination can be observed in the culture media utilized in IVF techniques **(Flowchart 2)**.

Flowchart 2: Standard operational protocol for sterile zones handling, management, and mobility.

```
┌─────────────────────────────────────────────────────────┐
│ Handling and preparing sperm in a separate room         │
│ should be accomplished with caution                     │
└─────────────────────────────────────────────────────────┘
                          ↓
┌─────────────────────────────────────────────────────────┐
│ The laboratory should be shielded from the outside      │
│ atmosphere to the greatest degree possible              │
└─────────────────────────────────────────────────────────┘
                          ↓
┌─────────────────────────────────────────────────────────┐
│ A washing room with a sufficient water supply should be │
│ attached to the laboratory for effective scrub control  │
└─────────────────────────────────────────────────────────┘
                          ↓
┌─────────────────────────────────────────────────────────┐
│ Visitors can change into new operation theaters (OTs)   │
│ gowns before accessing the laboratory                   │
└─────────────────────────────────────────────────────────┘
                          ↓
┌─────────────────────────────────────────────────────────┐
│ A non-toxic laboratory disinfectant (Oosafe) should be  │
│ used to wipe the floor, tabletops, and workstations at  │
│ regular intervals (preferable twice daily)              │
└─────────────────────────────────────────────────────────┘
                          ↓
┌─────────────────────────────────────────────────────────┐
│ To prevent contamination, all processing steps should   │
│ be performed in a laminar air hood                      │
└─────────────────────────────────────────────────────────┘
                          ↓
┌─────────────────────────────────────────────────────────┐
│ After each treatment, waste materials should be         │
│ disposed of accurately and promptly                     │
└─────────────────────────────────────────────────────────┘
                          ↓
┌─────────────────────────────────────────────────────────┐
│ The internal insulation of an older incubator is the    │
│ origin of repeated fungal infection. It is desirable    │
│ to get rid of the old incubator                         │
└─────────────────────────────────────────────────────────┘
                          ↓
┌─────────────────────────────────────────────────────────┐
│ Antibiotics used in media have bactericidal and         │
│ bacteriostatic properties that aid in infection         │
│ prevention                                              │
└─────────────────────────────────────────────────────────┘
```

MAINTENANCE OF ESSENTIAL PIECES OF EQUIPMENT AND CHECKPOINTS IN AN IVF LABORATORY

Laboratories usually have various pieces of equipment as shown in **Figure 7**.

It is prudent and necessary to conduct regular quality control inspections of all types of equipment. At the very least, on every day of operation, each piece of equipment should be scrutinized for appropriate functioning. **Table 5** enlists some common instruments and pieces of equipment and what to and when to monitor them. This form of equipment monitoring aids in identifying and repairing noncompliant equipment.

A logbook or registry with service/repair records should be kept with all equipment. All ART clinics should accomplish quality assessments through internal and external audit management and interprofessional scrutiny.

DISPOSABLES AND CONSUMABLES

The goal of quality control of equipment and consumables is to ascertain whether the products carried to the laboratory or culture possess any "toxic"

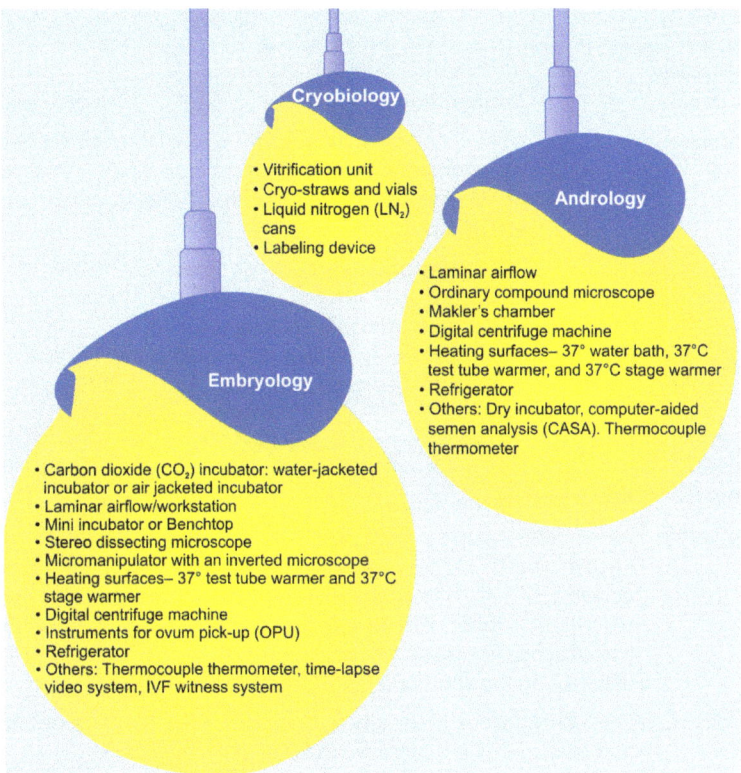

Fig. 7: Sections of the assisted reproductive technology (ART) laboratory and necessary equipment.

TABLE 5: List of equipment, parameters of QC, frequency of QC, and frequency of calibration.

Equipment	Parameters of QC	Frequency of QC	Frequency of calibration
Incubator	Temperature CO_2	Daily Daily	Once in a 3 month
Heating surfaces	Temperature	Daily	Once in a 3 month
Heating bath	Temperature Water level	Daily Daily	Once in a 3 month
Heating block	Temperature	Daily	Once in a 3 month
Microscope	Image quality	Daily	Once in a 3 month
CASA	Sperm count Motility (%) Vitality (%) Motility (%)	Daily Daily Daily Daily	Once in a year
Storage dewars	Liquid N_2 level	Daily	
Refrigerator	Temperature	Daily	Once in a 3 month
Heating, ventilation, and air conditioning system	Room temperature Room humidity	Daily Daily	Clean filters periodically

(CASA: computer-assisted sperm analysis; QC: quality control)

TABLE 6: Different disposables/consumables and their examination.

Disposables/consumables	Examination
Plasticware	It should be manufactured from reputable sources and distributed from them. The most crucial part is to have a grade of tissue culture certified as nontoxic using mouse embryo assay (MEA)
Culture media	The quality of culture media is dependent on the following: • The transport chain maintenance • The laboratory storage. Bear in mind that once best used, no media is acceptable

TABLE 7: The optimal condition for IVF and embryo development.

Parameters	Key role
Temperature	IVF gametes (oocytes, sperm, and embryos) depend principally on incubators (37°C) as they are sensitive to temperature. Long exposure at below 37°C leads to permanent meiotic spindle damage and fails to fertilize or abnormally fertilize. Using a warmer 37°C stage over a microscope (stereo and inverted), the test tube warmer assists in maintaining the appropriate temperature outside the incubator
Humidity	The mold infection in the laboratory is a common contaminant; thus, humidity control is imperative to avoid the infection
pH and osmolarity	The pH of the incubator should be managed to hold at 7.2–7.4 by specifying a CO_2 percentage (5–6%). The cultivation of oocytes in oil-overlaid culture media upholds osmolarity
Light	Since oocytes are more susceptible to light, they can only be screened and graded under microscopic light. Low-intensity light can be used to manipulate oocytes and embryos. Light with a wavelength of <480 nm has been revealed to detriment hamster oocytes in studies

Source: Hirao Y, Yanagimachi R. Detrimental effect of visible light on meiosis of mammalian eggs in vitro. J Exp Zool. 1978;206(3):365-9.

element. The users should ensure that any items bought by them have already been tested for toxicity with mouse embryo assay (MEA). Manufacturers examine all the products to make certain that they do not pose a risk prior to sale, as shown in **Table 6**.

The optimal condition for IVF and embryo development relies on a satisfactory physiochemical equilibrium, and it is dependent on the factors mentioned in **Table 7**.

MONITORING OF LABORATORY ENVIRONMENT

To monitor air quality, the center should validate high-efficiency particulate air (HEPA) filters consistent with the manufacturer's recommendations.

TABLE 8: Checkpoints in IVF laboratory.	
When to check?	**What to check?**
Daily checking	CO_2 cylinder, temperature, and humidity of laboratory, CO_2 concentration and temperature of incubators, Temperature of heating stage and test tube warmer, bubbles in the Teflon tubes of the micromanipulator, microscopes, liquid N_2 storage, overall cleaning—IVF OT, IVF laboratory and vicinity, and daily disposal of waste materials from the laboratory after each procedure is mandatory
Weekly checking	Liquid nitrogen level, the water level on the floor of an incubator, pH of the culture media, and fan of the incubator
Monthly checking	Changing of liquid paraffin of micromanipulator tubes, stock of all disposables and media, checking of UPS, and alarm system
Quarterly checking	Servicing and calibration of an incubator, servicing of all microscopes, servicing of the micromanipulator, servicing of all test tube warmers, and refrigerators if needed
Half-yearly checking	Change of filter of laminar airflow, change of CO_2 filters of an incubator, change of a filter of Coda tower
Annual checking	Record keeping and maintenance, and overall laboratory complex

(IVF: in vitro fertilization; OT: operation theater; UPS: uninterruptible power supply)

For laboratory desks, laminar airflow cabinets, incubators, and other areas where an aseptic environment is needed, air samples, and swabs must be assayed for the microbial count at least once every three months. For IVF laboratory quality control, some checkpoints are desirable that should be tracked as per the set standards on a regular, weekly, monthly, quarterly, half-yearly, and annualized basis; checkpoints in the laboratory setting should be monitored **(Table 8)**.

The monitoring of these laboratory checkpoints offers a shred of clear evidence if something goes wrong and that any equipment repair or calibration is necessary before the deadline.

RECORD KEEPING AND DOCUMENTATION

The outcomes should be measured periodically. The following should be analyzed sporadically in consultation with the clinical staff for a full assessment of the findings. All records should be held to demonstrate that quality monitoring has been carried out, and data can be validated later to determine and correct the cause of the problem (quality assurance/improvement task). As shown in **Box 1**, a standard laboratory should keep track of the mentioned documents.

LABORATORY STAFFING

Enough personnel should be available to conduct both andrology and embryology work in order to cover all of the functions stated in the guidelines. Even if no ART cases are conducted, the ART laboratory should have a set amount of work (primarily quality control functions) that must be accomplished in order to keep the laboratory running. To qualify as a technologist, employees must conduct a minimum of 30 complete protocols in accordance with ASRM guidelines. Moreover, at least two qualified embryologists should be present in a laboratory according to the ASRM guidelines **(Table 9)**. In compliance with ICMR guidelines, an ART team should have a proposed framework for education and staffing **(Table 10)**. It must have the requisite credentials or degrees and a deep understanding of its areas and commitments in ART.

OCCUPATIONAL TRAINING

All ART laboratory staff should receive research laboratory adroitness training from a clinical laboratory technologist course/program. Currently, there are master's degree courses in clinical embryology and numerous postgraduate diploma courses in India. The National Academy of Medical Science (NAMS), which is overseen by the Ministry of New Delhi's National

BOX 1: Protocol for record management and accurate documentation.
- Documentation of daily laboratory work experience, as well as all checkpoints (lab temperature and humidity, temperature of text tube warmer, stage warmer, and refrigerator, temperature and CO_2 percent of incubators, CO_2 cylinder pressure, LN_2 level check and filling) and instrument assessment study are critical for potential upgrade or alteration
- A file containing all consent forms or legal documents related to IUI, home collection, surrogacy, egg/sperm donation and adoption, embryo/sperm freezing continuation/discontinuation, embryo transfer, and so on
- Publication and research program records, which are essential for future advancement
- Documents pertaining to the license, registration, and so on
- Laboratory meeting minutes and documentation of next objective, etc.
- All SOPs should be compiled into a manual and kept in the laboratory, where they can be consulted

TABLE 9: Minimum number of embryologists per cycle as per ASRM guidelines.

Number of laboratory cycles	Minimum number of embryologists
1–150	2
151–300	3
301–600	4
>600	For an additional 200 cycles, 1 additional embryologist

TABLE 10: Educational and staffing structure for an ART team.

Staffing level	Academic qualification
Director	Postgraduate Degree or Diploma in Management and Administration, Life Science, Pharmacy/Pharmacology or Medicine from a recognized University
Incharge	Postgraduate Degree or Diploma in Obstetrics and Gynecologist
Gynecologist	Preferably Postgraduate Degree or Diploma in Obstetrics and Gynecologist
Andrologist	At least a degree (preferably a postgraduate degree) in Life Sciences or Medicine
Clinical embryologist	Postgraduate Degree in Life Science or Medicine
Counselor	At least a degree (preferably a postgraduate degree) in Social Sciences, Psychology, Life Sciences, or Medicine

Board of Examination, has launched a Fellowship in Reproductive Medicine that will comprise comprehensive training in infertility, including ART.

CODE OF PRACTICE

The ICMR guidelines state that a "code of practice" plays a vital role to perpetuate the standard of an ART clinic. It covers all aspects of the care given at the ART clinic. It primarily concerns the staff's ability to:
- Provide information to the patients
- Maintain confidentiality
- Take consent from the patient regarding each procedure

CONCLUSION

Although managing QA and QC is a challenging job, good team coordination will make it much easier. Internal audit and routine or occasional strict supervision of clinical and laboratory triggers are enhancing output. Continuous education, adequate preparation, optimal quality control practices, and internal and external audits boost the ART clinic's total standard.

SUGGESTED READING

1. Bento F, Esteves S, Agarwal A. In: Boston MA (Eds). Introduction to Quality Management in ART Clinics: A Practical Guide. New York: Springer Publishing Company; 2013. pp. 3-6.
2. Boone WR, Johnson JE, Locke AJ, Crane MM 4th, Price TM. Control of air quality in an assisted reproductive technology laboratory. Fertil Steril. 1999;71(1):150-4.
3. Centers for Disease Control and Prevention, Centers for Medicare and Medicaid Services. Medicare, Medicaid, and CLIA programs; laboratory requirements relating to quality systems and certain personnel qualifications. Final rule. Fed Regist. 2003;68(16):3639-714.

4. Charles L, Kissel C. Introduction of a Structured Training Course for Medical Doctors in Training in the Field of Reproductive Medicine. Obstetrics Frauenheilkd. 2004;64(2):160-3.
5. Dancet EAF, D'Hooghe TM, Spiessens C, Sermeus W, De Neubourg D, Karel N, et al. Quality indicators for all dimensions of infertility care quality: consensus between professionals and patients. Hum Reprod. 2013;28(6):1584-97.
6. Ectors FJ, Vanderzwalmen P, Van Hoeck J, Nijs M, Verhaegen G, Delvigne A, et al. Relationship of human follicular diameter with oocyte fertilization and development after in-vitro fertilization or intracytoplasmic sperm injection. Hum Reprod. 1997;12(9):2002-5.
7. European Society of Human Reproduction and Embryology (ESHRE), Special Interest Group of Embryology, Alpha Scientists in Reproductive Medicine. The Vienna consensus: report of an expert meeting on the development of ART laboratory performance indicators. Hum Reprod Open. 2017; 2017 (2): hox011.
8. Fabozzi G, Cimadomo D, Maggiulli R, Vaiarelli A, Ubaldi FM, Rienzi L. Which key performance indicators are most effective in evaluating and managing an in vitro fertilization laboratory? Fertil Steril. 2020;114(1):9-15.
9. Gardner DK, Weissman A, Howles CM, Shoham Z. Textbook of assisted reproductive technologies: Laboratory and clinical perspectives (Reproductive Medicine and Asst. Reproduction), 3rd edition. London: Informa Healthcare; 2009.
10. Gianaroli L, Plachot M, van Kooij R, Al-Hasani S, Dawson K, DeVos A, et al. ESHRE guidelines for good practice in IVF laboratories. Committee of the Special Interest Group on Embryology of the European Society of Human Reproduction and Embryology. Hum Reprod. 2000;15(10):2241-6.
11. Hirao Y, Yanagimachi R. Detrimental effect of visible light on meiosis of mammalian eggs in vitro. J Exp Zool. 1978;206(3):365-9.
12. Johnson L. Regulation of assisted reproductive treatment (ART) in Australia and current ethical issues. Indian J Med Res. 2014;140(Suppl 1):S9-12.
13. Kamini R. Principles & Practice Of Assisted Reproductive Technology (3 Vols), 1st edition. New Delhi: Jaypee Brothers Medical Publishers (P) Ltd; 2014.
14. Matson PL. Internal quality control and external quality assurance in the IVF laboratory. Hum Reprod. 1998;13(Suppl 4):156-65.
15. Mayer JF, Jones EL, Dowling-Lacey D, Nehchiri F, Muasher SJ, Gibbons WE, et al. Total quality improvement in the IVF laboratory: choosing indicators of quality. Reprod Biomed Online. 2003;7(6):695-9.
16. Ministry of Health and Family Welfare, Government of India. National Guidelines for Accreditation, Supervision and Regulation of ART Clinics in India. Indian Council of Medical Research National Academy of Medical Sciences (India); 2005. [online] Available from https://main.icmr.nic.in/sites/default/files/art/ART_Pdf.pdf [Last accessed July, 2022].
17. Nagy ZP, Varghese AC, Agarwal A. Practical manual of in vitro fertilization: advanced methods and novel devices. New York: Springer; 2016.
18. Nogueira D, Friedler S, Schachter M, Raziel A, Ron-El R, Smitz J. Oocyte maturity and preimplantation development in relation to follicle diameter in gonadotropin-releasing hormone agonist or antagonist treatments. Fertil Steril. 2006;85(3):578-83.
19. Olofsson JI, Banker MR, Sjoblom LP. Quality management systems for your in vitro fertilization clinic's laboratory: Why bother? J Hum Reprod Sci. 2013;6(1):3-8.
20. Practice Committee of Society for Assisted Reproductive Technology, Practice Committee of American Society for Reproductive Medicine. Revised minimum standards for practices offering assisted reproductive technologies. Fertil Steril. 2008;90(Suppl 5):S165-8.
21. Scott RT, Hofmann GE, Muasher SJ, Acosta AA, Kreiner DK, Rosenwaks Z. Correlation of follicular diameter with oocyte recovery and maturity at the time of transvaginal follicular aspiration. J In Vitro Fert Embryo Transf. 1989;6(2):73-5.

CHAPTER 33

Ovarian Hyperstimulation Syndrome

Bansi Shinde, Shashikant Umbardand

INTRODUCTION

Ovarian hyperstimulation syndrome (OHSS) is the most serious and potentially fatal iatrogenic complication of controlled ovarian stimulation (COS).[1,2] It represents with broad clinical and laboratory spectrum, ranging from mild to occasional serious and critical OHSS. It is commonly associated with increased ovarian volume and high serum estradiol (E2) levels with fluid shift to third spaces.

Though it's an iatrogenic condition, rarely spontaneous occurrence or familial predisposition is seen.

INCIDENCE

Mostly under reported.

Mild	8–23%
Moderate	<1–7%
Severe	<1–10%

Incidence of moderate to severe form may reach up to 20% in high-risk women.[3]

PATHOPHYSIOLOGY

Increased vascular permeability (VP) with loss of fluids, proteins and electrolytes in the third space is hallmark of OHSS.[4] Though extensively studied, exact etiology remains controversial.

High levels E2 were supposed to play key role in OHSS, but E2 did not cause circulatory dysfunction or exhibit direct vasoactive effects. Ajonuma et al. showed up-regulation of cystic fibrosis transmembrane conductance regulator (CFTR) by E2, leading to increased channel activity in most exocrine glands and peritoneal membrane causing excessive fluid shift.[5]

Variety of cytokines and growth factors are increased in OHSS (as per **Flowchart 1**). Many of these are proangiogenic and are responsible for neovascularization and increased endothelial permeability.

Flowchart 1: Pathophysiology of ovarian hyperstimulation syndrome (OHSS).

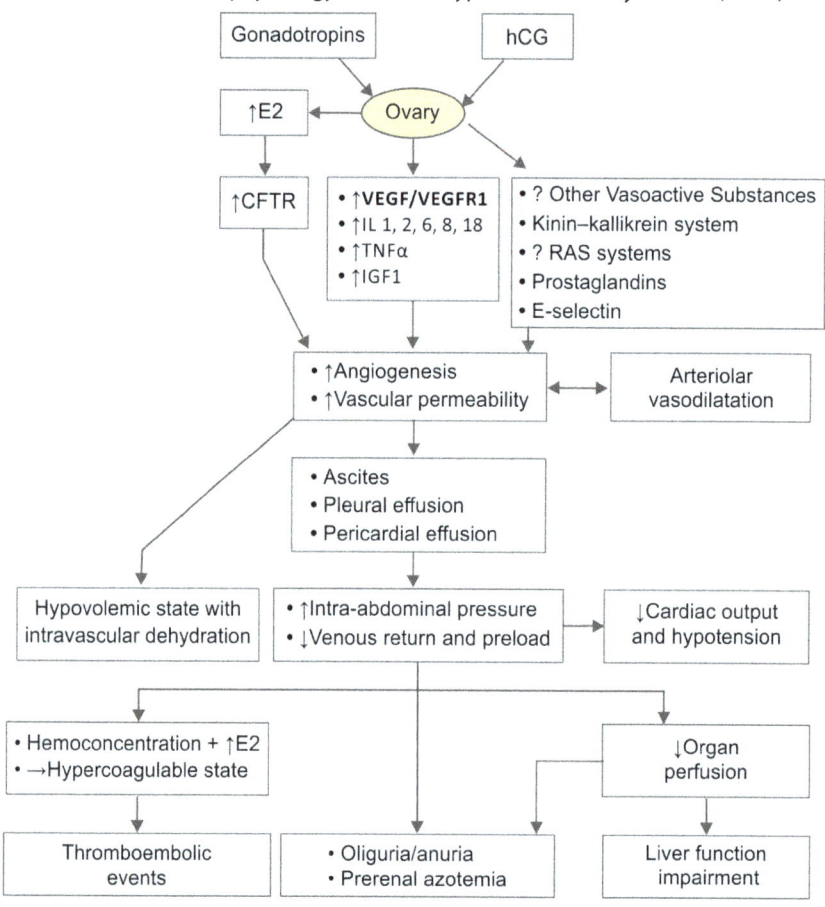

Current research suggests that human chorionic gonadotropin (hCG) and Vascular endothelial growth factor (VEGF) play critical role in OHSS. VEGF levels correlate with severity of OHSS and with-holding hCG administration will prevent OHSS. In humans, hCG has shown increased VEGF expression in granulosa lutein cells.[6] Recombinant VEGF created similar condition which was reversed by VEGF antiserum in study conditions. VEGF antiserum may prove revolutionary in OHSS treatment.

CLINICAL DIAGNOSIS

The important and most common symptoms are given in **Table 1**.

CLASSIFICATION

It is classified as per severity or onset of disease **(Table 2)**. Based on severity of disease, it will help the clinician to assess appropriate management plan.

TABLE 1: Most common symptoms and signs.

Clinical symptoms	Clinical signs	Laboratory findings
• Lower abdominal discomfort • Abdominal distension • Nausea/vomiting Breathlessness/cough • Diarrhea • Respiratory discomfort • Rapid weight gain • Oliguria/anuria	• Increased ovarian size • Ascites • Pleural effusion • Pericardial effusion • Low BP	• Hemoconcentration • Leukocytosis • Electrolyte imbalance • Deranged liver enzymes • ↓creatinine clearance • Hypoalbuminemia

TABLE 2: Classification as per severity or onset of disease.[7]

OHSS stage	Clinical features	Laboratory features
Mild	• Abdominal distention/discomfort • Mild nausea/vomiting/diarrhea • Mild dyspnea • Enlarged ovaries	No important alterations
Moderate	• Mild features + • USG evidence of ascites	• Hemoconcentration (Hct >41%) • Leukocytosis (>15,000/mL)
Severe	• Mild and moderate features + • Clinical evidence of ascites • Hydrothorax/Pleural effusion • Severe dyspnea • Oliguria/anuria • Intractable nausea/vomiting • Low blood/central venous pressure • Rapid weight gain (>1 kg in 24 hours) • Syncope • Severe abdominal pain • Venous thrombosis	• Severe hemoconcentration (Hct >55%) • WBC >25,000 mL • CrCl <50 mL/min • Cr >1.6 mg/dL • Na$^+$ <135 mEq/L • K$^+$ >5 mEq/L • Elevated liver enzymes
Critical	• Anuria/acute renal failure • Arrhythmia/pericardial effusion • Thromboembolism • Massive hydrothorax • Arterial thrombosis • Adult respiratory distress syndrome • Sepsis	Worsening of findings

Classification by Disease Onset

Early: 3–7 days after hCG trigger, Due to ovarian stimulation, always iatrogenic.

Late: >10 days after hCG trigger, due to endogenous hCG from early pregnancy. It is Last longer and likely more severe. Rarely, it can occur in nonstimulated cycles.

PREVENTION

Ovarian hyperstimulation syndrome being an iatrogenic complication every effort should be made for prevention. Due to controversial pathophysiology and few criteria of reliable value, *prevention is not always possible.*

- *Identify high-risk women (Box 1):* Think of alternative option in these patients like life style modification, use of oral ovulogens, laparoscopic ovarian drilling (LOD)
- *Stimulation protocols:*
  For IUI:
  - Aromatase inhibitors preferred over clomiphene citrate in hyper-responders.
  - Gonadotropins—use *chronic low dose protocol.*
  - Hyper-response (E2 >1,700 pg/mL or >6 dominant follicles)—convert to IVF/cancel cycle.
  - Ovum pick-up (OPU) will decrease granulosa cell mass and hence circulating proinflammatory cytokines.
    - Explain patient to keep abstinence to prevent late OHSS
    - Judicious use of ovulation induction/ovulogens/gonadotropins

  In ART:
  - *Step-down protocols* better over *step-up* in hyper-responders
  - *Antagonists protocol* significantly reduces risk of OHSS
  - Recombinant FSH or urinary products—does not make any difference
  - Mild stimulation protocol to be used
  - Proper cycle monitoring by frequent use of USG/E2 levels

BOX 1: High-risk factors.

- Previous history OHSS
- Age <33 years
- Lean patients
- PCOS
- AMH >3.36 ng/mL
- AFC >10–12 per ovary
- High E2 (>3,500 pg/mL for ART or >1,700 pg/mL for OI)
- Multifollicular development (>20 for ART or >6 for OI)
- More than 24 oocytes retrieved
- hCG luteal support
- Long GnRH-a protocols
- Pregnancy

- Continuation of GnRH-a for 7 days after hCG trigger in long agonist protocol.
- Single embryo transfer in high-risk patients.
- Use of progesterone for hCG for luteal phase support
- *Trigger modifications:*
  - hCG mimics the standard preovulatory LH surge; but have high affinity for LH receptors and long half-life
  - Reduction in standard dose of 10,000 IU of hCG to 3300–5000 IU as per E2 levels, does not reduce risk of OHSS.
  - rLH in doses of 5,000–30,000 IU induced successful ovulation. Compared to hCG there is decreased incidence of OHSS.
  - GnRHa induces endogenous LH/FSH surge; in ovaries with intact HPO axis. Short LH surge (24 hours), along with pituitary downregulation of GnRH-receptors lead to reduced LH support and early luteolysis
  - GnRHa trigger will not work or there will be suboptimal response in patients with low baseline FSH and LH levels, very low LH level on the day of trigger, prolonged use of OC pills or with suppressed HPO axis (as in long agonist protocol).
  - *Dual trigger or rescue hCG* will prevent luteolysis; but again, there is risk of moderate to severe OHSS.
- *Cycle cancellation:* Very effective in reduction of OHSS but rarely followed due to economic loss, psychological factors and emotional stress for all involved.
- *Coasting:*
  - Coasting means with-holding gonadotropins for variable time to decrease the E2 levels and risk of OHSS.
  - At present, there is no sufficient evidence that coasting decreases the risk of OHSS.
- *Cryopreservation:*
  - Elective cryopreservation of embryos will avoid endogenous hCG rise and late OHSS.
  - As per recent systematic reviews, cryopreservation prevents OHSS.[7]
- *Role of albumin:* Not useful for prevention.
- *Dopamine agonist:*
  - It is postulated that Dopamine agonists reduces VEGF production and subsequent OHSS.
  - Cabergoline is given as 0.5 mg/day from hCG administration for 8 days.
  - As per recent practicing guideline form ASRM, dopamine agonists reduce incidence of OHSS.[7]
- *Metformin:*
  - Insulin-sensitizer, given as 500 mg TDS or 850 mg SR BID, from ovarian downregulation until OPU.

- From 2006, multiple studies showed that it decreases risk of OHSS in PCOS patients
- *Aspirin:*
  - Low dose aspirin 100 mg/day given from day 1 of stimulation to day of pregnancy test.
  - Women taking aspirin has lower incidence of severe OHSS.
- *Calcium infusion:*
  - Calcium inhibits cAMP synthesis and cAMP-dependent renin secretion
  - Given as 10 mL of 10% calcium gluconate in 200 mL of normal saline on day of OPU and day 1, 2 and 3 post-OPU.
  - Decreased risk of OHSS in patients receiving calcium infusion
  - Recommendation for routine use needs further studies

  1. Luteal antagonist administration
  2. Glucocorticoid use (Prednisolone 10–30 mg/day)
  3. Luteal Letrozole
  4. High dose (200 mg/day) IM progesterone

  } Insufficient data at present to make any recommendations[7]

- *Kisspetin-54:* Hypothalamic peptide, potent stimulator of HPO axis, increases LH and FSH secretion, promising results, no OHSS, can be a molecule for future.
- *In vitro maturation of oocytes (IVM):* Can be the treatment option of future.

Best prevention plan at present
Use of milder stimulation protocol/antagonist protocols; preferably step-down
↓
Associated use of Metformin, Low dose aspirin
↓
Agonist trigger with associated use of dopamine agonist and? Calcium infusion
↓
Cryopreservation followed by frozen embryo transfer

PROGNOSIS

- Mild and moderate cases = Excellent prognosis
- Severe cases = Morbidity is clinically significant, and fatalities do occur
- Optimistic if adequate treatment is given

Causes of death: Hypovolemic shock, electrolyte imbalance, hemorrhage, thromboembolism. Estimated fatality rates are 1 per 400,000–500,000 stimulated cycles.

MANAGEMENT

- Should be individualized, taking into account risk factors and conception (Fig. 1)
- Treatment of OHSS depends on severity—OPD/IPD management
- Appropriate counseling and reassurance with verbal and written information about their condition
- Heightened clinical suspicion and early intervention are paramount to the reduction of morbidity and mortality.

Mild and Moderate Cases

- Managed as outpatients
- Record vital clinical parameters, weight, abdominal circumference, intake-urine output, CBC, LFT/RFT, S/E, USG-ascites, ovarian volume

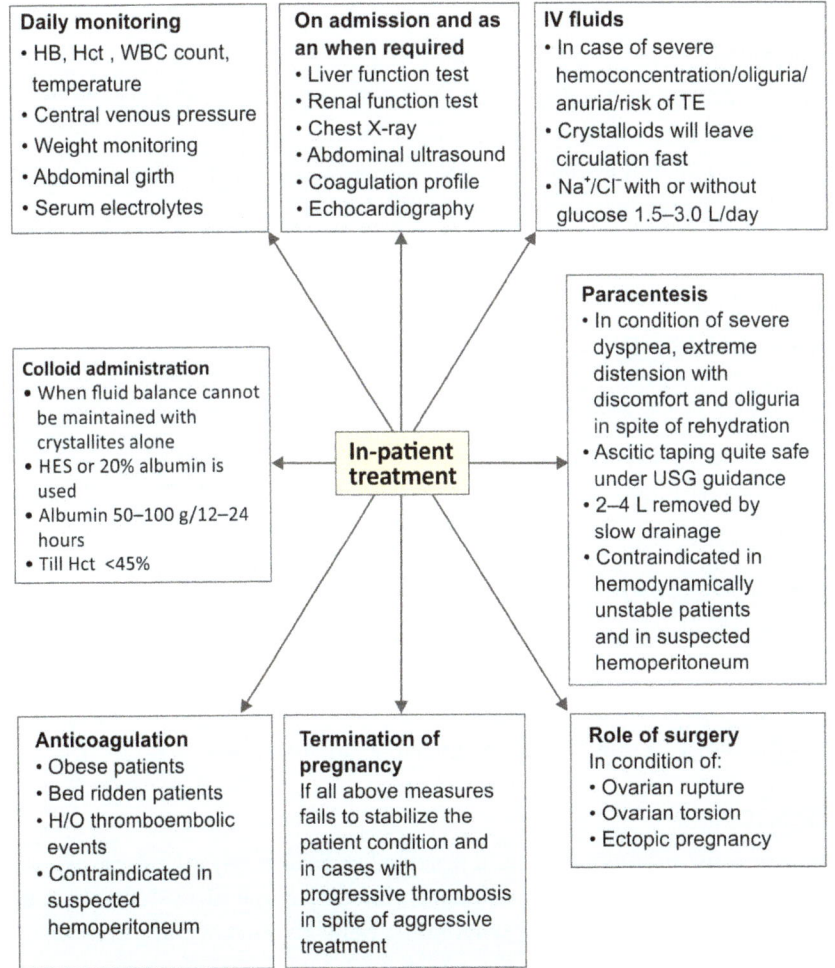

Fig. 1: Management of ovarian hyperstimulation syndrome (OHSS).

- Review every 2-3 days
- Usually self-limiting, resolves over a period of 10-12 days, if no conception
- Investigations repeated if the severity is worsening
- Hematocrit is a useful guide to the degree of intravascular volume depletion.

Clinicians and patients should be vigilant for signs of worsening OHSS. These include:
- Increasing abdominal distension and pain
- Shortness of breath
- Tachycardia or hypotension
- Reduced urine output (less than 1,000 mL/24 h) or positive fluid balance (>1,000 mL/24 h)
- Weight gain
- Increasing hematocrit (Hct >45%).

Pain Relief

- Nonsteroidal anti-inflammatory drugs (NSAIDs) should be avoided, may compromise renal function. Paracetamol is preferred.
- Severe pain may signal a complication such as ovarian torsion/rupture or ectopic pregnancy which is surgically managed.
- Possibility of pelvic infection should be considered.

Antiemetics

If nausea, vomiting.

Hydration/Fluid Therapy

- Encourage patients to drink to thirst,[7] reinforce fluid intake of 1-2 L.
- Encourage intake of fluids rich in proteins and electrolytes like fruit juices, soups.

Diet

Freshly prepared high protein diet preferred and increased fluid intake.

Activity

Physical activities should be minimal and avoid intercourse.

Urine Color

Color of urine is a very good and practical indicator denoting intravascular volume status.[8,9] Ask patients to report immediately if it turns darker in spite of adequate fluid intake. Early rehydration helps to prevent complications.

Severe and Critical OHSS

- Majority will need in-patient management
- Hospital admission should be considered for women who show the worsening signs mentioned earlier. Inpatient management helps in closer monitoring and multidisciplinary approach and early intervention.
- Patients with persistent dehydration and hemoconcentration despite adequate fluid replacement may need invasive hemodynamic monitoring.
- *Role of diuretics:* Diuretics should be avoided as they further deplete intravascular volume, but they may have a role in a multidisciplinary setting if oliguria persists despite adequate fluid replacement and drainage of ascites **(Flowchart 2)**.

Flowchart 2: Algorithm for intensive care of the patient with critical OHSS.[8]

Indications for Paracentesis
- Severe abdominal distension and abdominal pain secondary to ascites
- Shortness of breath and respiratory compromise secondary to ascites
- Oliguria despite adequate volume replacement, secondary to increased abdominal pressure causing reduced renal perfusion.

Intravenous Fluid Therapy
- If oral fluids cannot maintain hydration crystalloids are useful.
- Human albumin: Human albumin solution 25% may be used as a plasma volume expander in doses of 50–100 g, infused over 4 hours and repeated 4- to 12-hourly. Good diuresis and relief of symptoms observed after albumin infusion.

Careful maintenance of blood volume, correction of electrolyte imbalances, and relief of secondary complications of ascites and hydrothorax are generally sufficient to support the patient during the severe phase of ovarian hyperstimulation and will decrease thrombotic events.

The risk of thrombosis should be managed:
- Severe or critical OHSS, and moderate OHSS with predisposing risk factors for thrombosis should receive LMWH prophylaxis.
- Thrombosis can occur in the arteries (25%) and veins (75%).
- Thromboembolic incidence is in between 0.7 and 10% of cases of severe OHSS; frequently involving arterial system of upper body parts.
- Therefore, clinicians should remain vigilant of patients presenting with unusual symptoms such as dizziness, loss of vision and neck pain **(Table 1)**.
- *Pregnancies* complicated by OHSS may be at increased risk of preeclampsia, Preterm delivery, VTE.[10]

CONCLUSION

Ovarian hyperstimulation syndrome is an iatrogenic complication of COS. Hence, every treating physician must be aware of this syndrome—high risk factors, clinical features and preventive measures.

Milder hyperstimulation though, is a part of COS, with modified stimulation protocols, milder patient friendly stimulation, decreasing (preferably avoiding) hCG for trigger and use of GnRH-a trigger, options such as coasting, cycle cancellation, single embryo transfer and whenever required cryopreservation followed by FET will decrease the chances of severe and critical OHSS.

Thus, decreasing risk of OHSS along with early diagnosis and better management avoiding serious complication and eventually death of these patients will make ART more safe.

REFERENCES

1. Abramov Y, Elchalal U, Schenker JG. An epidemic of severe OHSS; a price we have to pay? Hum Reprod. 1999;14(9):2181-3.
2. Carlo CD, Savoia F, Ferrara C, Tommaselli GA, Bifulco G, Nappi C. Case Report: a most peculiar family with spontaneous, recurrent ovarian hyperstimulation syndrome. Gynecol Endocrinol. 2012;28(8):649-51.
3. Nastri CO, Ferriani RA, Rocha IA, Martins WP. Ovarian hyperstimulation syndrome: pathophysiology and prevention. J Assist Reprod Genet. 2010;27(2-3):121-8.
4. Tollan A, Holst N, Forsdahl F, Fadnes HO, Oian P, Maltau JM. Transcapillary fluid dynamics during ovarian stimulation for in vitro fertilization. Am J Obstet Gynecol 1990;162(2):554-8.
5. Ajonuma LC, Tsang LL, Zhang GH, Wong CHY, Lau MC, Ho LS, et al. Estrogen-induced abnormally high cystic fibrosis transmembrane conductance regulator expression results in ovarian hyperstimulation syndrome. Mol Endocrinol. 2005;19(12):3038-44.
6. Yamamoto S, Konishi I, Tsuruta Y, Nanbu K, Mandai M, Kuroda H, et al. Expression of vascular endothelial growth factor (VEGF) during folliculogenesis and corpus luteum formation in the human ovary. Gynecol Endocrinol. 1997;11(6):371-81.
7. Practice committee of American Society for Reproductive medicine. Prevention and treatment of moderate and severe ovarian hyperstimulation syndrome: a guideline. Fertil Steril. 2016;106(7):1634-47.
8. Levine Z, Navot D. Life-threatening forms of ovarian stimulation syndrome and intensive care of ovarian hyperstimulation syndrome patient. Ovarian Hyperstimulation Syndrome, 1st edition. Florida: CRC Press; 2006. pp. 169-77.
9. Kavouras SA. Assessing hydration status. Curr Opin Clin Nutr Metab Care. 2002; 5(5):519-24.
10. Schirmer DA 3rd, Kulkarni AD, Zhang Y, Kawwass JF, Boulet SL, Kissin DM. Ovarian hyperstimulation syndrome after assisted reproductive technologies: trends, predictors, and pregnancy outcomes. Fertil Steril. 2020;114(3):567-78.

34 | Recurrent Implantation Failure

Mohan Raut, Mugdha Raut

INTRODUCTION

Repeated embryo implantation failure is an extremely frustrating condition for both patients and clinicians and its treatment constitute one of the most difficult challenges in the field of in vitro fertilization (IVF).[1] The term "implantation failure" is used in case of two types of cases, patients who have never shown increased levels of human chorionic gonadotropin (hCG), and those who have increased hCG levels without any evidence of a gestational sac on ultrasonography (USG).[2] Implantation failure can apply to patients undergoing assisted reproductive technology (ART) and also in case of patients trying to conceive without any fertility treatment. However, in case of recurrent implantation failure (RIF), it is applicable only to patients undergoing ART.[3]

INCIDENCE

It has been reported that in healthy fertile women, spontaneous pregnancy is achieved in only about 25–40% cases in the first cycle when the pregnancy is planned.[4] In ART, the maximum implantation rate is between 40 and 60%.[5] 10% of couples undergoing IVF suffer from recurrent IVF failure.[6]

DEFINITIONS

It is difficult to give an exact definition of RIF as there are different criteria used by different centers.

Criteria used while defining RIF:
- Number of embryos transferred
- Number of embryos transfer (ET) procedures performed

Accordingly, there are various definitions of RIF as follows:
1. Patients with >12 embryos transferred in several procedures without achieving pregnancy (Coulam, 1995).[7]
2. Patients with 5–6 unsuccessful cycles, including frozen embryo transfer (FET). A total number of embryos transferred are between 10 and 15 (UK).

3. Failure to achieve pregnancy after three fresh ET procedures or three high grade embryos (Tan, 2005).[8]
4. Failure to achieve pregnancy after three or more unsuccessful transfers of high quality embryos or transfers of 10 or more embryos, in total in multiple transfers (PGD Consortium ESHRE).[9]
5. Failure to achieve pregnancy after eight or more transfers of eight cell embryos or five or more blastocyst transfers.[5]
6. Failure to achieve pregnancy after three single embryo transfer with good quality embryo (2006).[10]
7. Failure to achieve pregnancy after three or more ET or four embryos in a women >40 years of age (2014).[2]
8. *Recommendation of Istanbul Consensus:* Failure of implantation of good quality embryo. Evaluation of good quality embryo should include morphokinetic assessment and ploidy status.[11]

CAUSES

- *Multifactorial RIF:* Known causes are present. Anatomic defects in reproductive system, male factor, genetic abnormalities in embryo, endocrine disorders, diabetes, thyroid disorder, infection, antiphospholipid syndrome.
- *Endometrial RIF:* Presence of thin endometrium, >6 mm with impaired vascularity.
- *Idiopathic RIF:* Absence of factors from group A and B. There is impaired immunological interaction between endometrium and embryos.

INVESTIGATIONS

- Gametes/embryo assessment
- Assessment of endometrium
- Investigations for uterus and tubes
- Assessment of systemic factors

Gamete/Embryo Assessment

Oocytes

- Morphology (**Flowchart 1**)
    - Oocyte maturity
    - Nuclear maturity
    - Size, e.g., giant oocyte (Diameta)
    - Intracytoplasmic anomalies:
        - Incorporations
        - Retractile bodies
        - Central granulosus
        - Vacuolization

Flowchart 1: Oocyte morphology.

- Oocyte maturity
- Nuclear maturity
- Size (e.g., giant oocyte (diameta)
- Intracytoplasmic anomalies
  - Incorporztions
  - Retractile bodies
  - Central granulosus
  - Vacuolization
  - Smooth endoplasmic reticulum clusters
  - Perivitelline space granularity
  - First polar body morphology
  - Mitotic spindle

  - Smooth endoplasmic reticulum clusters
  - Perivitelline space granularity
  - First polar body morphology
  - Mitotic spindle
- Follicular fluid biochemical marker
  - Anti-Müllerian hormone (AMH)
  - Plasminogen activation inhibitor (PAI).

Higher levels of AMH and PAI are associated with increased implantation and live birth rates.

Sperm Assessment (Flowchart 2)

- DNA integrity
  - DNA fragmentation index (>27% is significant)
  - TUNEL assay (Deoxynucleotidyl transferase–mediated dUTP nick end labeling assay)
  - "Halo" test
  - Single-cell gel electrophoresis assay
  - Sperm chromatin structure assay (SCSA)
  - DNA breakage detection fluorescence in situ hybridization
  - Sperm chromatin dispersion assay (SCDA)
- Cytoplasmic assessment
  - Intracytoplasmic morphologically selected sperm injection (IMSI)
  - Detects degree and number of cytoplasmic vacuoles and facilitates selection of healthy sperms
- Apoptotic sperm detection
  - *Annexin V apoptosis assay:* It helps to exclude apoptotic sperms.

Embryo Assessment (Flowchart 3)

- **Morphology:**
  - D_3 embryo
    - Cell to cell contact
    - Cytoplasmic fragmentation

Recurrent Implantation Failure

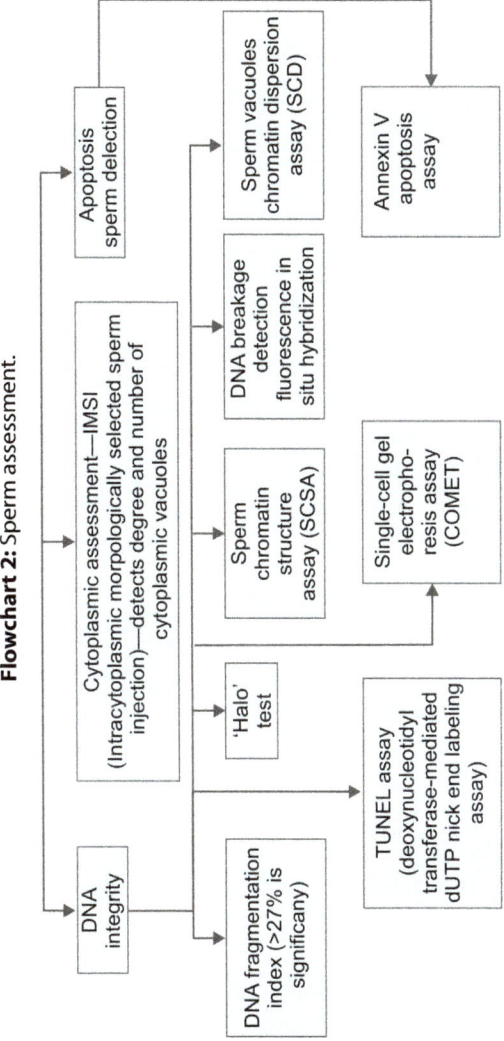

Flowchart 2: Sperm assessment.

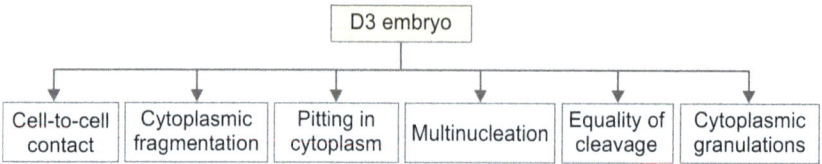

Flowchart 3: Embryo assessment.

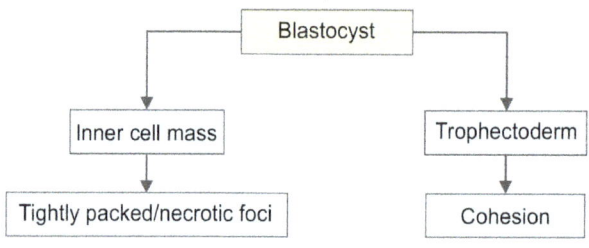

Flowchart 4: Blastocyst assessment.

- Pitting in cytoplasm
- Multinucleation
- Equality of cleavage
- Cytoplasmic granulations
- Blastocyst **(Flowchart 4)**
- Inner cell mask
  - Tightly packed
  - Necrotic foci
- Trophectoderm: Cohesiveness
- **Metabolites assessment (spent media)**
  - Glucose (higher uptake – good prognosis)
  - Pyruvate (higher uptake – good prognosis)
  - Amino acid turnover (greater turnover – poor prognosis)
- **Embryoscope**
  - For time-lapse video monitoring of embryo development
- **Prenatal genetic testing (PGT)**
  - PGT-A for aneuploidy
  - PGT-M for monogenic/single gene detected
  - PGT-SR for structured chromosomes rearrangements.

Assessment of Endometrium

Endometrial Biopsy (Flowchart 5)

- Histopathology (hormonal status)
- TB-PCR/Bactate culture.

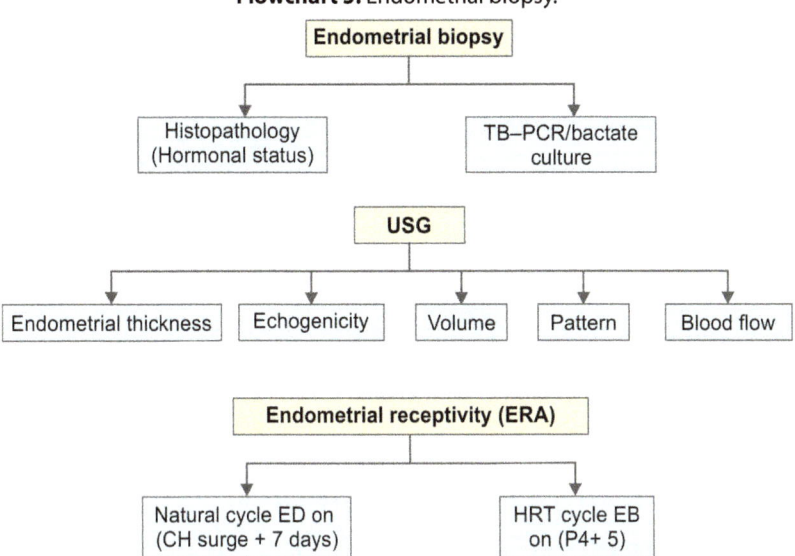

Flowchart 5: Endometrial biopsy.

Ultrasonography
- Endometrial thickness
- Echogenicity
- Volume
- Pattern
- Blood flow

Endometrial Receptivity (ERA)
- Natural cycle ED on (LH surge + 7 days)
- Hormone replacement therapy (HRT) cycle EB on (P4 +5).

Uterine Fluid Proteome
Women with RIF have altered uterine fluid proteins.

Metabolomics Study
- Semen
- Vaginal fluid.

Local Immunological Factors
- Immunohistochemistry: Endometrial NK cells (CD57)
- KIR genotype of endometrial NK cells
- Endometrial cytokines (Th1:Th2 ratio)
- Immune profiling of endometrium: Immune dysregulation.

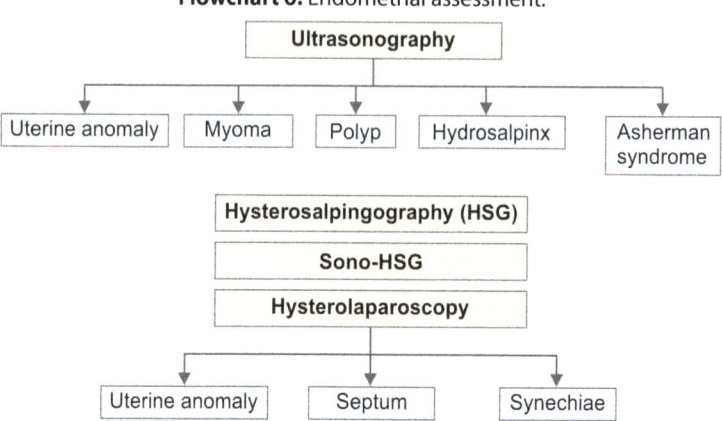

Flowchart 6: Endometrial assessment.

Uterus and Tubes Assessment (Flowchart 6)

- Ultrasonography
  - Uterine anomaly
  - Myoma
  - Polyp
  - Hydrosalpinx
  - Asherman syndrome
- Hysterosalpingography (HSG)
- Sono-HSG
- Hysterolaparoscopy
  - Uterine anomaly
  - Septum

Assessment of Systemic Factors

- Body mass index (BMI) measurement
- Systemic disease
  - Diabetes mellitus
  - *Thyroid disorders:* Hypothyroidism, hyperthyroidism, Hashimoto's thyroiditis
- Immunological: Autoimmune
  - Antiphospholipid antibodies (APLA), systemic lupus erythematosus (SLE), rheumatoid arthritis (RA).

TREATMENT (FLOWCHART 7)

- Uterus and adnexa
- Gametes/embryo
- Endometrium
- General treatment

Flowchart 7: Treatment.

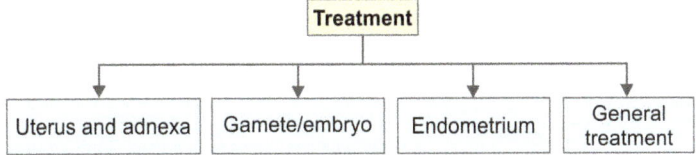

Uterus and Adnexa (Flowchart 8)

- Myomectomy
- Polypectomy
- Removal of intrauterine adhesions
- Treatment of adenomyosis
  - GnRH
  - Dienogest
- Septum resection.

Gametes or Embryo (Flowchart 9)

- Oocyte
  - Change in stimulation protocol [(↑gonadotropin and luteinizing hormone (LH)]
- Sperm
  - Antioxidants
  - IMSI
  - Testicular sperm extraction (TESE)
- Embryo
  - Blastocyst transfer
  - Assisted hatching
  - Embryo selection
    - PGT-A tested embryo
    - Metabolic analysis of spent media
  - Change in ET
    - Improved technique
    - Sequential transfer.

Endometrium (Flowchart 10)

- Loss of synchrony
  - Between stroma and glands
    - ERA
  - Between endometrium and embryos
    - Modification of ovulation stimulations protocols
- Thin endometrium
  - *Genetic:* Stem cell therapy
  - *Traumatic:* Stem cell therapy

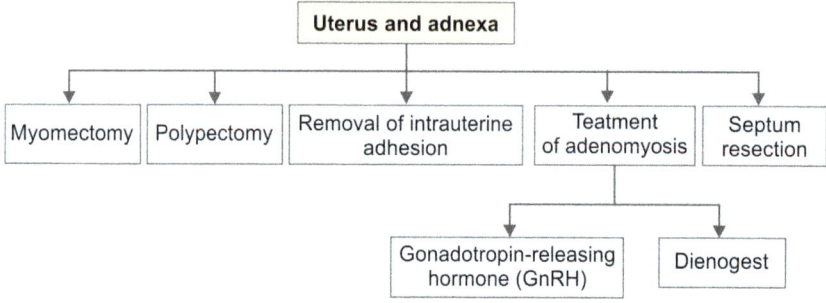

Flowchart 8: Uterus and adnexa.

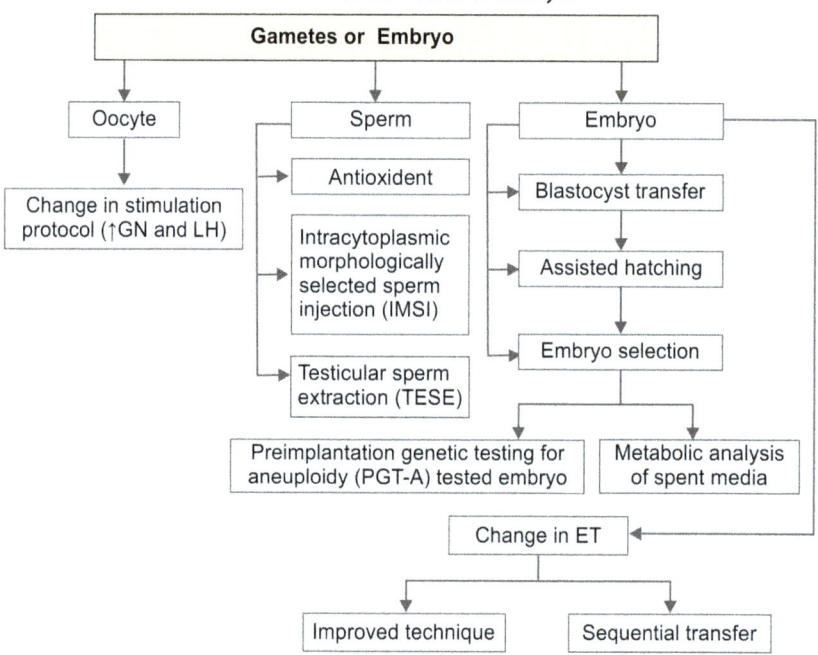

Flowchart 9: Gametes or Embryo.

- Vascular
  - Sildenafil
  - L-Arginine
- Endocrine
  - E2
- Immune problem
  - Immunotherapy
    - Granulocyte-colony stimulating factor (G-CSF)
    - Intravenous immunoglobulin (IVIg)
    - Intralipid
    - Lymphocyte immunization therapy (LIT)

Recurrent Implantation Failure

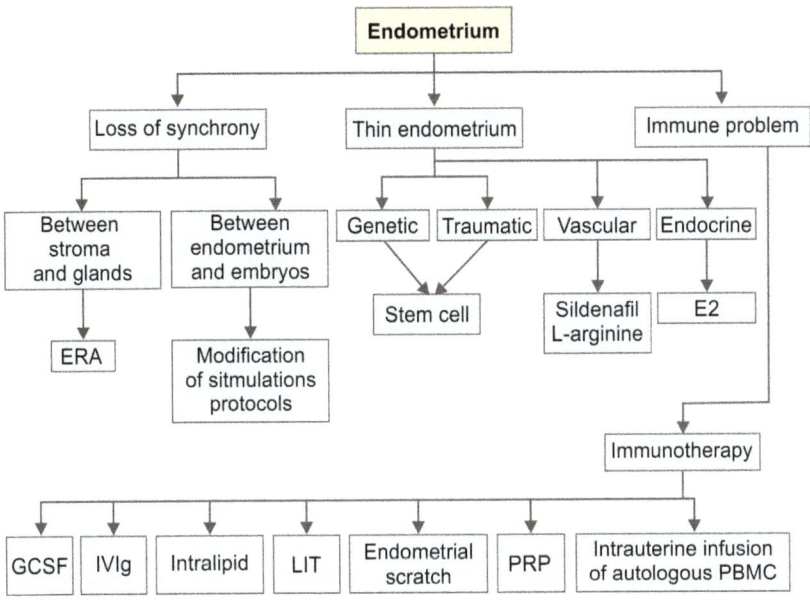

Flowchart 10: Endometrium.

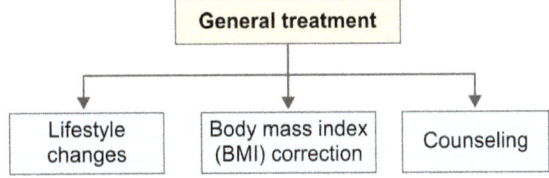

Flowchart 11: General treatment.

- Endometrial scratch
- Platelet-rich plasma (PRP)
- Intrauterine infusion of autologous peripheral blood mononuclear cells (PBMC).

General Treatment (Flowchart 11)

- Lifestyle changes
- BMI correction
- Counseling.

PROGNOSIS

The prognosis of RIF depends on the etiology and the criteria used for defining the condition. RIF in itself is not a diagnosis. It is very important to identify women who can succeed if they continue the IVF treatment and the subgroups who can be benefited by specific therapies. A study of 118 patients with RIF (failure to conceive after three ETs), found that 49% of women achieved live birth in a 5.5-year follow-up period.[12] This indicates that approximately 50% of RIF patients may not ultimately succeed. Hence, more work is required to develop and validate a diagnostic algorithm to identify the subgroups of women with better prognosis.

GUIDELINES

Canadian Fertility and Andrology Society Clinical Practice Guidelines (2020)[13]

Summary of recommendations:
A. May be offered
   1. Karyotype testing
   2. Preimplantation genetic thrombophilia workup
B. Limited to research settings only
   1. Serological and endometrial-immune testing
   2. Endometrial receptivity assays
   3. Empirical low molecular weight heparin
   4. Immunotherapy, intralipid, glucocorticoids, granulocyte colony stimulating factor
C. Not recommended
   1. Hysteroscopy if baseline ultrasound is normal
   2. Acquired and congenital
   3. Sperm DNA fragmentation index
   4. Screening for chronic endometritis
   5. Endometrial injury in the preceding menstrual cycle
   6. Aspirin.

REFERENCES

1. Busnelli A, Somigliana E, Cirillo F, Baggiani A, Levi-Setti PE. Efficacy of therapies and interventions for repeated embryo implantation failure: a systematic review and meta-analysis. Sci Rep. 2021;11(1):1747.
2. Coughlan C, Ledger W, Wang Q, Liu F, Demirol A, Gurgan T, et al. Recurrent implantation failure: definition and management. Reprod Biomed Online. 2014;28(1):14-38.
3. Bashiri A, Halper KI, Orvieto R. Recurrent implantation failure-update overview on etiology, diagnosis, treatment and future directions. Reprod Biol Endocrinol. 2018;16:121.
4. Gnoth C, Godehardt D, Godehardt E, Frank-Herrmann P, Freundl G. Time to pregnancy: results of the German prospective study and impact on the management of infertility. Hum Reprod. 2003;18(9):1959-66.
5. Rinehart J. Recurrent implantation failure: definition. J Assist Reprod Genet. 2007;24(7):284-7.
6. Coughlan C, Ledger W, Wang Q, Liu F, Demirol A, Gurgan T, et al Recurrent implantation failure: definition and management. Reprod Biomed Online. 2014;28(1):14-38.

7. Coulam CB. Implantation failure and immunotherapy. Hum Reprod. 1995; 10(6):1338-40.
8. Tan BK, Vandekerckhove P, Kennedy R, Keay SD. Investigation and current management of recurrent IVF treatment failure in the UK. BJOG. 2005;112(6):773-80.
9. Thornhill AR, deDie-Smulders CE, Geraedts JP, Harper JC, Harton GL, Lavery SA, et al. ESHRE PGD Consortium 'Best practice guidelines for clinical preimplantation genetic diagnosis (PGD) and preimplantation genetic screening (PGS)'. Hum Reprod. 2005;20(1):35-48.
10. Margalioth EJ, Ben-Chetrit A, Gal M, Eldar-Geva T. Investigation and treatment of repeated implantation failure following IVF-ET. Hum Reprod. 2006;21(12):3036-43.
11. Alpha Scientists in Reproductive Medicine and ESHRE Special Interest Group of Embryology. The Istanbul consensus workshop on embryo assessment: proceedings of an expert meeting. Hum Reprod. 2011;26(6):1270-83.
12. Koot YEM, Saxtorph MH, Goddijn M, de Bever S, Eijkemans MJC, Wely MV, et al. What is the prognosis for a live birth after unexplained recurrent implantation failure following IVF/ICSI? Hum Reprod. 2019;34(10):2044-52.
13. Shaulov T, Sierra S, Sylvestre C. Recurrent Implantation Failure: A CFAS Guideline. Reprod BioMed Online. 2020;41(5):819-33.

35 | Thin Endometrium

Nandita Palshetkar, Rohan Palshetkar

INTRODUCTION

Endometrium is a dynamic and regenerative tissue which undergoes changes throughout the cycle. Two hormones, namely estrogen and progesterone produced by the ovary have a significant role in bringing about the changes in the endometrium.

According to Radiological Society of North America, the endometrium is thinnest during menstruation ranging from 2 to 4 mm in thickness. During proliferative phase (6–14 days) it thickens to 5–8 mm. As ovulation occurs, the endometrium can be as thick as 11 mm.[1]

Alteration in gene expression, endometrial architecture causes changes in the endometrial composition. All these components together form the "window of implantation". This window is the period when the embryo has the best opportunity to implant in the endometrium.

The impact of thin endometrium has been a long-standing topic of debate as *how thin is this?*

El Touchy et al. and Richer et al. in a study reported the minimum thickness of endometrium required for embryo transfer to be 7 mm. However, some studies take the cut-off as 8 mm **(Table 1; Figs. 1 and 2)**.[2,3]

CAUSES

- Asherman syndrome
- Clomiphene citrate—prolonged use

TABLE 1: Endometrial thickness and number of pregnancies.[4]

Endometrial thickness	No. of cases (n = 100)	No. of pregnancies (n = 40)	Percentage (%)
<8 mm	4	0	0
8–10 mm	41	20	50
10–12 mm	25	10	25
12–14 mm	20	9	22.5
>14 mm	10	1	2.5

Thin Endometrium

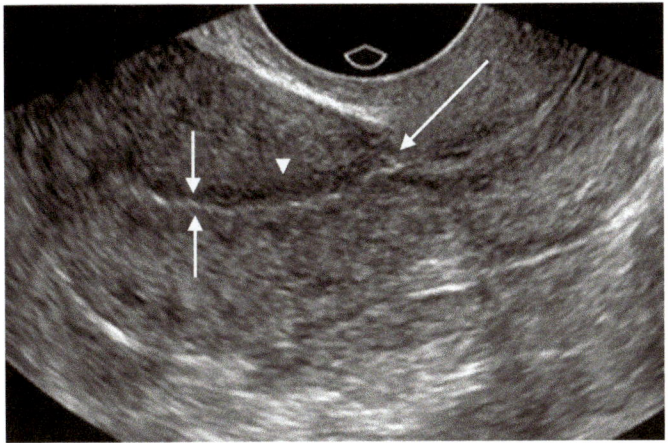

Fig. 1: Sonographic finding of thin endometrium.

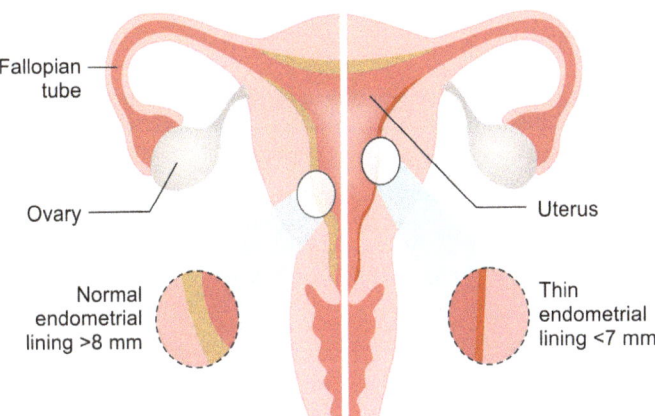

Fig. 2: The development of normal thin endometrium.

- Postpartum endometritis
- Septic abortion
- Pelvic radiation
- Chemotherapy
- In-utero diethylstilbestrol (DES)
- Hypothalamic hypogonadism
- Fibroids
- Müllerian anomalies
- Hyperandrogenemia
- Premature ovarian insufficiency
- Iatrogenic
- Idiopathic

DIAGNOSIS

Ultrasound-transvaginal

The endometrium should be measured in the long axis or sagittal plane, ideally on transvaginal scanning, with the entirety of the endometrial lining through to the endocervical canal in view.

Transvaginal sonography (TVS) is the ideal method. One should visualize the endometrial lining in its entirety throughout to the endocervical canal.

Doppler Ultrasound

For improving implantation rate, the endometrial should have an optimum blood flow. Miwa et al., concluded that when the blood supply to the endometrium is ideal, the growth is also ideal. Decreased vascular endothelial growth factor (VEGF) expression, impedance of flow of the uterine radial arteries and low epithelial growth are responsible for a thin endometrium **(Tables 2 and 3)**.

TABLE 2: Prerequisite for a good endometrial growth.

A good uterine blood flow is important for endometrial growth

Estrogen produces a vasodilatory effect on uterine arteries	RI and PI of uterine arteries are decreased if levels of estradiol is high	Any resistance to blood flow impairs glandular growth, which results decrease in VEGF, in turn causes poor blood flow to endometrium

(PI: pulsatility index; RI: resistive index)

TABLE 3: Applebaum uterine scoring system for reproduction (USSR).

Parameters	Determination	Score
Endometrial thickness (mm)	<7	0
	7–9	2
	10–14	3
	>14	1
Endometrial layering	• No layering	0
	• Hazy 5-line appearance	1
	• Distinct 5-line appearance	3
Endometrial motion (no. of myometrial contractions in 2 minutes (real-time)	<3	0
	≥3	3
Myometrial echogenicity	• Course, inhomogeneous	1
	• Relatively homogeneous	2

Contd...

Contd...

Parameter	Determination	Score
Uterine artery Doppler flow (PI)	2.99–3.0	0
	2.49	1
	<2	2
Endometrial blood flow in zone 3	• Absent	0
	• Present but sparse	2
	• Present multifocally	5
Myometrial blood flow (Grayscale)	• Absent	0
	• Present	2

MANAGEMENT

There are several agents which are studied and are available for improving the endometrial thickness. The hormonal adjuvant estrogen has been the most promising of all the agents.

There are other agents and procedures that may be used for the treatment of thin endometrium such as human chorionic gonadotropin (hCG), Vitamin E, Aspirin, endometrial scratching, stimulated cycles, pentoxifylline, granulocyte colony-stimulating factor (G-CSF), sildenafil and even stem cell therapy.[5,6]

Estrogen

Being a hormone dependent tissue, the endometrium proliferates in response to estrogen, which further induces the production of progesterone receptors.

The endometrium depends on estrogen for growth. As the endometrium grows, it causes the production of progesterone receptors. According to Steer et al., adding estrogen is the most logical step in improving thin endometrium.[7] There are several preparations of estrogen available in the market. Oral estradiol valerate (EV), estradiol transdermal patch and gel and newly available estradiol hemihydrates (EH) (oral and transdermal).

Several studies have been performed to determine which estrogen is the most effective in improving the endometrial thickness and bringing about a higher pregnancy rate. Kundan et al. demonstrated EH as a better option for optimal endometrial growth.[8] Over the years, oral administration of EV has been the best and most widely used method for improving endometrial thickness. When estradiol valerate is given for a longer period of time with COH cycles, it improved the mean endometrial thickness from 6.7 to 8.6 mm as well as significant increase of pregnancy rate (38.5 vs. 4.3%).[9,10]

Transdermal and vaginal use of estrogen has also shown improved endometrial thickness and higher pregnancy rate. Also, there is an ongoing debate of constant dose administration versus increasing dose of estradiol. However, there have been studies that there is no statistical significance in

OPR or LBR for increasing or constant dose or through different routes of administration (oral or transdermal).[11]

Sildenafil

Sildenafil acts as a type 5-specific phosphodiesterase inhibitor hence augments the vasodilatory effects of nitric oxide by preventing the degradation of cGMP. Nitric oxide (NO) relaxes vascular smooth muscle through a cGMP-mediated pathway. Sildenafil citrate improves the uterine artery blood flow and the sonographic endometrial thickening in patients with a prior assisted reproductive cycle failing due to poor endometrial response.[12]

Sildenafil is given in the dose of 25 mg twice daily orally or vaginally starting from day 1 and discontinued 48–72 hours prior to embryo transfer. Taka saki et al. found that vaginal sildenafil increases the endometrial thickness from 7.1 to 9.4 mm with 50% pregnancy rates in IVF cycles.[13]

Low-dose Human Chorionic Gonadotropin

Several studies have shown the effectivity of low-dose hCG in increasing the endometrial thickness and hence its receptivity. Luteinizing hormone (LH)/hCG receptors are present in the endometrium and positive interaction is seen when hCG is injected during the follicular phase.

A low dose of hCG 150 IU can be administered on day 8 or day 9 of estrogen administration subcutaneously for 7 days. TVS performed on days 14 to 15 showed 20% improvement of endometrial thickness.[14] Another study by Robab et al. also concluded that adding hCG to conventional preparation method was an effective protocol to achieve improved endometrial thickness and favorable pregnancy outcomes.[15]

Low-dose Aspirin

Higher pregnancy rate and better endometrial pattern were achieved in patients with thin endometrium after aspirin administration. Aspirin therapy could not significantly increase the endometrial thickness and the resistance of uterine and ovarian flow.

Patients with a thin endometrium achieved a higher pregnancy rate (PR) and a more receptive endometrium when aspirin was added to their treatment cycle. A study showing effects in endometrium in a group receiving aspirin and non-aspirin group showed a better morphology and PR when aspirin was added. They also concluded that there was no statistical significance in the endometrial thickness and blood flow.[16] About 75–81 mg of aspirin is the dose recommended for use.

L-arginine

L-arginine is a NO-donor and relaxes vascular smooth muscles of endometrium and it has been shown to decrease the resistive index.[17]

TABLE 4: Evaluation of the role G-CSF in thin endometrium.[20-22]

Study	Dose of GCSF	Duration of therapy	Results
Nobert Gleicher et al., 2011	1 mL 30 MU (300 μg)	2–7 days before embryo transfer (ET) by ET catheter	Dramatic improvement in endometrial thickness all four patients conceived with one intramural ectopic pregnancy
Y Kim et al., 2012	1 mL 30 MU (300 μg)	On the day of hCG injection	Significantly higher endometrial thickness (85% showed improvement), implantation and ongoing pregnancy rate
Maryam Eftekhar, 2014	1 mL 30 MU (300 μg)	12th–13th day of cycle but repeated once more if endometrial thickness below 7 mm within 48–72 hours	• No difference in endometrial thickness • Chemical pregnancy rate and clinical pregnancy rate were found to be better (39.30 vs. 14.30% and 32.10 vs. 12.00%, respectively)

Granulocyte Colony-stimulating Factor

It is a cytokine that stimulates neutrophilic granulocyte differentiation and proliferation, it may induce endometrium proliferation and growth, thus improve pregnancy outcome. Infusion of G-CSF in endometrial cavity is a safe and probably effective method to increasing endometrial thickness for patients with thin and unresponsive endometrium.

In the recent years, the effectiveness of G-CSF as a potential agent for increasing endometrial thickness has been studied and results were found to be favorable. Furthermore, it seems that this effect was associated with a higher potential of pregnancy **(Table 4)**.[18]

The route of G-CSF can be subcutaneous or intrauterine where 300 μg/mL of G-CSF is administered on the day of oocyte retrieval or 5 days before embryo transfer. TVS is done after 48 hours to assess the endometrial thickness and if the desired thickness of 7 mm is not achieved a second dose can be given. Intrauterine administration is done using an intrauterine insemination (IUI) catheter under USG guidance.[19]

PLATELET-RICH PLASMA

Platelet-rich plasma (PRP) is a new treatment option which has been suggested (Chang et al., 2015).[23] Blood is collected from the patients' peripheral vein. PRP is made from the blood collected. It contains VEGF, cytokines, epidermal growth factor, transforming growth factor and platelet derived growth factor. These factors help in the development of the endometrium 0.3–0.5 mL of PRP can be injected into the uterine cavity but using a catheter (IUI or ET). PRP was done on day 11–12 and repeated again on day 13–14.[24-26]

ENDOMETRIAL SCRATCHING

Few studies have reported improvement in endometrial thickness following endometrial scratching done in the luteal phase of one cycle prior to the in vitro fertilization (IVF) cycle. It is a low cost technique, done using a small catheter of 3 mm width, known as "Pipelle" in patients who have under gone repeated failed attempts of IVF. The mechanical disruption to the endometrium modulates the genetic expression of factors important for implantation. It causes release of growth factors, hormones and proinflammatory cytokines, which makes the newly formed lining more receptive to the implanting embryo.

A Cochrane analysis performed by Nastri et al.[27] compared 14 studies including 1,063 patients and found higher rates of pregnancies and live births group undergoing endometrial scratching.

STEM CELL THERAPY

The endometrial stem cells are present in both basalis and functionalis layers of the human endometrium and these cells play a key role in regenerating endometrial lining during each menstrual cycle.

Taylor et al. suggested that hematopoietic and nonhematopoietic bone marrow derived stem cells may help in proliferation of the endometrium.[28] In cases of thin endometrium, there a few papers which have reported success. In a case of Asherman syndrome, stem cells were isolated from the bone marrow and injected into the uterine cavity. The thickness of the endometrium improved to 8 mm and a clinical pregnancy post-IVF was achieved.[29]

CONCLUSION

Endometrial growth plays a crucial role in receptivity of endometrium and implantation of pregnancy. Poor endometrial development leads to poor pregnancy rates, however it is not the sole predictor of pregnancy occurrence. Endometrial pattern, blood flow and recently endometrial receptivity analysis (ERA) is playing a promising role in predicting endometrial receptivity. Estradiol has been the gold standard for treatment of thin endometrium. Vaginal sildenafil is also coming up as a reasonable first-line treatment. GCSF can be regarded as a second-line management. Stem cell therapy appears to be a promising method in refractory cases.

REFERENCES

1. Radiological Society of North America. What to know about endometrial thickness (Danielle Dresden). Medical News Today; 2019.
2. El-Toukhy T, Coomarasamy A, Khairy M, Sunkara K, Seed P, Khalaf Y, et al. The relationship between endometrial thickness and outcome of medicated frozen embryo replacement cycles. Fertil Steril. 2008;89(4):832-9.

3. Richter KS, Bugge KR, Bromer JG, Levy MJ. Relationship between endometrial thickness and embryo implantation, based on 1,294 cycles of in vitro fertilization with transfer of two blastocyst-stage embryos. Fertil Steril. 2007;87(1):53-9.
4. Ng EHY, Chan CCW, Tang OS. The role of endometrial and subendometrial vascularity measured by three-dimensional power Doppler ultrasound in the prediction of pregnancy during frozen thawed embryo transfer cycles. Hum Reprod. 2006;21(6):1612-7.
5. Miwa I, Tamura H, Takaaki A, Yamagata Y, Shimamura K, Sungio N. Pathophysiology features of "thin endometrium". Fertil Steril. 2009;91(4):998-1004.
6. Lebovitz O, Orvieto O. Treating patients with "thin" endometrium - an ongoing challenge. Gynaecol Endocrinol. 2014;30(6):409-14.
7. Steer CV, Tan SL, Dillion D, Mason BA, Campbell S. Vaginal Color Doppler assessment of uterine artery impedence correlates with immunohistochemical markers of endometrial receptivity required for implantation of an embryo. Fertil Steril. 1995;63(1):101-8.
8. Kundun VI, Kalyani KI, Anjum AS. Prospective randomized comparative trail between estradiol hemihydrates and estradiol valerate for endometrial preparation in frozen–thawed embryo transfer cycles. Fertil Steril ARSM; 2020.
9. Demir B, Dilbaz S, Cinar O, Ozdegirmenci O, Dede S, Dundar B, et al. Estradiol supplementation in intracytoplasmic sperm injection cycles with thin endometrium. Gynecol. Endocrinol. 2013;29(1):42-5.
10. Chen MJ, Yang JH, Peng FH, Chen SU, Ho HN, Yang YS. Extended estrogen administration for women with thin endometrium in frozen-thawed in-vitro fertilization programs. J Assist Reprod Genet. 2006;23(7-8):337-42.
11. Madero S, Rodriguez A, Vassena R, Vernaeve V. Endometrial preparation: effect of estrogen dose and administration route on reproductive outcomes in oocyte donation cycles with fresh embryo transfer. Hum Reprod. 2016;31(8):1755-64.
12. Zinger M, Liu JH, Thomas MA. Successful use of vaginal sildenafil citrate in two infertility patients with Ashermann's syndrome. J Womens Health (Larchmt). 2006;15(4):442-4.
13. Takasaki A, Tamura H, Miwa I, Taketani T, Shimamura K, Sugino N. Endometrial growth and uterine blood flow: a pilot study for improving endometrial thickness in patients with a thin endometrium. Fertil Steril. 2010;93(6):1851-8.
14. Papanikolaou EG, Kyrou D, Zervakakou G, Paggou E, Humaidan P. "Follicular HCG endometrium priming for IVF patients experiencing resisting thin endometrium. A proof of concept study". J Assist Reprod Genet. 2013;30(10):1341-5.
15. Davar R, Miraj S, Mojtahedi MF. Effects of adding human chorionic gonadotropin to frozen thawed embryo transfer cycles with history of thin endometrium. Int J Reprod Biomed. 2016;14(1):53-6.
16. Hsieh YY, Tsai HD, Chang CC, Lo HY, Chen CL. Low-dose aspirin for infertile women with thin endometrium receiving intrauterine insemination: a prospective, randomized study. J Assist Reprod Genet. 2000;17(3):174-7.
17. Ledee-Batnille N, Oliviness F, Lefaix JL, Chaouat G, Frydman R, Delanian S. Combined treatment by pentoxifylline and tocopherol for recipient women with a thin endometrium enrolled in a oocyte donation programme. Hum Reprod. 2002;17(5):1249-53.
18. Tehraninejad E, Tanha FD, Asadi E, Kamali K, Aziminikoo E, Rezayof E. G-CSF intrauterine for thin endometrium, and pregnancy outcome. J Fam Reprod Health. 2015;9(3):107-12.
19. Singal S, Sharma RK, Ahuja N. GCSF in patients with thin endometrium–subcutaneous or intrauterine? Fertil Sci Res. 2020;7(1):43.
20. Gleicher N, Vidali A, Barad DH. Successful treatment of unresponsive thin endometrium. Fertil Steril. 2011;95(6):2123.e13-7.

21. Kim YY, Jung YH, Jo JD, Kim MH, Yoo YJ. Kim S. The effect of transvaginal endometrial perfusion with G-CSF. Fertil Steril. 2012;98(3):S183.
22. Eftekar M, Sayadi M, Arabjahvani F. Transvaginal perfusion of G-CSF for infertile women with thin endometrium in frozen ET program: A non-randomized clinical trial. Iran J Reprod Med. 2014;12(10):661-6.
23. Chang Y, Li J, Chen Y, Wei L, Yang X, Shi Y, et al. Autologous platelet-rich plasma promotes endometrial growth and improves pregnancy outcome during in vitro fertilization. Int J Clin Exp Med. 2015;8(1):1286-90.
24. Kim H, Shin JE, Koo HS, Kwon H, Choi DH, Kim JH. Effect of Autologous Platelet-Rich Plasma Treatment on Refractory Thin Endometrium during the Frozen Embryo Transfer Cycle: a Pilot Study. Front Endocrinol (Lausanne). 2019;10:61.
25. Chang Y, Li J, Wei LN, Pang J, Chen J, Liang X. Autologous platelet-rich plasma infusion improves clinical pregnancy rate in frozen embryo transfer cycles for women with thin endometrium. Medicine (Baltimore). 2019;98(3):e14062.
26. Nagireddy S, Reddy NS, Daniel GM, Srinivasan SN, Katneni L. Autologous PRP for management of thin endometrium in frozen embryo transfer cycles: would it improve the outcome. Fertil Steril. 2019;112(3):E418-9.
27. Nastri Co, Lensen SF, Gibreel A, Raine-Fenning N, Ferriani RA, Bhattacharya S. Endometrial injury in women undergoing assisted reproductive technique. Cochrane Database Syst Rev. 2015;(3):CD009517.
28. Taylor HS. Endometrial cells derived from donor stem cells in bone marrow transplant recipients. JAMA. 2004;292(1):81-5.
29. Nagori CB, Panchal SY, Patel H. Endometrial regeneration using autologous adult stem cells followed by conception by in vitro fertilization in a patient of severe Asherman's syndrome. J Hum Reprod Sci. 2011;4(1):43-8.

CHAPTER 36

Recurrent Pregnancy Loss

Sushma Deshmukh, Ashutosh Thole, Shashikant Raghuwanshi

INTRODUCTION

Loss of pregnancy at any stage is emotionally traumatic for a couple and repetition of such losses is devastating for a couple and frustrating for the doctor. It becomes more painful in spite of a large standard battery of investigations; it turns out to be negative. Though there are many known and unknown causes, we need to evaluate the couple thoroughly and proper counseling will help in resolution of their grief.

SPECTRUM AND DEFINITION

Recurrent pregnancy loss (RPL) is defined as the loss of two or more pregnancies.[1] It excludes ectopic, molar pregnancies and implantation failure. Its incidence is around 1-2%. The study by Emma Rasmark Roepke et al. suggested that the incidence of RPL has increased during last 10 years.[2]

ETIOLOGY

Many studies demonstrated multiple reasons for RPL. But in fact, there exist a small number of accepted etiologies for RPL which we can evaluate. Causes are: genetics 5%, immunological 20-50%, hormonal 17-20%, anatomical 12-16%, hematological in small subset of patients, infective 0.5-1.5%, miscellaneous—emerging concept, unexplained 30-40%.

The common established causes include uterine anomalies, antiphospholipid syndrome, hormonal and metabolic disorders, and cytogenic abnormalities. Other etiologies are chronic endometritis, inherited thrombophilias, luteal phase deficiency, and high sperm DNA fragmentation levels.

Even after evaluation half of all cases will remain unexplained or idiopathic. Elderly women, obesity, excessive alcohol consumption, and smoking are few risk factors associated with RPL.

Genetic Causes

Chromosomal causes accounts for 50% of first trimester losses. Abnormalities can be in total chromosomal number or structural abnormalities.

Abnormal Chromosomal Number

- It may involve autosomes or sex chromosomes. There can be trisomies (50%), monosomy X (20%), triploidy (15%), and tetraploidy (5%).
- Trisomy can occur in any chromosome.
- Trisomy 13, 18, and 21 (compatible with life).
- Trisomy 16 is the most common in abortus and it is usually maternal.
- Triploidy, tetraploidy—molar pregnancy.

Structural Abnormalities

It includes, balanced chromosomal translocations, inversions, sex chromosome mosaicism. 50% of structural abnormalities are inherited. The most commonly observed rearrangements are reciprocal translocation, Robertsonian translocation, inversion. Sex chromosome mosaicism includes single gene disorders like X-linked (thalassemia major) and inherited thrombophilia.

Incidence: First trimester—75-90%, second trimester—15%, third trimester—5%.

Evaluation:
- Karyotype, chromosomal microarray (CMA), fluorescence in situ hybridization (FISH) analysis, microRNA analysis, next generation sequencing (NGS), and preimplantation genetic testing (PGT).
- *Fetal karyotyping:* It is recommended by the Royal College of Obstetricians and Gynecologists (RCOG) and the American Society for Reproductive Medicine (ASRM). Patients can be provided an accurate diagnosis and better prognostication regarding future pregnancy. It relieves couples' anxiety.
- *Parental karyotyping:* Parental chromosomal abnormalities, especially balanced reciprocal or Robertsonian translocations as well as inversions, insertions, and mosaicism. It is recommended by the ASRM and the European Society of Human Reproduction and Embryology (ESHRE).

Autoimmune Causes

The autoimmune causes of recurrent pregnancy loss are antiphospholipid syndrome and thrombophilia.

Antiphospholipid Syndrome

Autoimmune syndrome has important role in RPL. Antiphospholipid (aPL) antibodies are heterogeneous group of antibodies of which the most common are anticardiolipin (aCL) and lupus anticoagulant (LAC). It is well accepted and most treatable cause of RPL. It causes placental thrombosis, infarction which may results in preembryonic, embryonic or fetal loss.

TABLE 1: Clinical and laboratory findings in reproductive autoimmune syndrome.

	Antiphospholipid syndrome (APS)	**Reproductive autoimmune failure syndrome (RAFS)**

Clinical features	• Thrombosis (≥1 unexplained venous or arterial thrombosis, including stroke)
	• Autoimmune thrombocytopenia
	• Recurrent pregnancy loss
	  – ≥1 consecutive and otherwise unexplained fetal deaths (≥10 weeks)
	  – ≥3 consecutive and otherwise unexplained pre-embryonic or embryonic pregnancy losses
		• Fetal growth retardation (<34 weeks)
		• Severe preeclampsia
		• Obstetric complications (abruption placenta, chorea gravidarum, herpes gestationis, HELLP syndrome)
		• Unexplained infertility
		• Endometriosis
		• Recurrent pregnancy loss
		  – ≥1 consecutive and otherwise unexplained fetal deaths (≥10 weeks)
		  – ≥3 consecutive and otherwise unexplained pre-embryonic or embryonic pregnancy losses

Laboratory findings	• Anticardiolipin antibodies (ACA) (>20 GPL or MPL units) • Lupus anticoagulant (LAC)	• Antiphospholipid (aPL) antibodies • LAC • Gammopathy (usually polyclonal, mostly IgM) • Antinuclear antibodies • Organ-specific autoantibodies (antithyroid)

(HELLP: hemolysis, elevated liver enzymes, and low platelets)

Diagnosis: Diagnosis of aPL made by presence of one clinical and one laboratory criteria which must be positive on two occasions in 3 months apart **(Table 1)**.

What to test:
- Lupus anticoagulant
- Factor V Leiden [polymerase chain reaction (PCR)]
- Protein C activity
- Protein S activity
- Anticardiolipin antibodies—IgG and IgM
- Antiphosphatidylserine (aPS)
- Anti-β2-glycoprotein (If aCL positive but <40 GPL)

Management:
- *Preconception:*
  • Minimize/eliminate thrombotic risk factors
  • Initiate prenatal vitamins and calcium + vitamin D
  • Report early on a positive pregnancy test

TABLE 2: Suggested anticoagulation doses.

Prophylactic regimens	First trimester	Second trimester	Third trimester
Unfractionated heparin (UFH)	5,000 U twice daily	7,500–10,000 U twice daily	10,000 U twice daily
Low molecular weight heparin (LMWH)	Weight based (initial prenatal weight)		
	<50 kg	50–90 kg	91–130 kg
Enoxaparin	20 mg daily	40 mg daily	60 mg daily
Dalteparin	2,500 units daily	5,000 units daily	7,500 units daily
Therapeutic regimens	Initial dose	Adjusted target	
UFH	10,000 units twice daily	aPTT 1.5–2.5 6 hours after injection	
LMWH			
Enoxaparin	1 mg/kg twice daily		
Dalteparin	200 units/kg daily		
Warfarin (postpartum only)		Target INR 2.0–3.0	

Source: Adapted from Malvasi A, Tinelli A, Di Renzo GC. Management and Therapy of Early Pregnancy Complications. Cham, Switzerland: Springer; 2016.

- *During pregnancy:*
    - Patients with RPL—low dose aspirin (LDA) 75–150 mg/day + prophylactic UFH/LMWH
    - Patients with prior thrombosis—shift from warfarin to LDA + therapeutic UFH/LMWH.
    - Common dosing regimens for anticoagulation in pregnancy are reviewed in **Table 2**.
    - *Warfarin:*
        - Avoid in first trimester—teratogenic effects
        - Benefits—lower cost, lower risk of osteoporosis, and no injections
        - Shift to heparin in third trimester
    - *Other therapies for patients refractory to LDA + heparin:*
        - Hydroxychloroquine
        - I/V immunoglobulin
        - Plasma exchange

Labor and delivery:
- Schedule delivery
- Stop heparin 12 hours prior to labor
- Stop aspirin 7 days prior
- Restart heparin 12 hours postdelivery

Postpartum: Thromboprophylaxis for 6 weeks.

Anatomical Factors in Recurrent Pregnancy Loss

Anatomical uterine abnormalities associated with RPL are:
- Congenital (Müllerian) abnormalities
- Acquired—leiomyoma, polyp, and intrauterine adhesions
- Cervical incompetence.

The most common assessment tool is transvaginal ultrasound in secretory phase for better visualization of the endometrium. USG helps in diagnosis of uterine fibroids, polyps, and duplication of uterus. 3D/4D ultrasonography is more accurate and can reliably differentiate between septate **(Figs. 1A and B)** and bicorporeal uteri.[3-5] Renal anomalies are associated in 20-30% of cases.

Hysterosalpingography (HSG): HSG delineates the interior of the uterine cavity. USG and HSG form a very effective screening tool for evaluation of RPL.

Saline infusion sonography (SIS) **(Fig. 2):** Along with interior contour it gives assessment of length and width of a uterine septum, while planning the

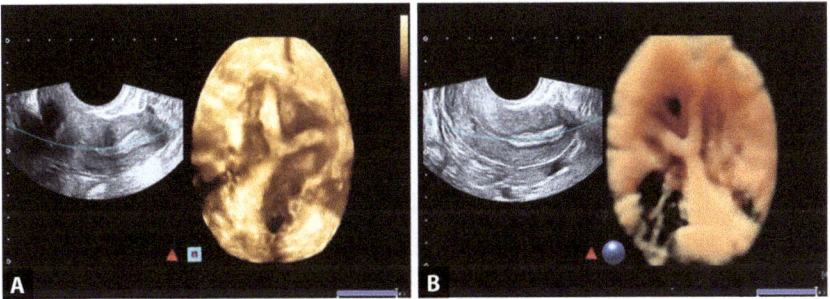

Figs. 1A and B: Septate uterus: 4D images.
Courtesy: Dr Sandeep Mahajan.

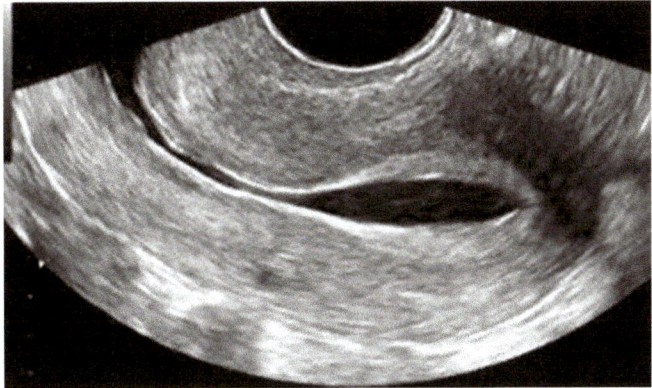

Fig. 2: Saline infusion sonography.

surgical resection.[6,7] SIS is highly accurate in diagnosing and categorizing congenital uterine anomalies (CUAs).[8]

Magnetic resonance imaging (MRI): MRI provides excellent delineation of both internal and external uterine contours and can differentiate septate from bicorporeal uteri.

Hysteroscopy combined with laparoscopy is gold standard. Hysteroscopy allows diagnosis and simultaneous treatment of intrauterine lesions. Concomitant laparoscopy helps to diagnose and to guide the limit of surgery. Diagnosis and treatment can be done with office hysteroscopy as an outpatient department (OPD) procedure.

Sonoembryoscopy and uterine Doppler US is under evaluation, currently we do not have enough evidence to recommend it in routine investigation of RPL.[9]

Congenital Uterine Anomalies (Fig. 3)

Its prevalence is 12.3% in patients of miscarriage, and 24.5% in patients with miscarriage and infertility.[10] Uterine anomalies need not always results in pregnancy loss and many women with such abnormalities results in normal obstetrical outcome. Impaired vascularization and cavity distortion may be the possible reasons for miscarriages. 75% of these are septate (ESGE U2) and arcuate uteri (ESGE U1c). Restoration of a normal cavity is the basis of surgical management in these patients.

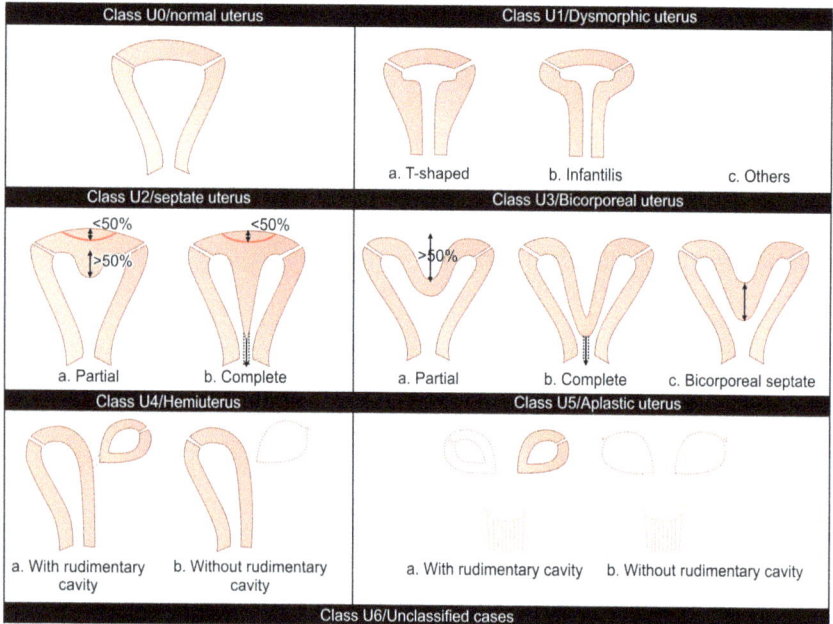

Fig. 3: ESHRE + ESGE classification of uterine anomalies.

The European Society of Human Reproduction and Embryology (ESHRE) and the European Society for Gynecological Endoscopy (ESGE) have established a common working group with the name CONUTA (CONgenital UTerine Anomalies)—New updated classification system.

Septate uterus (class U2): Uterus has normal outline and an internal indentation at the fundal midline exceeding 50% of the uterine wall thickness. It occurs due to abnormal absorption of the midline septum. In some studies, the endometrium covering the septum showed differences in histologic composition and gene expression compared with the normal uterine wall.[11] The degree of septation varies from a partial midline septum with one cervix to complete septation with two cervical openings.

Among the all CUA, uterine septae is the most common cause of pregnancy loss and easiest of all to treat. There is risk for spontaneous abortion (21-44%) and preterm delivery (12-33%)[11-14] in these patients, although no clear biological basis for impaired reproductive outcome in these affected patients has been found.[11]

Post-treatment reproductive outcome is good with operative hysteroscopy. The goal of the procedure is to reduce the septal surface area by incision or resection of septum. Surgery can be done with scissors' **(Figs. 4A and B)**, resectoscope, versapoint or laser with good success rates and infrequent complications.

Patients can attempt conception 2 months postoperatively.[15] Uterine rupture during pregnancy has been reported rarely; therefore, a trial of labor is generally recommended.[16]

Bicorporeal utreus (class U3): It is characterized by the presence of an external indentation at the fundal midline exceeding 50% of the uterine wall thickness. U3a—partial bicorporeal uterus, U3b—complete bicorporeal uterus, and U3c—partial subseptate uterus (ESGE ESHRE classification above). Patients

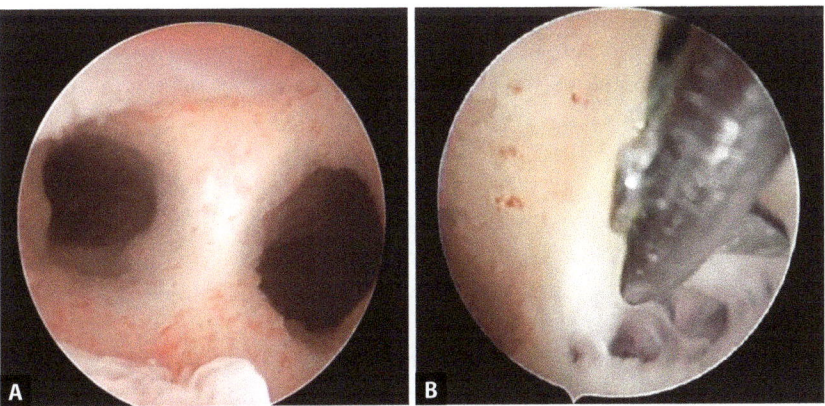

Figs. 4A and B: Septum and resection with scissors.

with partial bicorporeal uterus are not at increased risk of adverse obstetrical outcome. Patients with more severe bicorporeal uteri may or may not have an adverse pregnancy outcome. Strassman procedure is rarely performed. Metroplasty is not recommended for bicorporeal uterus with normal cervix.

Hemiuterus (class U4): Rudimentary horn may or may not have cavity and it may be communicating or noncommunicating. Pregnancy loss may be associated with reduced uterine volume along with compromised vascularity. The higher prevalence of incompetent cervix has led some authors to recommend that cervical cerclage be placed to improve obstetrical outcome. Women with hemiuterus and no previous history of second trimester loss or premature birth should be managed expectantly with frequent follow-ups.

Arcuate uterus (class U1c): Mild concave indentation of endometrial cavity at midline fundus gives uterus an arcuate configuration. It has nearly similar reproductive outcome as of normal uterus. Treatment is usually expectant.

Acquired Uterine Abnormalities

Uterine fibroids: In a review, submucous fibroid increases the risk of miscarriage from 22 to 47%.[17] Submucous leiomyoma can impede normal implantation.[17,18]

Hysteroscopic myomectomy is the procedure of choice for submucous myomas. The American Association of Gynecologic Laparoscopist (AAGL) practice guidelines concluded that at least in selected patients, submucous myomectomy may reduce the risk of spontaneous abortion.[19]

Endometrial polyps: A significant proportion (27%) of endometrial polyps regressed spontaneously within 1 year, specifically smaller polyps (<1 cm).[20] There is no clear evidence of its association with pregnancy loss. Hysteroscopic removal can be considered for larger polyps (>1 cm) in women with RPL without any other known cause for RPL.[19-21]

Intrauterine adhesions (IUA): Hysteroscopy is mainstay in diagnosis and treatment of adhesions. Hysteroscopic removal of adhesions with scissors **(Fig. 5)** is recommended,[19-22] but recurrence is of concern. Nonsurgical options like stem cell therapies are being explored but need confirmation before being applied clinically.[23]

Cervical Incompetence

These patients present with history of painless, recurrent second trimester losses, or preterm deliveries with no or minimal uterine activity. There is lack of uniform diagnostic criteria and objective tests to diagnose this condition. It can be congenital or acquired.

Cervical cerclage has been used to prevent late second trimester losses or preterm births. Various methods such as McDonalds, Shirodkar, and transabdominal are defined in literature. Cerclage should be performed at

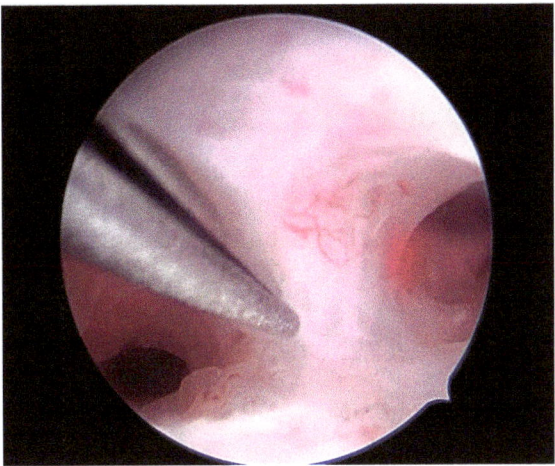

Fig. 5: Intrauterine adhesiolysis with scissors.

13-16 weeks of gestation after ultrasound evaluation of fetus for viability and exclusion of apparent anomalies in the fetus.

A recent review on cerclage concludes that benefits of cerclage are limited, but advisable in a women with three prior adverse events, and those with a short cervix (<25 mm) who have had a prior preterm birth.[24]

ENDOCRINE ETIOLOGIES

In the pregnancy, there are physiological alterations at the boundary between mother and fetus which causes endocrinal and metabolic changes influencing growth and development of the fetus. Endocrine disorders such as polycystic ovary syndrome (PCOS), luteal phase defect (LPD), diabetes mellitus, thyroid disease, and hyperprolactinemia are contributing approximately 8–12% of RPL.

Recurrent pregnancy loss in PCOS occurs in 40–50% of total pregnancies.[25]

Maternal obesity has been reported as an independent risk factor for miscarriage.[26] Obesity is also associated with PCOS, insulin resistance leading to RPL.

Luteal phase defect is due to inadequate production of progesterone by the corpus luteum and endometrial maturation is insufficient for proper placentation.[27] Studies suggested that progesterone causes downregulation of Th1 cytokines and upregulation of Th2 cytokines to maintain pregnancy. In the presence of progesterone, lymphocytes release progesterone-induced blocking factor in pregnancy which also shift balance toward Th2 dominance.[28] When the progesterone levels are below 12 ng/mL, there is abnormal luteal phase and increased risk of miscarriage.

Thyroid hormone influences normal ovulation by regulating granulosa and luteal cells.[29] Hypothyroidism (overt and subclinical) associated with adverse fetal outcome. Thyroid autoimmunity is also associated with recurrent miscarriage (RM), preterm delivery, and neonatal respiratory distress syndrome in euthyroid women.[30,31]

IDIOPATHIC FACTORS

The etiology of RPL is unknown in at least 40% of cases. Due to lack of information about its etiology, idiopathic recurrent pregnancy loss (iRPL) has become challenging reproductive problem worldwide.

- Vascular endothelial growth factor (VEGF) gene polymorphisms in women with RM demonstrating that the *-1154G/A* VEGF gene polymorphism is associated with idiopathic recurrent abortions. The risk of RPL was lower in the carriers of the G allele than in women carrying the A allele.[32]
- Few studies suggested the relationship between DNA fragmentation in the male gamete and idiopathic RPL. Men with higher DNA fragmentation index (DFI) are infertile whereas men with lower DFI (26%) can conceive but may land up with RPL. Thus sperm DFI should be evaluated in couples experiencing idiopathic RPL.[33] Study by E. Rajcan-Separovic et al. shows that paternal array comparative genomic hybridization (CGH) analysis is useful for detecting copy number variants (CNVs) in cases of RPL.[34]
- Preimplantation genetic diagnosis improves pregnancy outcome for women with idiopathic RPL, especially those with more than two previous losses, and >35 years of age, and that improvement is not affected by fertility status.[35]

COMPLETE EVALUATION AND COUNSELING

- Routine laboratory evaluation
- Thorough hormonal workup and treatment
- PCOS evaluation and lifestyle management
- Overt hypothyroidism arising before conception or during early gestation should be treated with levothyroxine in women with RPL
- Though there is insufficient evidence of LPD, it should be treated.
- 3D/4D sonography to rule out anatomical causes
- Karyotyping of partners with RM is mandatory, karyotype of products of conception. About 5% of couples with recurrent spontaneous miscarriage (RSM) are carriers of balanced translocations. The chance of RSM where one of the partners is a carrier of balanced translocation is 30%. Amniocentesis is advised at 16 weeks for karyotyping and level II USG at 16–18 weeks. Can also use donor sperm, oocyte, and apply preimplantation genetic diagnosis (PGD).
- Evaluation for antiphospholipid antibodies (APLA)
- Thrombophilia panel for factor V Leiden, prothrombin
- Sperm DNA integrity assay—DFI >30% will have poor fertility.
- Counseling plays important role.

CONCLUSION

Over the years, treatments such as surgical correction of uterine anomalies or aspirin and heparin for antiphospholipid syndrome are considered as evidence based. These therapies helped to improve RPL. But almost half of the cases are put under unexplained variety and being treated with progesterone, anticoagulation, immunomodulatory empirically. Apart from all above modalities of management, we need to consider the psychological aspect of the couple due to RPL. Thus for successful outcome along with recommended therapies, clinics should take the psychosocial needs of couples into account.

REFERENCES

1. ESHRE Guideline Group on RPL; Bender Atik R, Christiansen OB, Elson J, Kolte AM, Lewis S, et al. ESHRE guideline: recurrent pregnancy loss. Hum Reprod Open. 2018;2018:(2):hoy004.
2. Rasmark Roepke E, Matthiesen L, Rylance R, Christiansen OB. Is the incidence of recurrent pregnancy loss increasing? A retrospective register-based study in Sweden. Acta Obstet Gynecol Scand. 2017;96(11):1365-72.
3. Raga F, Bonilla-Musoles F, Blanes J, Osborne NG. Congenial Müllerian anomalies: diagnostic accuracy of three-dimensional ultrasound. Fertil Steril. 1996;65:523.
4. Troiano RN, McCarthy SM. Mullerian duct anomalies: imaging and clinical issues. Radiology. 2004;233:19.
5. Bermejo C, Martínez Ten P, Cantarero R, Diaz D, Pérez Pedregosa J, Barrón E, et al. Three-dimensional ultrasound in the diagnosis of Müllerian duct anomalies and concordance with magnetic resonance imaging. Ultrasound Obstet Gynecol. 2010;35:593.
6. Soares SR, Barbosa dos Reis MM, Camargos AF. Diagnostic accuracy of sonohysterography, transvaginal sonography, and hysterosalpingography in patients with uterine cavity diseases. Fertil Steril. 2000;73:406.
7. Alborzi S, Dehbashi S, Parsanezhad ME. Differential diagnosis of septate and bicornuate uterus by sonohysterography eliminates the need for laparoscopy. Fertil Steril. 2002;78:176.
8. Devi Wold AS, Pham N, Arici A. Anatomic factors in recurrent pregnancy loss. Semin Reprod Med. 2006;24:25-32.
9. Robberecht C, Pexsters A, Deprest J, Fryns JP, D'Hooghe T, Vermeesch JR. Cytogenetic and morphological analysis of early products of conception following hystero-embryoscopy from couples with recurrent pregnancy loss. Prenat Diagn. 2012;32:933-42.
10. Chan YY, Jayaprakasan K, Zamora J, Thornton JG, Raine-Fenning N, Coomarasamy A. The prevalence of congenital uterine anomalies in unselected and high-risk populations: a systematic review. Hum Reprod Update. 2011;17:761.
11. Rikken J, Leeuwis-Fedorovich NE, Letteboer S, Emanuel MH, Limpens J, van der Veen F, et al. The pathophysiology of the septate uterus: a systematic review. BJOG. 2019;126:1192.
12. Grimbizis GF, Camus M, Tarlatzis BC, Bontis JN, Devroey P. Clinical implications of uterine malformations and hysteroscopic treatment results. Hum Reprod Update. 2001;7:161.
13. Ludmir J, Samuels P, Brooks S, Mennuti MT. Pregnancy outcome of patients with uncorrected uterine anomalies managed in a high-risk obstetric setting. Obstet Gynecol. 1990;75:906.

14. Heinonen PK. Complete septate uterus with longitudinal vaginal septum. Fertil Steril. 2006;85:700.
15. Candiani GB, Vercellini P, Fedele L, Carinelli SG, Merlo D, Arcaini L. Repair of the uterine cavity after hysteroscopic septal incision. Fertil Steril. 1990;54:991-4.
16. Angell NF, Tan Domingo J, Siddiqi N. Uterine rupture at term after uncomplicated hysteroscopic metroplasty. Obstet Gynecol. 2002;100:1098-9.
17. Klatsky PC, Tran ND, Caughey AB, Fujimoto VY. Fibroids and reproductive outcomes: a systematic literature review from conception to delivery. Am J Ostet Gynecol. 2008;198:357-66.
18. Simpson JL. Causes of fetal wastage. Clin Obstet Gynecol. 2007;50:10-30.
19. Jaslow CR. Uterine factors. Obstet Gynecol Clin North Am. 2014;41:57-86.
20. Lieng M, Istre O, Sandvik L, Qvigstad E. Prevalence, 1-year regression rate, and clinical significance of asymptomatic endometrial polyps: cross-sectional study. J Minim Invasive Gynecol. 2009;16:465-71.
21. Salim S, Won H, Nesbitt-Hawes E, Campbell N, Abbott J. Diagnosis and management of endometrial polyps: a critical review of the literature. J Minim Invasive Gynecol. 2011;18:569-81.
22. Kodaman PH, Arici A. Intra-uterine adhesions and fertility outcome: how to optimize success? Curr Opin Obstet Gynecol. 2007;19:207-14.
23. Santamaria X, Cabanillas S, Cervello I, Arbona C, Raga F, Ferro J, et al. Autologous cell therapy with CD133+ bone marrow-derived stem cells for refractory Asherman's syndrome and endometrial atrophy: a pilot cohort study. Hum Reprod. 2016;31:1087-96.
24. Story L, Shennan A. Cervical cerclage: an established intervention with neglected potential? Eur J Obstet Gynecol Reprod Biol. 2014;176:17-9.
25. Chakraborty P, Goswami SK, Rajani S, Sharma S, Kabir SN, Chakravarty B, et al. Recurrent pregnancy loss in polycystic ovary syndrome: role of hyperhomocysteinemia and insulin resistance. PLoS One. 2013;8(5):e64446.
26. Bellver J, Rossal LP, Bosch E, Zúñiga A, Corona JT, Meléndez F, et al. Obesity and the risk of spontaneous abortion after oocyte donation. Fertil Steril. 2003;79:1136-40.
27. Graham JD, Clarke CL. Physiological action of progesterone in target tissues. Endocr Rev. 1997;18:502-19.
28. Szekeres-Bartho J, Balasch J. Progestagen therapy for recurrent miscarriage. Hum Reprod Update. 2008;14:27-35.
29. Wakim AN, Polizotto SL, Buffo MJ, Marrero MA, Burholt DR. Thyroid hormones in human follicular fluid and thyroid hormone receptors in human granulosa cells. Fertil Steril. 1993;59:1187-90.
30. De Vivo A, Mancuso A, Giacobbe A, Moleti M, Maggio Savasta L, De Dominici R, et al. Thyroid function in women found to have early pregnancy loss. Thyroid. 2010;20:633-7.
31. Lata K, Dutta P, Sridhar S, Rohilla M, Srinivasan A, Prashad GR, et al. Thyroid autoimmunity and obstetric outcomes in women with recurrent miscarriage: A case-control study. Endocr Connect. 2013;2:118-24.
32. Papazoglou D, Galazios G, Papatheodorou K, Liberis V, Papanas N, Maltezos E, et al. Vascular endothelial growth factor gene polymorphisms and idiopathic recurrent pregnancy loss. Fertil Steril. 2005;83(4):959-63.
33. Kumar K, Deka D, Singh A, Mitra DK, Vanitha BR, Dada R. Predictive value of DNA integrity analysis in idiopathic recurrent pregnancy loss following spontaneous conception. J Assist Reprod Genet. 2012;29(9):861-7.
34. Rajcan-Separovic E, Diego-Alvarez D, Robinson WP, Tyson C, Qiao Y, Harvard C, et al. Identification of copy number variants in miscarriages from couples with idiopathic recurrent pregnancy loss. Hum Reprod. 2010;25(11):2913-22.
35. Garrisi JG, Colls P, Ferry KM, Zheng X, Garrisi MG, Munné S. Effect of infertility, maternal age, and number of previous miscarriages on the outcome of preimplantation genetic diagnosis for idiopathic recurrent pregnancy loss. Fertil Steril. 2009;92(1):288-95.

CHAPTER 37

Application of Stem Cells in Infertility

Sunita Tandulwadkar, Nilesh Balkawade

INTRODUCTION: WHAT ARE STEM CELLS?

The body is made up of about 200 different kinds of specialized cells such as muscle cells, nerve cells, fat cells, and skin cells. All cells in the body come from stem cells. Stem cells are undifferentiated "blank" cells that do not yet have begun to develop into specialized tissue and organs. Once the differentiation pathway of a stem cell has been decided, it can no longer become another type of cell on its own.

Under certain physiologic or experimental conditions, they can be induced to become tissue- or organ-specific cells with special functions.

- *Self-renewal:* Stem cells can renew themselves almost indefinitely. This is also known as proliferation.
- *Differentiation:* Stem cells have the special ability to differentiate into cells with specialized characteristics and functions.
- *Unspecialized:* Stem cells themselves are largely unspecialized cells which then give rise to specialized cells.

CHARACTERISTICS OF MESENCHYMAL STEM CELL

The Mesenchymal and Tissue Stem Cell Committee of the International Society for Cellular Therapy introduced criteria for mesenchymal stem cells (MSCs).[1]

1. MSCs should be *plastic-adherent* when preserved in standard cell culture media.
2. MSCs should have a *specific gene expression pattern* with expression of the surface molecules CD73, CD90, and CD105, and without the expression of CD11b, CD14, CD19, CD34, CD45, and CD79a.
3. MSCs should have the *ability to differentiate into various cell types*, including adipocytes, osteoblasts, and chondroblasts, in cell culture conditions **(Table 1)**.

STEM CELL HARVEST AND INFUSION

Stem cells can be isolated from several human organs such as bone marrow, umbilical cord, and adipose tissue. Bone marrow is a rich source of stem cells.

TABLE 1: Association between miRNAs and different MSCs and their effects on the female reproductive system.[2]

MSCs			
	BMSCs	miR-21	Inhibition of GCs apoptosis by targeting PDCD4 and PTEN
		Exosomai miR-644-5P	Inhibition of GCs apoptosis by targeting P53
		Exosomal miR-144-5P	Inhibition of GCs apoptosis by targeting PTEN
	AFSCs	Exosomai miR-10a	Inhibition of GCs apoptosis by targeting BIM
		Exosomai miR-146a	Inhibition of GCs apoptosis by targeting of IRAKI and TRAF6
	PMSCs	miR-222	Increasing PMSCs apoptosis by targeting BCL2L11

(AFSCs: amniotic fluid stem cells; BCL2L11: B-Cell Lymphoma 2 Like 11; BIM: Bcl-2-Like Protein 11; BMSCs: bone marrow stromal cells; GCs: granulosa cells; IRAK1: interleukin-1 receptor-associated kinase 1; MSCs: mesenchymal stem cells; PDCD4: programmed cell death protein 4; PMSCs: placenta mesenchymal stem cells; PTEN: phosphatase and tensin homolog; TRAF6: TNF receptor-associated factor 6)

These stem cells are called autologous hematopoietic stem cells and they are considered to be adult stem cells. These cells can be easily harvested from the bone marrow of hip bone of the patient undergoing the stem cell infusion. With the latest nontouch, digital technology, stem cells can be isolated from the bone marrow of an individual within 30 minutes in the most sterile conditions. Since there is no hospitalization, no cut and no surgery, immediate mobilization is possible, and it becomes a patient friendly method of procedure.

Role of Stem Cells in Infertility

Decreasing semen parameters and premature ovarian failure have become a global concern. For both male and female partners experiencing infertility, current treatment options rely solely on the premise that both partners produce functional haploid gametes. For those couples where one partner is unable to produce a functional gamete, no treatment options are available other than the use of donor gametes. Stem cells are coming up as a miraculous therapy in various conditions, including infertility.

Review of literature shows that more than of 11,400 published studies have investigated the potential use of stem cell as an effective therapy for several conditions leading to both male and female infertility.

AZOOSPERMIA

It is found in 20% of men who seek infertility treatment.
Types of azoospermia are:
- Obstructive (sperm is blocked from exiting the testicle)
- Nonobstructive (sperm is not produced at all).

The testis has both exocrine and endocrine functions. The exocrine function involves the continuous production of spermatozoa, which are released from the testis, transported through the excurrent ducts, and eventually ejaculated. The endocrine activity consists of the secretion of testosterone, which is necessary to maintain secondary sexual characteristics, accessory sex organs, and spermatogenesis.

REFRACTORY ENDOMETRIUM

For successful conception, apart from healthy embryo, we need excellent endometrium so as to have healthy dialogue between embryo and endometrium.

The human endometrium is a dynamic remodeling tissue undergoing >400 cycles of regeneration, differentiation, and shedding during woman's reproductive years. Endometrial thickness is the key factor in the implantation of the embryo and in the achievement of pregnancy. Endometrial grows about 1–2 mm every other day. Ideally, at the time of ovulation, the endometrium would be about 8 mm or more in thickness. There is no officially accepted definition of a thin endometrium, which results in a lower rate of full-term pregnancy. The commonly accepted cutoff is <7 mm on the day of luteinizing hormone (LH) surge or human chorionic gonadotropin (hCG) administration.[3]

The prevalence of this pathology is 0.5% of infertile women undergoing assisted reproductive treatments.[4]

Asherman's syndrome is an uncommon gynecological disorder caused by the destruction of the endometrium due to repeated or aggressive curettages and/or endometritis.[5] As a result, there is loss of functional endometrium in many areas. The uterine cavity is obliterated by intrauterine adhesions, leading to amenorrhea, infertility, recurrent pregnancy loss, etc. It causes adhesion and fibrosis of the endometrium such that there is very little healthy endometrium for implantation. Refractory endometrium too, offers very limited treatment options.

A normal uterine cavity and endometrial lining are necessary in order to conceive and maintain a pregnancy. The only therapeutic modality available for such women is surrogacy.

Bone marrow stem cells contribute for endometrium regeneration. On the basis of these facts, bone marrow stem cells can be used for regeneration of damaged endometrium. Endometrium is dynamic, cyclically regenerating tissue, a unique model of physiological angiogenesis in adult. Angiogenesis results in either sprouting a new vessel through recruitment of local endothelial cells from neighboring blood vessel and/or by endothelial progenitor cells circulating in blood after release from bone marrow. Endometrial angiogenic stem cells isolated from autologous adult stem cells could regenerate injured endometrium not responding to conventional treatment for Asherman's syndrome. Endometrial regeneration using autologous adult stem cells followed by conception through in vitro fertilization in a patient of severe Asherman's syndrome is shown by Nagori et al. in 2011.[6]

Woman with severe Asherman's syndrome treated with autologous bone marrow derived stem cells from endometrial regeneration led to a successful implantation.[7,8] Bone marrow stem cells exert their influence by the secretion of massive amount of growth factors and cytokines to result in a therapeutic outcome called "trophic" activity. It is known that stem cells secrete bioactive molecules that:
- Inhibit apoptosis and limit the field of damage or injury
- Inhibit scarring or fibrosis at the site of injury
- Stimulate angiogenesis
- Stimulate the mitosis of tissue-specific and tissue-intrinsic progenitors[9,10]

Tandulwadkar et al. published a study in which it is mentioned that even autologous intrauterine platelet rich plasma instillation for suboptimal endometrium in frozen embryo transfer cycles tends to improve the outcomes in form of endometrial thickness and vascularity.[11]

PREMATURE OVARIAN FAILURE

During the lifetime, a numerically fixed pool of oocytes is committed for the fertility. This original pool would account in woman for approximately 106 oocytes in puberty, but the number declines with aging until exhaustion at menopause.

Premature ovarian failure (POF) is the loss of function of the ovaries before age 40. It is associated with sex steroid deficiency, amenorrhea, infertility, and elevated serum gonadotropins.[12] In majority of the cases, underlying cause is not identified.[13] 10% of women undergoing IVF show diminished ovarian reserve, though the incidence is increasing by the day. However, pregnancy rate remains low despite a plethora of interventions and is associated with high pregnancy loss.

In adolescents, it would seem that the more common causes of POF include cytogenetic abnormalities involving the X chromosome, ovarian dysfunction occurring in association with other autoimmune endocrine disturbances, and chemotherapy and/or radiation therapy given for any of a number of malignancies.[14]

Known causes include:
- Genetic aberration which could involve the X chromosome and autosomes.
- *Autoimmune ovarian damage:* Antiovarian antibodies are reported in POF by several studies.
- Iatrogenic following surgical radiotherapeutic or chemotherapeutic interventions as in malignancies.
- Environmental factors such as viral infection and toxins for which no clear mechanism is known.[15]

M Edessy had injected bone marrow derived mesenchymal stem cells into the ovaries, via laparoscopy in 10 patients. Endometrial fractional biopsy was histopathologically (HP) and immunohistochemically (IH), stained and evaluated according to Edessy stem cells score (ESS).

After transplantation two cases (20%) (ESS = 5 and 6) resumed menstruation after 3 months, one of them (10%) (Case no 5) (ESS = 6) got pregnancy after 11 months and delivered a healthy full-term baby. The two menstruating cases showed focal secretory changes after being atrophic endometrium in case no. 5 and distorted proliferative endometrium in case no. 10.[16]

Several researchers in Eunice Kennedy Shriver National Institute of Child Health and Human Development, US (January 2017) and Hospital University La Fe (September 2014) have confirmed the presence of ovarian stem cells, as well as bone marrow derived stem cells that have been able to colonize the ovaries and have folliculogenesis.[17]

The first baby of autologous stem cell therapy in POF is a reality and hope. The first stem cell baby "Zein Rajani", is a mature living female, 38 weeks, 3.3 kg.[16] In 2018, Gupta et al. reported the world's first successful case of application of autologous bone marrow-derived stem cell therapy (ABMDSCT) in a 45-year-old female to give successful birth to a healthy baby.[18] In 2020, Tandulwadkar et al. published a pilot study of 20 patients in patient-oriented strategies encompassing individualized oocyte number (POSEIDON) groups 3 and 4. The study group underwent laparoscopic/transvaginal intraovarian instillation of autologous bone marrow-derived stem cells (ABMDSCs) combined with platelet-rich plasma (PRP) and the outcome was analyzed.[19] Primary outcome was antral follicle count (AFC) and mature metaphase II (MII) oocytes and secondary outcome was anti-Müllerian hormone (AMH) levels and number of Grade A and B embryos frozen on day 3. After 6 weeks of intraovarian instillation ABMDSCs mixed with PRP, patients were reassessed for AFC and AMH and their response to subsequent controlled ovarian stimulation (COS) cycle was observed. Statistically significant improvement was seen in AFC, MII oocytes, and Grade A and Grade B embryos. AMH was also increased in some patients, but the result was not statistically significant. They concluded that intraovarian instillation of ABMDSCs combined with PRP is safe and it optimized the recruitment of existing dormant primordial follicles to improve oocyte yield and hence the number and quality of embryos after COS in POSEIDON Group 3 and 4 poor responders.[20]

Stem cell therapy seems to be a promising approach. Nonetheless, in order to safely recruit it in clinical application toward treating ovarian insufficiency in the context of infertility, it should be highlighted that it is equally imperative to consider both strengths and weaknesses.

Not only this, stem cells have also been used in treating myocardial infarction and multiple sclerosis.[21,22]

REGULATION OF RESEARCH IN INDIA

The clinical research environment in India is currently undergoing a tremendous flux, with regulators coming under severe criticism from the press, public, and the elected government.[9]

There are the new Indian Council for Medical Research–Department of Biotechnology (ICMR-DBT) draft guidelines on stem cell research, and the Central Drugs Standard Control Organization (CDSCO) draft on compensation toward injury due to participation in clinical research that are responses to several questions that face us today.[10,12]

ETHICAL CONCERNS

The ethical guidelines for biomedical research on human subjects were published by the ICMR in 2000. However, their recommendations are nonbinding. At the same time, the Drugs Controller General has issued binding regulations on good clinical practices (GCP) for clinical research in India (2001), based on World Health Organization (WHO) standards, and it is reported that programs to train clinicians in GCP are proliferating around the country (Kahn 2006).[16]

While statutory laws have been strengthened in 2014, prospects for their implementation remain weak, given embedded challenges of putting healthcare laws and professional codes into practice.[23]

The guidelines propose a system of review and monitoring of the field based on a National Apex Committee (NAC) for Stem Cell Research and Therapy and, at the institutional level, Institutional Committees for Stem Cell Research and Therapy. All research, including clinical trials, would require the prior approval of, and be registered with, the NAC. Prohibited areas of research include reproductive cloning, implantation of a human embryo into the uterus after *in vitro* manipulation, and transfer of human blastocysts generated by somatic cell nuclear transfer (SCNT) into a human or nonhuman uterus.[16,24]

As stem cell science moves from the laboratory to the clinic and the experimental treatment of patients, in India it does so in a governance vacuum. The ICMR has approved the national guidelines for Stem Cell Research, revised by ICMR in November 2017. Approval for clinical trials to be sought from Institutional Ethics Committee (IEC) and National Apex Committee for Stem Cell Research and Therapy (NAC-SCRT).

REFERENCES

1. Dominici M, Le Blanc K, Mueller I, Slaper-Cortenbach I, Marini F, Krause D, et al. Minimal criteria for defining multipotent mesenchymal stromal cells. The International Society for Cellular Therapy position statement. Cytotherapy. 2006;8:315-7.
2. Zhang C. The roles of different stem cells on premature ovarian failure. Curr Stem Cell Res Ther. 2020;15:473-81.
3. Ching-Shwun Lin. Advances in stem cell therapy for erectile dysfunction, Advances in andrology. London: Hindawi Publishing Corporation; 2014.
4. Senturk LM, Erel CT. Thin endometrium in assisted reproductive technology. Curr Opin Obstet Gynecol. 2008;20(3):221-8.
5. Yu D, Wong YM, Cheong Y, Xia E, Li TC. Asherman syndrome—one century later. Fertil Steril. 2008;89(4):759-79.
6. Nagori CB, Panchal SY, Patel H. Endometrial regeneration using autologous adult stem cells followed by conception by in vitro fertilization in a patient of severe Asherman's syndrome. J Hum Reprod Sci. 2011;4(1):43-8.
7. Greenberg SH, Lipshultz LI, Wein AJ. Experience with 425 subfertile male patients. J Urol. 1978;119:507-10.
8. Sigman M, Lipshulz LI, Howard SS. In: Lipshulz LI, Howard SS (Eds). Infertility in the Male, 3rd edition. St. Louis: Mosby; 1997. pp. 173-93.
9. Male Infertility Best Practice Policy Committee of the American Urological Association; Practice Committee of the American Society for Reproductive Medicine. Report on optimal evaluation of the infertile male. Fertil Steril. 2006;86(5 Suppl 1): S202-9.
10. Jarvi K, Lo K, Fischer A, Grantmyre J, Zini A, Chow V, et al. CUA Guideline: The workup of azoospermic males. Can Urol Assoc J. 2010;4(3):163-7.
11. Tandulwadkar SR, Naralkar MV, Surana AD, Selvakarthick M, Kharat AH. Autologous intrauterine platelet-rich plasma instillation for suboptimal endometrium in frozen embryo transfer cycles: a pilot study. J Hum Reprod Sci. 2017;10:208-12.
12. NIH Consensus Conference Impotence. NIH Consensus Development Panel on Impotence. JAMA. 1993;270:83-90.
13. Albersen M, Shindel AW, Mwamukonda KB, Lue TF. The future is today: emerging drugs for the treatment of erectile dysfunction. Expert Opin Emerg Drugs. 2010;15:467-80.
14. Rebar RW. 2008. Premature ovarian "failure" in the adolescent. Ann N Y Acad Sci. 2008;1135:138-45.
15. Chang SH, Kim CS, Lee KS, Kim H, Yim SV, Lim YJ, et al. Premenopausal factors influencing premature ovarian failure and early menopause. Maturitas. 2007;58:19-30.
16. Edessy M, Hosni HN, Shady Y, Waf Y, Bakr S, Kamel M. Autologous stem cells therapy, the first baby of idiopathic premature ovarian failure. Acta Medica Int. 2016;3(1):19-23.
17. ClinicalTrials.gov. (2012). Ovarian Stem Cells From Women With Ovarian Insufficiency. [online]. Available from https://clinicaltrials.gov/ct2/show/record/NCT01702935 [Last accessed July, 2022].
18. Mittal S. Stem cell research: The India perspective. Perspect Clin Res. 2013;4(1):105-7.
19. Gupta S, Lodha P, Karthick MS, Tandulwadkar SR. Role of Autologous Bone Marrow-Derived Stem Cell Therapy for Follicular Recruitment in Premature Ovarian

Insufficiency: Review of Literature and a Case Report of World's First Baby with Ovarian Autologous Stem Cell Therapy in a Perimenopausal Woman of Age 45 Year. J Hum Reprod Sci. 2018;11(2):125-30.
20. Tandulwadkar S, Karthick MS. Combined Use of Autologous Bone Marrow-derived Stem Cells and Platelet-rich Plasma for Ovarian Rejuvenation in Poor Responders. J Hum Reprod Sci. 2020;13(3):184-90.
21. Nagori CB, Panchal SY, Patel H. Endometrial regeneration using autologous adult stem cells followed by conception by in vitro fertilization in a patient of severe Asherman's syndrome. J Hum Reprod Sci. 2011;4(1):43-8.
22. Tiwari SS, Raman S. Governing stem cell therapy in India: regulatory vacuum or jurisdictional ambiguity? New Genet Soc. 2014;33(4):413-33.
23. Zhang C. The roles of different stem cells on premature ovarian failure. Curr Stem Cell Res Ther. 2020;15:473-81.
24. Yu D, Wong YM, Cheong Y, Xia E, Li TC. Asherman syndrome—one century later. Fertil Steril. 2008;89(4):759-79.

CHAPTER 38

Algorithms for Artificial Intelligence in Reproductive Medicine

Leena Patankar, Amit Patankar

INTRODUCTION

There is rapid development in the field of assisted reproductive technology (ART) but even today there is a lack in the methods of judging the quality of the eggs, the sperm and the embryos accurately. It is difficult to predict the probability of a successful pregnancy for each patient and identify the cause of failure. The quality of embryos is the most critical factor for the success of in vitro fertilization (IVF). Embryo selection methods using a single parameter or algorithm have not been identified.

The term *artificial intelligence (AI)* was first coined by John McCarthy in 1955. AI is defined as the ability of machines to learn and display intelligence, which is in stark contrast to the natural intelligence demonstrated by humans and animals.

Advances in AI applications are constantly promoted by the increasing amount of data available in reproductive medicine.

Recently, AI is used mainly in the following areas:
- Select and predict the sperm cell to improve the success rate of treatment
- Assess the quality of embryos and oocytes and establish a useful ART prediction model and predict the outcome[1] (**Fig. 1**).

ROLE OF ARTIFICIAL INTELLIGENCE IN REPRODUCTIVE MEDICINE

Figure 1 describes the role of AI in reproductive medicine[1]:
- Big data include electronic medical records (EMRs) and other data.
- EMRs can capture data from various ways and the data is analyzed using AI such as machine learning and natural language processing (NLP). The machine learning (ML) method attempts to cluster the features of patients and predict the outcome of diseases by analyzing structured data such as medical imaging and genetic data. The NLP method extracts and processes meaningful information from unstructured clinical data, such as EMRs, to complement the structured data.

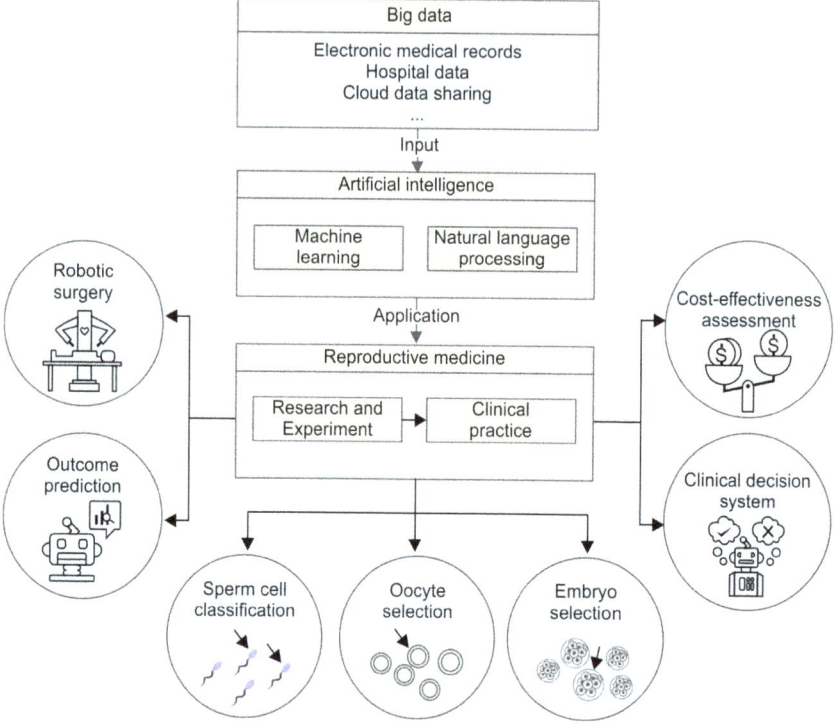

Fig. 1: The role of artificial intelligence (AI) in reproductive medicine.

- AI has been used in the many aspects of reproduction, from research and experiment to clinical practice.
- This schematic presentation in **Figure 1** shows the seven main applications of AI in reproductive medicine.

WORKFLOW OF ARTIFICIAL INTELLIGENCE IN REPRODUCTIVE MEDICINE (FLOWCHART 1)

Flowchart 1 describes the role of AI in reproductive medicine[1]:
- The first step is the collection of data.
- The data includes EMRs, hospital data and cloud data sharing.
- The second step is data preprocessing.
- The third step is the selection of the appropriate model.
- The data is analyzed using AI methods such as ML and NLP.
- Then the training dataset is used to train the model.
- The final steps include the evaluation and validation of the model.

Decision Tree Algorithm (Flowcharts 2 and 3; Table 1)

Flowchart 2 shows a decision tree model diagram with AMHR2 and LIF[2]:
- The model first separates cumulus cells samples upon AMHR2 expression (high or low) and then upon LIF expression (high or low).

Algorithms for Artificial Intelligence in Reproductive Medicine

Flowchart 1: Workflow of artificial intelligence (AI) in reproductive medicine.

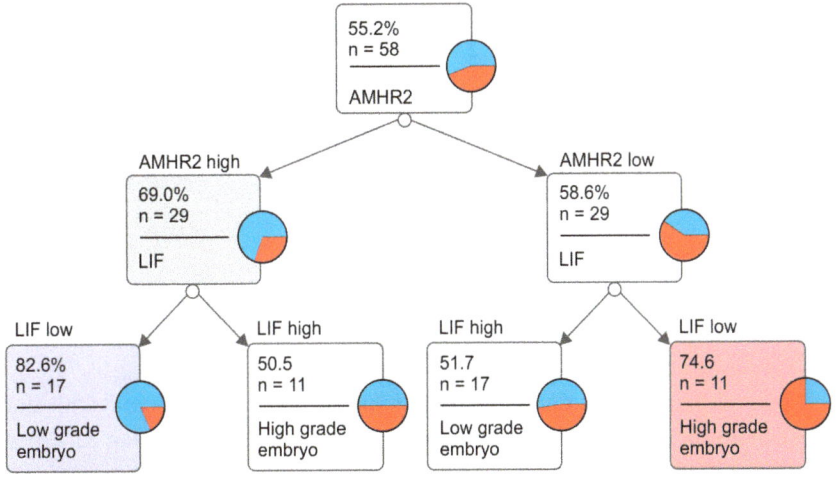

Flowchart 2: Decision tree algorithm.

(AMHR2: anti-Müllerian hormone receptor type 2; LIF: leukemia inhibitory factor)

- The blue color represents low quality embryos and red color represents high quality embryos.
- A combination of high AMHR2 and low LIF CC expression leads to an 82.6% possibility of developing a low-quality embryo, and combination of low AMHR2 and low LIF CC expression leads to 74.6% possibility of developing high quality embryos.

Flowchart 3: Decision tree for the selection of embryos.

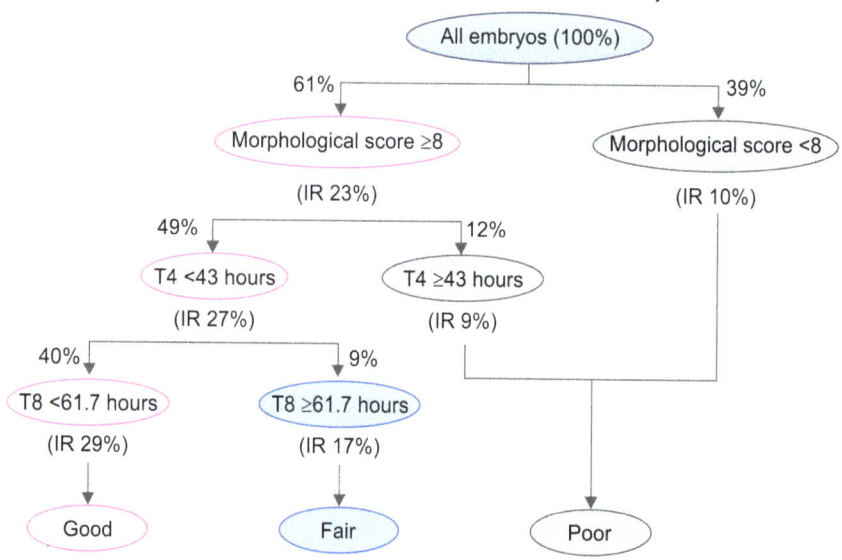

TABLE 1: Different algorithms in reproductive medicine.[1]			
Algorithm	**Advantages**	**Limitations**	**Application**
Decision tree	• Easy to interpret and understand • Can be combined with other techniques to improve the performance • Used as a White box model	Risk of overfitting (if the model is too complex and suitable for the training data, it is called overfitting)	Cost-effectiveness assessment of elective oocyte cryopreservation and embryo transfer

This data mining and decision tree model was based on classical embryo morphology and morphokinetics.

Flowchart 3 shows decision tree for the selection of embryos[3] with the highest implantation potential by means of the classical morphological score and morphokinetic parameters.

Among embryos with better morphological scores, morphokinetics permits deselection of embryos with the lowest implantation potential.

Random Forest Algorithm[1] (Tables 2 and 3)

- Hafiz et al. (2017)[4] used several data mining techniques to predict the implantation outcome of IVF and intracytoplasmic sperm injection (ICSI).

TABLE 2: Use of random forest algorithm.

Algorithm	Advantages	Limitations	Application
Random forest	• Corrects the problem of overfitting in the Decision Tree • More accurate than results predicted using an individual model	Need a large amount of maintenance work	Prediction of the outcome of IVF and ICSI

TABLE 3: Experimental results of random forest algorithm.

	AUC (%)	Accuracy (%)
SVM	57 ± 1.51	68.3 ± 1.05
Adaboost	47.52 + 4.5	66.99 + 2.85
RPART	82.05 ± 2.34	83.56 ± 0.99
RF	84.23 ± 0.91	83.96 ± 0.62
1 NN	50 ± 0	64.84 ±1.46

(AUC: areas under the ROC curve; Adaboost: Adaptive boosting; 1-NN: one-nearest-neighbor; RPART: recursive partitioning; RF: random forest; SVM: support vector machines)

- They collected and analyzed the data from 486 patients.
- Compared with other classifiers, RF and recursive partitioning (RPART) have achieved better prediction results [(areas under the ROC curve (AUC)—84.23% and 82.05%, respectively] **(Table 3)**.

Naïve Bayes Classifier Algorithm

Flowchart 4 illustrates the structure[5] of the Bayesian network as well as the **Table 4** describing the classification performance showing that this manually built Bayesian classifier returned 18 false negative and 2 false positive, with a general accuracy of 68.25% with 95.55% of specificity and no-implantation predictive value of 70.49% **(Table 4 and Flowchart 4)**.

Figure 2 (R Wang, 2019)[1] shows the researchers obtained human semen samples from eight healthy donors and acquired the quantitative phase maps of the sperm samples by using the diagram of the optical system.

Then they used a program to extract the phase map and features. Finally, the dataset obtained was used to train a two-class SVM classifier **(Table 5 and Fig. 2)**.

Decision tree model demonstrating how SVM equations are sequentially applied to CASA track parameters to identify sperm motility patterns[6] as shown in **Flowchart 5**.

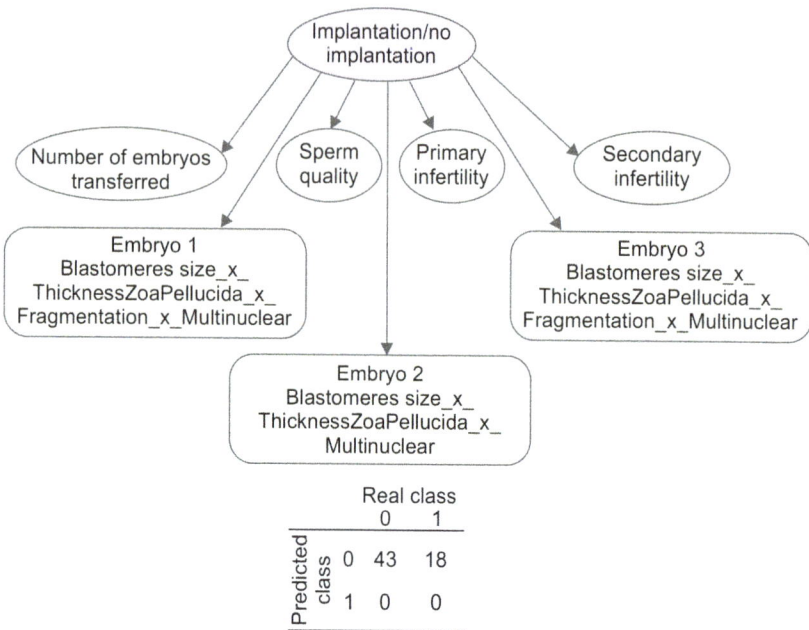

Flowchart 4: Naïve Bayes classifier algorithm.

TABLE 4: Use of Naïve Bayes classifier algorithm.[5]

Algorithm	Advantages	Limitations	Application
Naïve Bayes classifier	• Fast • Easy to train and understand • Perform well on small training datasets	• Problems occur if the input variables are related • Input variables must be statistically independent	Prediction of the implantation outcome of individual embryos based on no of embryos transferred

Figure 3 shows Girela et al.,[7] created an artificial neural network (ANN) model to produce a decision support system that can help predict the semen parameters based on the data collected by the questionnaires and can support the traditional diagnosis[5] **(Table 6, Fig. 3)**.

Flowchart 4 shows challenges associated to the use of ML/AI algorithms[8]:
- Data should be labeled accurately and unbiased
- ML/AI algorithms should be generalizable and avoid overfitting
- Algorithms should be validated in independent cohorts and continuously updated
- Algorithms need to be translated and adopted into clinical practice.

Algorithms for Artificial Intelligence in Reproductive Medicine — 351

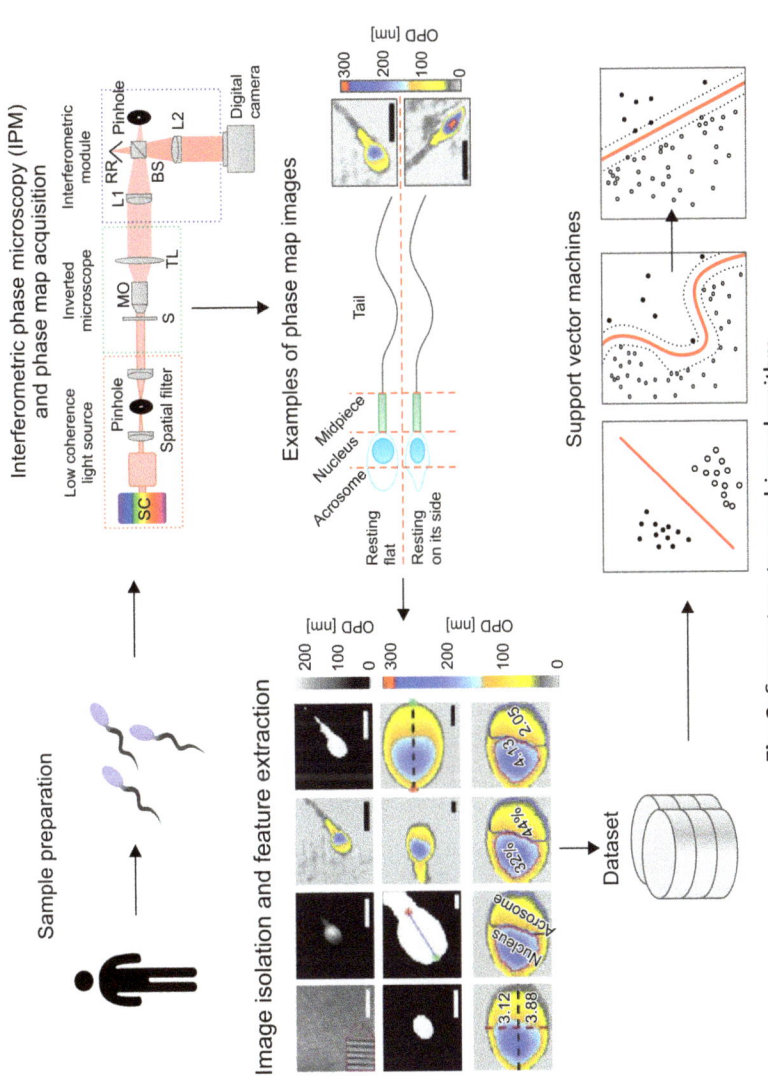

Fig. 2: Support vector machines algorithm.

TABLE 5: Use of support vector machines algorithm.[1]

Algorithm	Advantages	Limitations	Application
Support vector machines (SVMS)	• Perform well on nonlinear problems • Less risk of error • Powerful model with accurate prediction	• Difficult to train • Difficult to interpret and understand	• Classification of sperm cell • Embryo selection

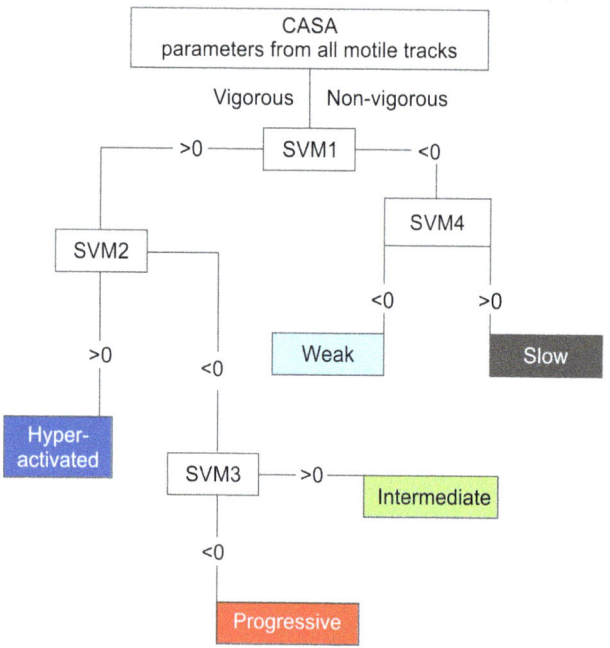

Flowchart 5: CASA track parameters to identify sperm motility patterns.

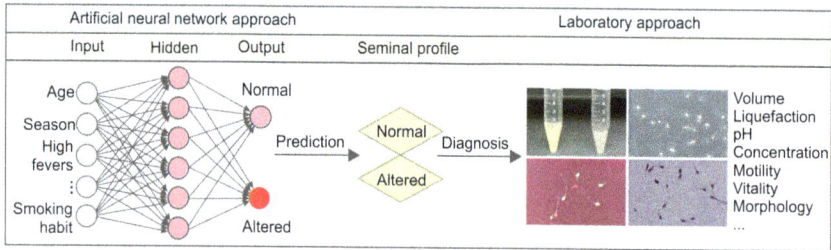

Fig. 3: Neural network and deep learning.

Algorithms for Artificial Intelligence in Reproductive Medicine

TABLE 6: Importance of neural network and deep learning algorithm.[1]

Algorithm	Advantages	Limitations	Application
Neural network and deep learning	• Algorithms can be adjusted to accommodate new problems quickly • Tolerate noise and missing values in data • Rapid development and broad prospect	• Require massive datasets to train the model • Highly demanding hardware (computing power) for training • Black box. Difficult to understand and interpret	Construction of a predictive model for the outcome of assisted reproductive technology (ART)

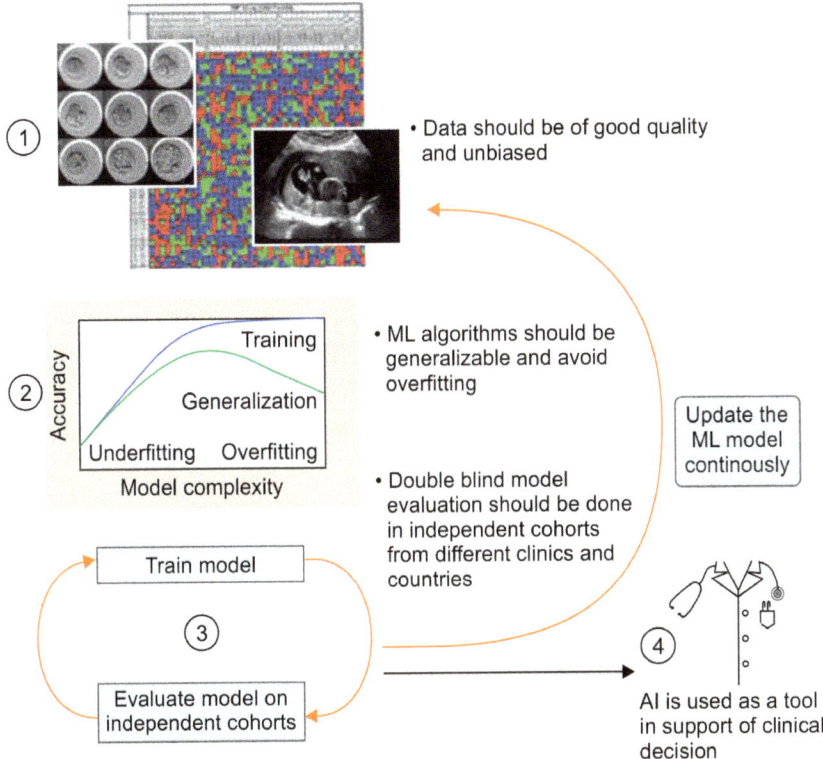

Fig. 4: Limitations of the use of machine learning and big data in the infertility sector.

CONCLUSION

With the correct application, AI is likely to improve the pregnancy outcomes as well as the patient care in infertile patients. However, at this stage it has some limitations as well as challenges.

Over the time, with more and more efforts and research, application of *artificial intelligence* will definitely improve. Undoubtedly AI has a place in reproductive medicine. With so much of data available and increasing demands for precision we are not far away from the era where artificial intelligence will no longer be a luxury but necessity.

REFERENCES

1. Wang R, Pan W, Jin L, Li Y, Geng Y, Gao C, et al. Artificial intelligence in reproductive medicine. Reproduction. 2019;158(4):R139-R154.
2. Devjak R, Burnik Papler T, Verdenik I, Fon Tacer K, Vrtačnik Bokal E. Embryo quality predictive models based on cumulus cells gene expression. Balkan J Med Genet. 2016;19(1):5-12.
3. Carrasco B, Arroyo G, Gil Y, Gómez MJ, Rodríguez I, Barri PN, et al. Selecting embryos with the highest implantation potential using data mining and decision tree based on classical embryo morphology and morphokinetics. J Assist Reprod Genet. 2017;34(8):983-90.
4. Hafiz P, Nematollahi M, Boostani R, Namavar Jahromi B. Predicting implantation outcome of in vitro fertilization and intracytoplasmic sperm injection using data mining techniques. Int J Fertil Steril. 2017;11(3):184-90.
5. Morales DA, Bengoetxea E, Larranaga P, Garcia M, Franco Y, Fresnada M, et al. Bayesian classification for the selection of in vitro human embryos using morphological and clinical data. Comput Methods Programs Biomed. 2008;90(2):104-16.
6. Goodson SG, White S, Stevans AM, Bhat S, Kao CY, Jaworski S, et al. CASAnova: a multiclass support vector machine model for the classification of human sperm motility patterns. Biol Reprod. 2017;97(5):698-708.
7. Girela JL, Gil D, Johnsson M, Gomez-Torres MJ, De Juan J. Semen parameters can be predicted from environmental factors and lifestyle using artificial intelligence methods. Biol Reprod. 2013;88(4):99.
8. Preprints. Big Data and Artificial Intelligence (AI) are poised to Transform Infertility Healthcare (Polanski I); 2020. [online] Available from https://www.preprints.org/manuscript/202010.0356/v2. [Last accessed June, 2022].

CHAPTER 39

Sperm Selection Technique

Shilpa Bhendarkar Joshi, Indrajeet Mulik, Sandip Nikhade, Rajvi Mehta

INTRODUCTION

The trend in increasing infertility in the last few decades is leading to greater utilization of assisted reproductive technology (ART). Given the pressure of getting positive pregnancy outcomes, there is an urge to improve the selection technique of gametes. The quality of sperm samples is one of the major determining factors in successful assisted reproduction, so there is a lot of emphasis on sperm separation and selection techniques with newer techniques of intrauterine insemination (IUI) and intracytoplasmic sperm injection (ICSI).

NEED OF SPERM PREPARATION

- Spermatozoa prepared by simple washing is at risk of contributing defective genome to the embryo and this may lead to increased developmental failure of ART-derived embryo after the 8-cell stage.
- The World Health Organization (WHO) recommends sperm separation from seminal fluid:
  - To limit the damage from leukocytes
  - To reduced reactive oxygen species (ROS) induced DNA damage
  - To increase sperm motility
  - To decrease the number of apoptotic sperms
  - To increase sperm plasma membrane integrity
  - To reduce debris

Choice of sperm preparation method depends on the following factors:
- Total motile count
- The ratio between motile/immotile sperm
- Volume of ejaculate
- Presence of antibodies/agglutination

SPERM PREPARATION TECHNIQUES

Swim-up Technique (Fig. 1 and Table 1)

Based on the active movement of spermatozoa from the prewashed cell pellet into an overlying medium (using an incubation period of 60 minutes).

Density-gradient Technique

The ejaculate is placed on top of a high-density media and is centrifuged for 15–30 minutes. Highly motile spermatozoa move actively in the direction of sedimentation and hence penetrate the media quicker than poorly motile or immotile sperms. Thus, highly motile sperm cells are enriched in a soft pellet at the bottom (**Fig. 2 and Table 2**).

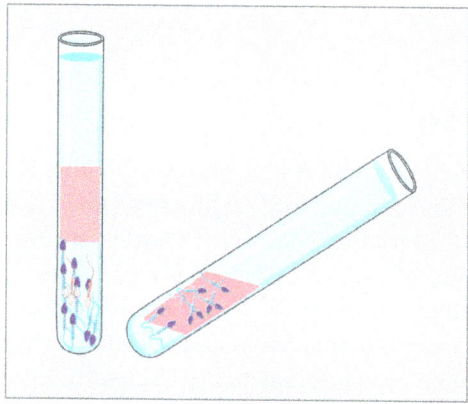

Fig. 1: Swim-up technique.

TABLE 1: Advantages and disadvantages of the swim-up technique.

Sr. No.	Advantages	Disadvantages
1.	Easy	Only for normozoospermic ejaculate
2.	Cost-effective	Low yield
3.	Very clean fraction	Prone to ROS-induced damage
4.	Good recovery in a highly motile sperm sample	Increase damage due to chromatin condensation

(ROS: reactive oxygen species)

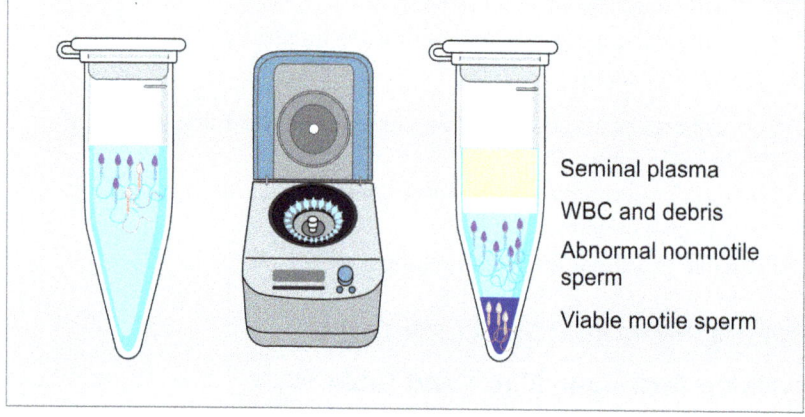

Fig. 2: Density-gradient technique.

TABLE 2: Advantages and disadvantages of density-gradient technique.

Sr. No.	Advantages	Disadvantages
1.	Leads to a good yield	Time-consuming
2.	Reduce ROS and leukocytes significantly	Risk of endotoxins
3.	Good for oligozoospermia	Widely used for ICSI/IVF

(ICSI: intracytoplasmic sperm injection; IVF: in vitro fertilization; ROS: reactive oxygen species)

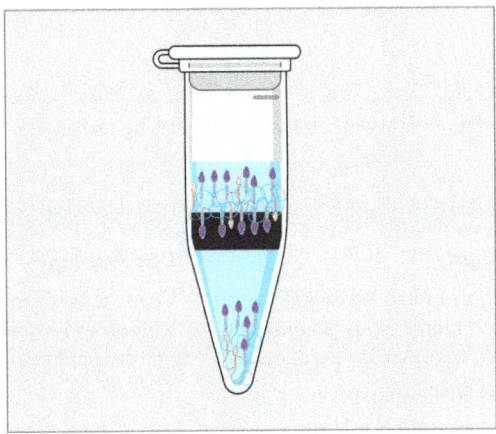

Fig. 3: Glass wool filtration technique.

TABLE 3: Advantages and disadvantages of glass wool filtration technique.

Sr. No.	Advantages	Disadvantages
1.	Simple to perform	Very expensive, filters tend to get dirty
2.	Good for asthenia/oligozoospermia	
3.	Good yield	
4.	Do not require prewash	
5.	Significantly reduces (90%) ROS and leukocytes	

(ROS: reactive oxygen species)

Glass Wool Filtration Technique

Motile spermatozoa are separated from immotile sperm cells utilizing densely packed glass wool fibers **(Fig. 3 and Table 3)**.

Magnetic Activated Cell Sorting Separation Technique

This technique separates nonapoptotic sperms from apoptotic sperms utilizing paramagnetic annexin V-conjugated microbeads. Annexin V shows

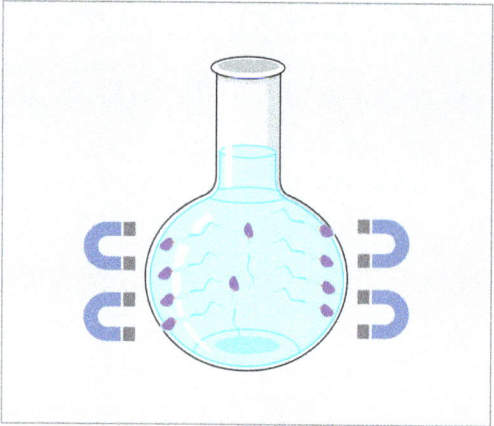

Fig. 4: Magnetic activated cell sorting technique.

Sr. No.	Advantages	Disadvantages
1.	Gives highly motile and viable sperms with good morphology via reducing apoptotic sperms/DNA fragments	Needs to be used in conjunction with other techniques such as density gradient to remove debris
2.	Improves fertilization potential of sperm when used in ICSI and cryopreservation	
3.	Good for oligoasthenozoospermia	
4.	Rapid, convenient, and noninvasive	

TABLE 4: Advantages and disadvantages of MACS technique.

(DNA: deoxyribonucleic acid; ICSI: intracytoplasmic sperm injection; MACS: magnetic activated cell sorting)

a high affinity to phospholipids and phosphatidylserine (PS) of the inner plasma membrane of the sperm. Hence, it eliminates spermatozoa with externalized PS (due to apoptosis) **(Fig. 4 and Table 4)**.

Zeta Potential Technique

Mature structurally and functionally intact sperms possess a greater non-electric negative charge due to membrane glycoproteins, thereby resulting in the more negative zeta potential of semen samples in healthy sperms **(Fig. 5 and Table 5)**.

Hyaluronic Acid-binding Test

- Based on the fact that the hyaluronic acid (HA) structure of the cumulus oophorus surrounding the oocyte plays the main role in the selection of functional sperm.

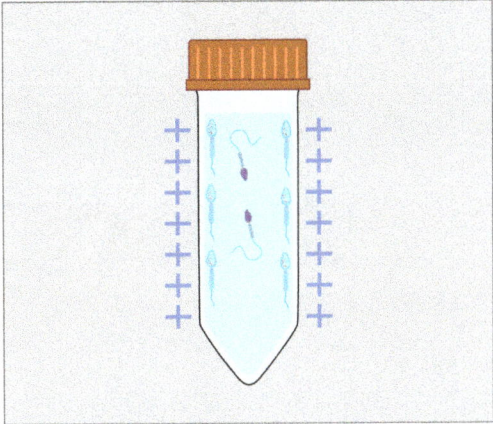

Fig. 5: Zeta potential technique.

TABLE 5: Advantages and disadvantages of zeta potential technique.

Sr. No.	Advantages	Disadvantages
1.	Simple and inexpensive	Not useful for testicular and epididymal sperm aspirates as they lack the charge on the sperm membrane surface
2.	Permits rapid recovery of sperm with improved parameters, normal DNA integrity, morphology and motility, thus improves the outcome of ICSI	

(DNA: deoxyribonucleic acid; ICSI: intracytoplasmic sperm injection)

- Hyaluronic acid bound sperms are:
  - Mature and normal in morphology and highly motile
  - No cytoplasmic residue
  - No DNA degradation
  - No acrosomal reaction
  - Less prone to chromosomal aneuploids
- Hence, physiological intracytoplasmic sperm injection (PICSI) is developed as a novel method for the selection of HA-bound spermatozoa where hyaluronan microdot is added in a PICSI dish, and in the incubation period of 5–10 months; we get mature sperm **(Fig. 6)**.

Advantages

- Increase in fertilization rate.
- Reduced chromosomal aberrations and hence increase the success of intracytoplasmic sperm injection (ICSI).
- Decrease chances of aneuploidies, thus the abortion rate.
  An overall increase in pregnancy rate and take-home baby rate.

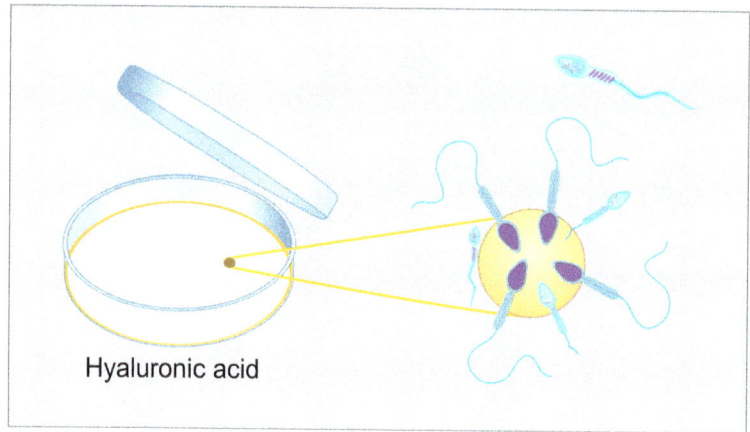

Fig. 6: Physiological intracytoplasmic sperm injection (PICSI) technique.

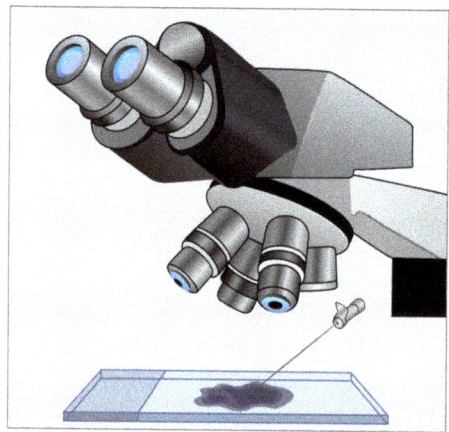

Fig. 7: Intracytoplasmic morphologically selected sperm inject (IMSI) technique.

Intracytoplasmic Morphologically Selected Sperm Inject (Fig. 7)

It is an advanced form of ICSI where spermatozoa are preselected before the procedure based on classification according to motile sperm organelle morphology examination (MSOME) **(Table 6)**.

Indications of Intracytoplasmic Morphologically Selected Sperm Inject

- Teratozoospermia
- Recurrent implantation failure after conventional IVF/ICSI absence of blastocysts in the previous cycle
- High DNA fragmentation

TABLE 6: Classification of motile sperm organelle morphology examination (MSOME) spermatogram.

Sr. No.	Classification	Form	Vacuole*	Grade	Selection type
1.	Class 1	Normal form	No vacuole	Grade 1	Normal spermatozoa (selected in IMSI)
2.	Class 2	Normal form	Maximum 2 small vacuoles	Grade 2	
3.	Class 3	Normal form	Atleast 1 big vacuole or >2 small vacuoles	Grade 3	
4.	Class 4	Abnormal form	Vacuoles	Grade 4	

*Vacuoles are associated with DNA damage.

TABLE 7: Sperm scoring.

Sr. No.			Score
1.	Head	• Normal of 2 axes • Normal of 1 axis • Abnormal of 2 axes	3 1 0
2.	Acrosome	• Normal • Abnormal	1 0
3.	Vacuole	• Absent • 1 small • >1 small	2 1 0
4.	Basis	• Normal • Abnormal	2 0
5.	Insertion	• Normal • Abnormal	1 0
6.	Cytoplasmic droplets	• Normal • Abnormal	1 0
Total			**12**

Limitations

- *Severe teratozoospermia:* Impossible to select class I and II spermatozoa **(Table 7)**.
- *Severe oligospermia and azoospermia:* Selection of sample size is very limited **(Fig. 8)**.

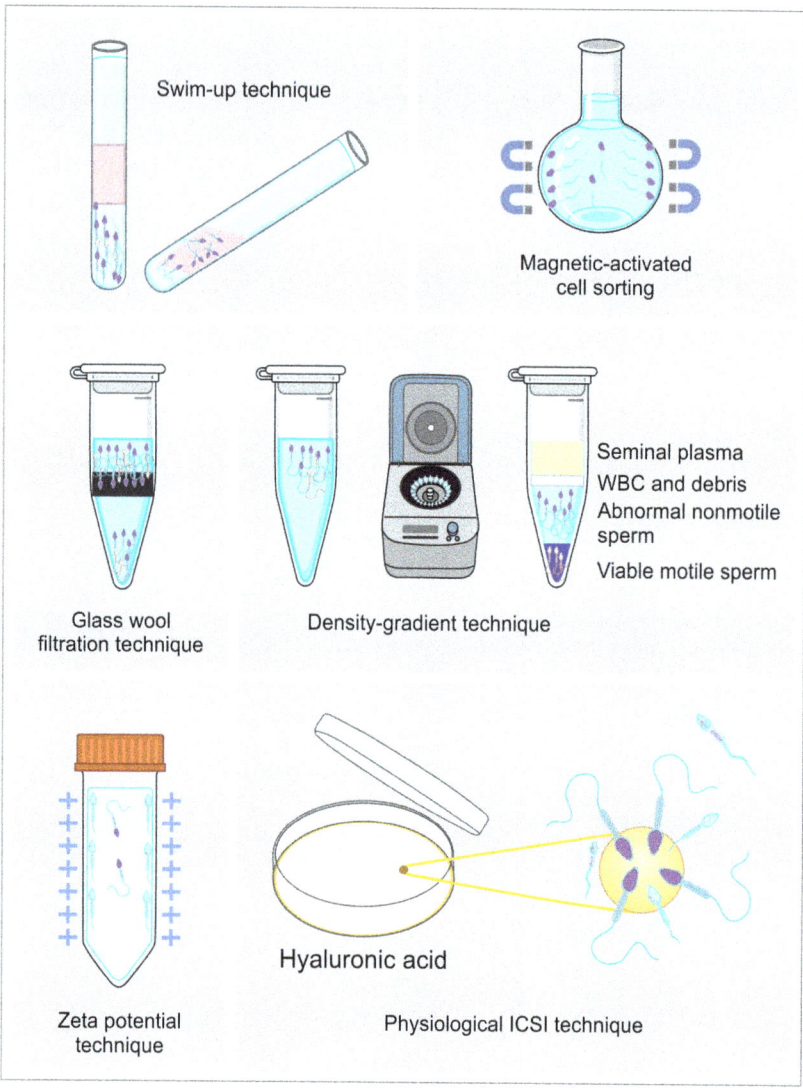

Fig. 8: Summary of sperm selection techniques.
Source: Created by BioRander

MICROFLUIDICS FOR SPERM SORTING (FUTURE PROSPECTS)

This is a new technology based on the microfluidics principle, which is used for semen analysis, sperm quantification, and sorting. Devices are made up of microscale parts for fluid delivery and separation of particles called as lab on chip (LOC) devices or micrototal analysis systems. Available devices are Qualisperm sorter and ZyMot sperm separation devices **(Table 8)**.

TABLE 8: Advantages and disadvantages of microfluidics sperm sorting.

Sr. No.	Advantages	Disadvantages
1.	Can process very small volume of sample (mL to nL), so reduces expenses of the reagent	Commercialization of system very difficult
2.	Improved sperm recovery	Not user friendly
3.	Bypass centrifugation	Highly sophisticated devices
4.	No sperm DNA damage	
5.	Improves >80% DNA integrity and isolates from independent motility	

CONCLUSION

Protocol to optimize sperm preparation and sperm selection significantly improves the outcome of ART in terms of decrease abortion rates, increase normal pregnancy rate, and take-home baby rate.

SUGGESTED READING

1. Academy of Clinical Embryologists. (2021). ACE Newsletter. [online] Available from https://www.theaceorg.in/wp-content/uploads/2021/05/ACEnewsletter-FINAL.pdf [Last accessed April, 2022].
2. Gardner DK, Weissman A, Howles CM, Shoham Z. Textbook of Assisted Reproductive Techniques, Volume 1: Laboratory Perspectives, Chapter 9. Boca Raton: CRC Press; 2018. pp. 117-23.
3. Gardner DK, Weissman A, Howles CM, Shoham Z. Textbook of Assisted Reproductive Techniques, Volume 1: Laboratory Perspectives, Chapter 5. Boca Raton: CRC Press; 2018. p. 50.
4. https://www.ncbi.nlm.nih.gov/pmc/articles/PMC4349780/
5. Miller D, Pavitt S, Sharma V, Forbes G, Hooper R, Bhattacharya S, et al. Physiological, hyaluronan-selected intracytoplasmic sperm injection for infertility treatment (HABSelect): a parallel, two-group, randomised trial. Lancet. 2019;393:416-22. [online] Available from https://www.thelancet.com/journals/lancet/article/PIIS0140-6736(18)32989-1/fulltext [Last accessed April, 2022].
6. Oseguera-López I, Ruiz-Díaz S, Ramos-Ibeas P, Pérez-Cerezale S. (2019). Novel Techniques of Sperm Selection for Improving IVF and ICSI Outcomes. [online] Available from https://www.frontiersin.org/articles/10.3389/fcell.2019.00298/full [Last accessed April, 2022].
7. Rao KA. Principles and Practice of Assisted Reproductive Technology, Volume 1, 5th edition, Chapters 4 and 5; 2018.pp.57-76.
8. Rao KA. Principles and Practice of Assisted Reproductive Technology, Volume 3, 5th edition, Chapter 90; 2018.pp.1184-94.
9. Rao KA. Principles and Practice of Assisted Reproductive Technology, Volume 3, 5th edition, Chapter 107. 2018;108:1364-73.
10. Rao KA. Principles and Practice of Assisted Reproductive Technology, Volume 3, 5th edition, Chapter 122. 2018;1531.
11. World Health Organization. (2010). WHO laboratory manual for the examination and processing of human semen, Fifth edition, chapters 1 and 2, pages 1-10. [online] Available from https://www.who.int/docs/default-source/reproductive-health/srhr-documents/infertility/examination-and-processing-of-human-semen-5ed-eng.pdf [Last accessed April, 2022].

40 | Selecting Best Embryo for Transfer

Vijay Mangoli, Neelam Bhise

INTRODUCTION

Avoiding multiple gestations has always been the priority of an assisted reproductive technology (ART) specialist. Over the period, due to improvements in stimulation protocols and upgradations in laboratory aspects, in vitro fertilization (IVF) treatment cycles have resulted in more competent embryos.[1]

Morphological assessment remains the most widely used criteria for selecting embryo for transfer. Though there is a positive correlation between morphological assessment and implantation rate, recent advances in embryology research shows that selection of embryo(s) on the basis of morphology on the day of transfer has its limitations.[2,3]

Creation of good quality embryos needs effective patient specific stimulations, optimum culture conditions, and an experienced and well-versed embryologist who can correlate various aspects of embryogenesis.

CRITERIA FOR EMBRYO SELECTION BASED ON MORPHOLOGY

Embryo selection should be looked upon as a continuous process rather than a single observation. The selection criteria begin with selecting optimum sperm and oocytes. The definition of common terminology and standardization of laboratory practice related to embryo morphology assessment will result in more effective comparisons of treatment outcomes. Alpha scientist European Society of Human Reproduction and Embryology (ESHRE) workshop held in 2011 stated standardized embryo grading which is widely followed.[4]

Selection Based on Morphology— Under Inverted Microscope

Sperm Morphology

Recent studies indicate that during embryogenesis, sperm contributes much more than its presumed role of mere contribution of genetic material.[5]

Therefore, it is important to segregate and provide maximum morphologically normal sperms from the raw semen sample during conventional IVF, and practically select an optimum single sperm during intracytoplasmic sperm injection (ICSI) procedure. Advent of procedures such as microfluidics sperm sorting and magnetic assisted cell sorter (MACS) may improve selection of high-quality sperm subpopulations by targeting highly motile sperm with lesser DNA fragmented sperms **(Fig. 1)**.[6]

Oocyte Morphology

Numerous publications reported morphological variations in the oocytes and resulting embryos from IVF cycles and their effect of pregnancy outcome.[7,8]

Following ovarian stimulation, oocytes are aspirated during the process of ovum pick-up. A mature metaphase II oocyte is expected from a follicle **(Figs. 2A and B)**.

However, a variety of oocytes can be retrieved which are less likely to result in implantable embryos and should be avoided while selecting best embryo for transfer **(Figs. 3A to F)**.

Zygote Morphology

When a sperm enters the ooplasm, a series of events follow in a well-regulated and time bound manner.

16-20 hours: Postinsemination, a healthy fertilized oocyte displays two pronuclei with 3-8 polarized nucleoli **(Fig. 4)**. Here again, zygote with abnormal fertilization like polyploidy is not uncommon **(Fig. 5)**.

Embryo Morphology

In 1991, during annual meeting of ESHRE at Paris, Professor Edwards gave an earnest advice to all budding embryologists—"*Embryologists, observe the embryos!!*" It has an immense deep meaning. A meticulous observation of growing embryos can reveal a lot more information than its theoretical counterpart. Embryos with maximum implantation potential display an overall correlation between embryo stage and postinsemination duration **(Tables 1 and 2)**. (Day of insemination = day 0).

Blastocyst Transfer Policy Based on Embryo Selection

The center should adapt "only blastocyst transfer" policy if it has established satisfactory optimum culture conditions in terms of blastocyst formation.

The logic behind this policy is—why transfer early cleavage stage embryos with the guesswork of—at least one of them will reach blastocyst, when we have ability to practically convert eligible embryo to the blastocyst stage.

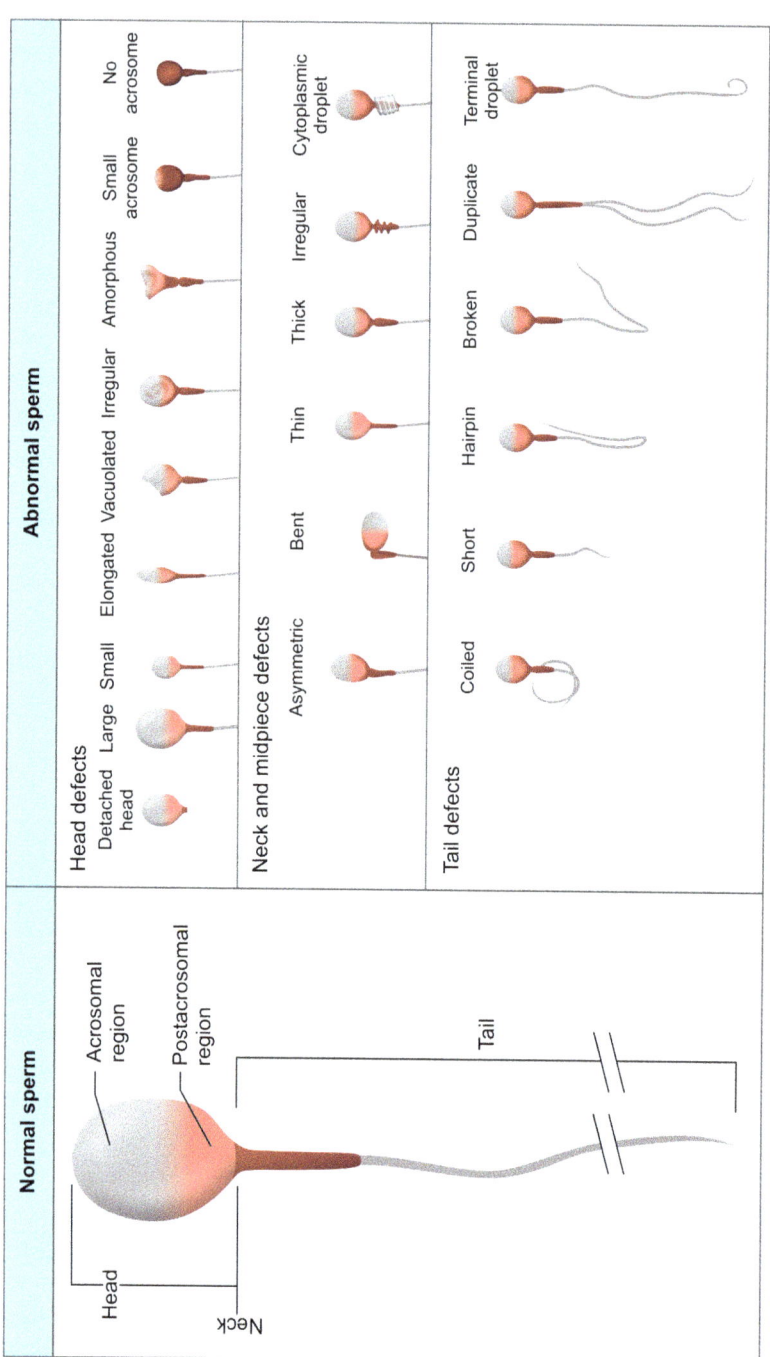

Fig. 1: Sperm morphology.

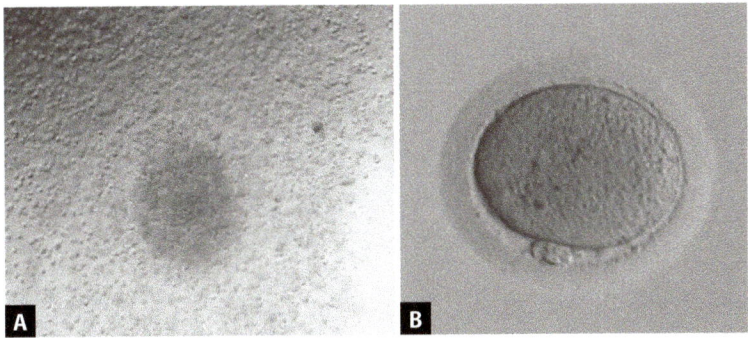

Figs. 2A and B: (A) Mature oocyte (cellular criteria); (B) Mature oocyte (nuclear criteria).
Source: Fertility Clinic, Mumbai

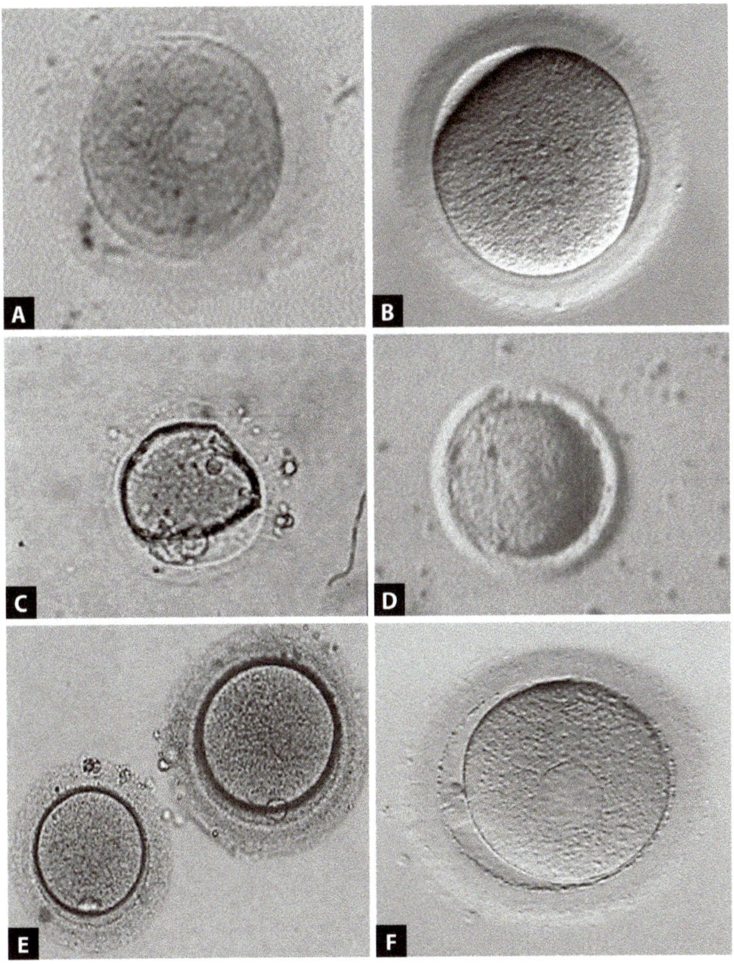

Figs. 3A to F: Stages of oocyte. (A) Immature (GV stage); (B) Intermediate (MI stage); (C) Postmature; (D) Atretic; (E) Giant oocyte; (F) Oocyte with smooth endoplasmic reticulum (SER)
Source: Fertility Clinic, Mumbai

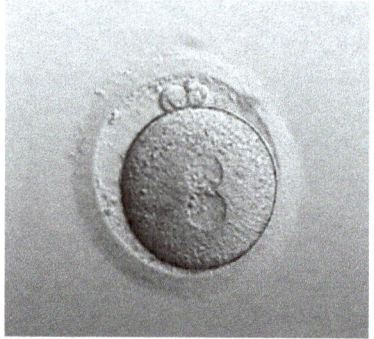

Fig. 4: Two pronuclei.

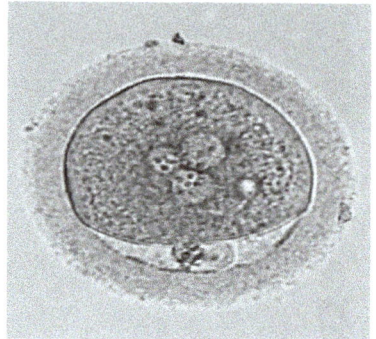

Fig. 5: Polyploidy.

TABLE 1: Growth pattern of embryos.

Normal growth pattern of healthy embryo:
1. Day 1 (22–24 hours)—2 cells (**Fig. 6**)
2. Day 2 (36–50 hours)—4–6 cells (**Fig. 7**)
3. Day 3 (60–75 hours)—8–16 cells (**Fig. 8**)
4. Day 4 (80–100 hours)—Morula/compacted (**Fig. 9**)
5. Day 5 (120–140 hours)—Blastocyst (**Fig. 10**)

TABLE 2: ESHRE consortium—Istanbul Consensus: Cleavage stage embryo grading.

Grade	*1*	*2*	*3*
Cell number	7–8 celled	7–8 celled	7–8 celled or less than that
Fragmentation	No fragmentation/<10% fragmentation	10–25% fragmentation	>25% fragmentation
Symmetry	Even cell size	Even cell size	Uneven cell size
Images			

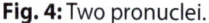

Especially, when it has been clearly shown that probability of live birth rates (LBRs) with a single blastocyst is much higher than transferring a single or two cleavage stage embryos (**Table 3**).[9,10]

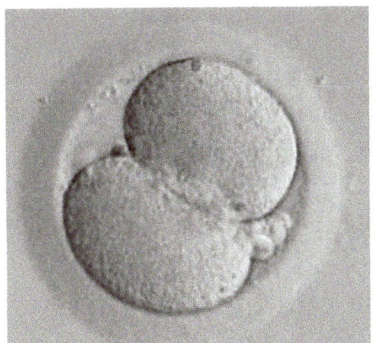

Fig. 6: 2-cell stage.
Source: Fertility Clinic, Mumbai

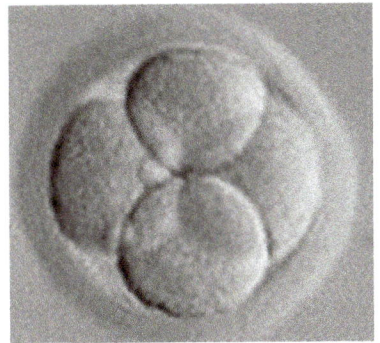

Fig. 7: 4-cell stage.
Source: Fertility Clinic, Mumbai

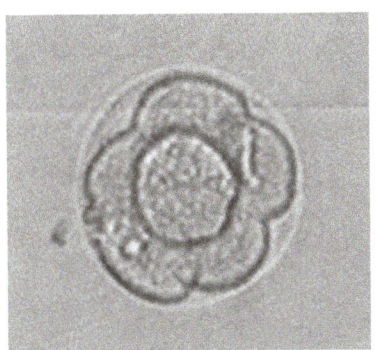

Fig. 8: 8-cell stage.
Source: Fertility Clinic, Mumbai

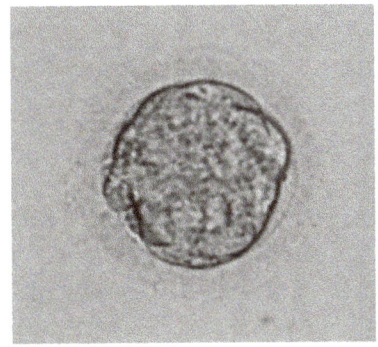

Fig. 9: Morula/compacted stage.
Source: Fertility Clinic, Mumbai

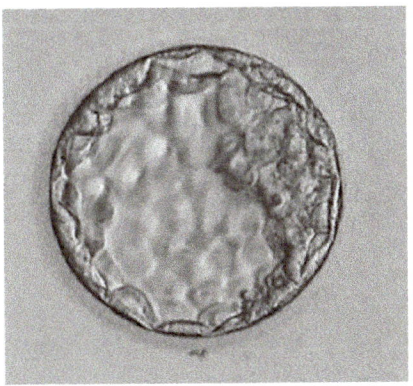

Fig. 10: Blastocyst.
Source: Fertility Clinic, Mumbai

TABLE 3: Blastocyst grading.[6]

Expansion grade	1	2	3	4	5	6
Blastocyst development and stage status	Blastocoel cavity less than half the volume of the embryo	Blastocoel cavity more than half the volume of the embryo	Full blastocyst cavity, completely filling the embryo	Expanded blastocyst cavity layer than the embryo, with thinning of the shell	Embryo has expanded and split open the zona	Embryo has completely hatched from the zona
Images						

Trophectoderm (TE) grade — *Trophectoderm quality*

A — Many smooth cells, forming a cohesive layer
B — Irregular cell layer, forming a loose epithelium
C — More irregular cell layer

ICM grade — *Inner cell mass quality*

A — Well-defined clump of cells
B — Several cells, loosely grouped
C — Very few cells

Moving toward Single Embryo Transfer with Optimum Embryo Selection

If it is possible to select the embryo having maximum implantation potential, the policy of single embryo transfer (SET) may be adapted successfully. The decision of SET is crucial and is effective under specific circumstances.[11]

These are the situations where a center can consider switching over to SET:
- Consistent multiple pregnancies even with only 2 embryos transferred
- Patients below 35 years of age with indications like tubal factor
- Patient with proven fertility
- If clinically patient is unfit to bear multiple pregnancies
- If the center has established very effective embryo freezing program, then center can offer SET without compromising overall pregnancy rate, and
- While transferring embryos in surrogates.

Selection Based on Morphology and Morphokinetics—Using Time-lapse Technology

A built-in camera is fitted in the incubator that takes photographs of each embryo cultured in special dishes at specified intervals. The biggest advantage of time-lapse is—it enables an embryologist to monitor individual growth pattern of all embryos continuously. These observations can be pivotal in taking decision to select the most appropriate embryo based on their behavioral patterns **(Figs. 11A to I)**.[12]

Selection Based on Metabolic Activities: Metabolomics

Metabolomics is the study of metabolites intake or excretion of zygotes and embryos of the culture medium in which they are cultivated. This measurement compilation can be applied to assisted conception by obtaining and examining the metabolic profiles of biofluids associated with oocytes, follicular fluid (FF) and embryos (culture medium or blastocoel fluid) for biomarkers of oocyte/embryo quality. Though appear promising, the concept is still impractical due to complexity and cost involved.[13]

Selection Based on Chromosomal Normalcy

A patient not becoming pregnant even after transferring morphologically optimum embryos is a common experience. Recent studies show that the main cause in such scenarios is extent of aneuploidy in the transferred embryos. *V Phan* had published data in 2013 that as high as up to 62.7% grade I blastocysts can be aneuploid.[14] However, based on evidences of mosaic patterns ESHRE published data in 2017 that even blastocysts declared as "abnormal" may result in normal pregnancy.[15] Therefore, large RCTs are required to reach a conclusive opinion about the utilization of preimplantation genetic testing for aneuploidy (PGT-A) in ART.

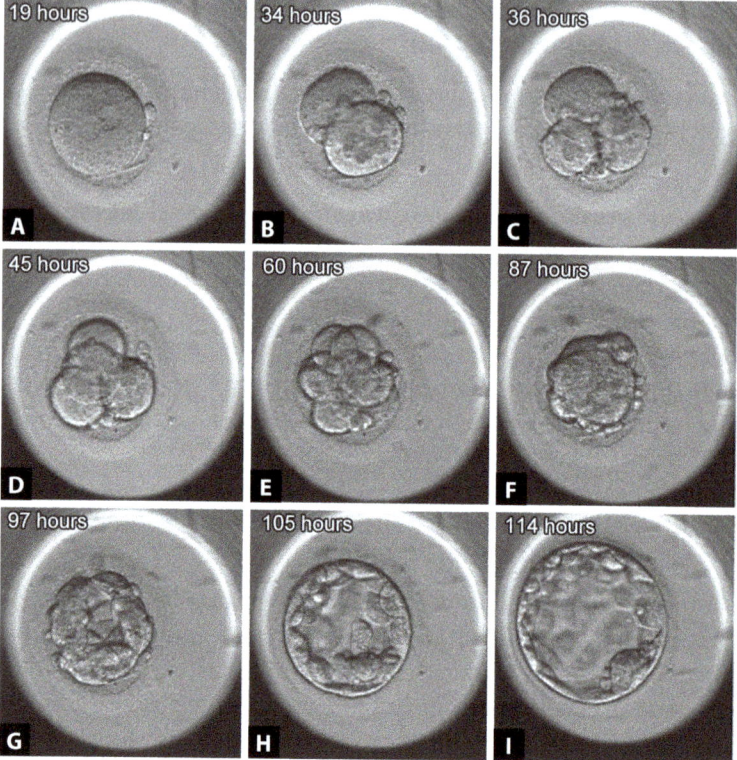

Figs. 11A to I: Time-lapse imaging.
Source: Cambridge University Press

Presently, invasive techniques of blastomere or trophectoderm biopsies are applied to understand chromosomal status of the embryos. Noninvasive chromosomal screening (NICS) is a noninvasive genetic test for identifying chromosomal aneuploidy by analyzing free DNA extracted from blastocyst spent culture media. It causes no damage to embryos and avoids loss of embryo biopsy samples occurred during conventional PGT-A test. The process is yet to be standardized and current concordance rate is about 85%. While PGT-A can give more specification into smaller mutations and translocations, noninvasive screening can give better embryo implantation rates by way of screening and guiding which embryo to select for transfer **(Table 4)**.[16]

Selection Based on Artificial Intelligence

Artificial intelligence (AI) is increasingly being utilized in assessing embryo quality based on static images of blastocyst being fed to the software which scrutinizes and compares this image with millions of blastocysts that gave rise to pregnancies. Though still in the primitive stage, in near future, AI

TABLE 4: Blastocyst spent culture media—free DNA testing (NICS).

Interpretation	Advantages	Limitations
Positive: Tested embryo has one or more chromosomes with gain/loss of an entire chromosome, known copy number variation (CNV) larger than 10 Mb or unknown CNV larger than 50 Mb	High accuracy noninvasive genetic test for identifying chromosomal aneuploidy with no risk of embryo loss	*Limitation:* Single gene mutations and small deletions/duplications may not be identified by NICS
Negative: No chromosomal aneuploidy detectable by NICS	Detects known CNV larger than 10 Mb OR Unknown CNV larger than 50 Mb	Parental disomy; ploidy may not be detected
Nonconclusive: No conclusive result	Better implantation rate in comparison to PGT-A tested embryos	

(NICS: noninvasive chromosomal screening; PGT-A: preimplantation genetic testing for aneuploidy)

maybe increasingly utilized in many aspects of ART from patient monitoring for response and quality control to assess the implantation potential of embryos. One major limitation of AI is—the static images of growing embryos are captured using camera placed at one angle. The embryo being spherical in shape, the information through one angle observation can be misleading. This aspect needs to be addressed otherwise incorrect information will be fed to the software that may result in misleading interpretations.[17]

Critical evaluation of embryogenesis to select embryos with maximum implantation potential along with an efficient cryopreservation program can be effectively employed to reduce multiple pregnancies and time interval for the patient to conceive.

REFERENCES

1. Desai NN, Goldstein J, Rowland DY, Goldfarb JM. Morphological evaluation of human embryos and derivation of an embryo quality scoring system specific for day 3 embryos: a preliminary study. Hum Reprod. 2000;15(10):2190-6.
2. Girard JM, Simorre M, Leperlier F, Reignier A, Lefebvre T, Barrière P, et al. Association between early βhCG kinetics, blastocyst morphology and pregnancy outcome in a single-blastocyst transfer program. Eur J Obstet Gynecol Reprod Biol. 2018;225:189-93.
3. Khosravi P, Kazemi E, Zhan Q, Malmsten JE, Toschi M, Zisimopoulos P, et al. Deep learning enables robust assessment and selection of human blastocysts after in vitro fertilization; 2019. NPJ Digit Med. 2019;2:21.
4. Alpha Scientists in Reproductive Medicine and ESHRE Special Interest Group of Embryology. The Istanbul consensus workshop on embryo assessment: proceedings of an expert meeting. Hum Reprod. 2011;26:1270-83.

5. Sharma U. Paternal contributions to offspring health: role of sperm small RNAs in intergenerational transmission of epigenetic information. Cell Dev Biol. 2019;7:215.
6. Pedrosa ML, Furtado MH, Ferreira MCF, Carneiro MM. Sperm selection in IVF: the long and winding road from bench to bedside. JBRA Assist Reprod. 2020;24(3):332-9.
7. Parisi F, Rousian M, Koning AHJ, Willemsen SP, Steegers EAP, Steegers-Theunissen RPM. Effect of human embryonic morphological development on fetal growth parameters: the Rotterdam Periconceptional Cohort (Predict Study). Reprod Biomed Online. 2019;38(4):613-20.
8. Vijay M, Ranjana M. Morphological assessment of oocytes and embryos. In: Rao K, Carp H, Fisher R (Eds). Principles and Practice of Assisted Reproductive Technology, 1st edition. New Delhi: Jaypee Brothers Medical Publishers (P) Ltd; 2014.
9. Hansotia M, Desai S, Mangoli V, Mangoli R, Koli T. Blastocyst transfer—A way ahead. Int J Gynaecol Obstet. 2000;70:B-15.
10. Su W, Xu J, Arhin SK, Liu C, Zhao J, Lu X. The feasibility of all-blastocyst-culture and single blastocyst transfer strategy in elderly women: a retrospective analysis. Biomed Res Int. 2020;2020:5634147.
11. Dahan MH, Tannus S. Believing that transferring more embryos will result in increased pregnancy rates: a flawed concept: a SWOT analysis. Middle East Fertil Soc J. 2020;25(32):9.
12. Ludin K, Park H. Time-lapse technology for embryo culture and selection. Upsala J Med Sci. 2020;125(2):77-84.
13. Garcia-Dominguez X, Diretto G, Frusciante S, Vicente JS, Marco-Jiménez F. Metabolomic analysis reveals changes in preimplantation embryos following fresh or vitrified transfer. Int J Mol Sci. 2020;21:7116.
14. Phan V, Littman E. Correlation between aneuploidy and blastocyst quality. Fertil Steril. 2013;100(3):S525-6.
15. Fiorentino F. The transfer of chromosomally "abnormal" embryos can still result in pregnancy in IV. Geneva: ESHRE Annual meeting; 2017.
16. Leaver M, Wells D. Non-invasive preimplantation genetic testing (niPGT): the next revolution in reproductive genetics? Hum Reprod Update. 2020;26(1):16-42.
17. Zaninovic N, Rosenwaks Z. Artificial Intelligence in human in vitro fertilization and embryology. Fertil Steril. 2020;114(5):914-20.

CHAPTER 41

What is New in In Vitro Fertilization?

Bindu Chimote, Kalpana Jetha, Shravani Welekar, Rooprekha Waghmare

INTRODUCTION

In vitro, the fertilization technique has proved to be a ray of hope for countless childless couples across the globe. The constant endeavor to enhance take-home baby rates has prompted several technological advances in this field, especially in the past decade. Newer developments have largely focused on improving laboratory culture conditions [culture media (CM)], designing novel criteria for the selection of best sperm [physiological intracytoplasmic sperm injection (PICSI)], and employing sophisticated techniques [time lapse, assisted hatching, preimplantation genetic testing/screening (PGT/S)] that allow the selection of euploid embryos leading to the birth of a healthy baby. This chapter attempts to discuss the latest know-how in in vitro fertilization (IVF) and to provide a practical algorithm for all practicing infertility specialists, clinicians, as well as embryologists.

LABORATORY CULTURE CONDITIONS (CULTURE MEDIA)

The combination of proper laboratory ambient air quality, incubator settings, media temperature, pH, and specific nutrients within the media constitute the laboratory culture conditions that provide an ideal growth environment for the embryos.

Culture media comprise a complex nutrient solution that supports cell growth and is the key component of artificial reproductive techniques. CM are developed for creating an environment that closely resembles the natural composition of the oviduct and uterine fluids needed for developing the embryo. CM are composed mainly of basic salt solutions, carbohydrates (glucose, lactate, and pyruvate), and amino acids. The major part, i.e., 99% of CM are water with high purity. Albumin or synthetic serum in concentrations of 5–20% (w/v or v/v) is also an integral part of media.[1]

Currently, two types of media are available commercially: (1) single step media and (2) sequential media. Sequential media uses back to nature principle and consists of fertilization media, cleavage media, and blastocyst media which are sequentially used from day one embryo to a blastocyst stage (with increasing glucose concentration). Single step media is used continuously from fertilization to the blastocyst stage with the approach "let the embryo choose".

For handling gametes outside the incubators, i.e., for flushing follicles and micromanipulation; media containing a phosphate buffer or HEPES organic buffer is used. pH in the range of 7.2–7.4 is maintained by a bicarbonate/CO_2 buffer system. Paraffin oil is used to overlay media to preserve osmolality when embryos are taken out of the incubator for microscopic assessment. The perfect conditions for embryo culture cannot yet be defined with a microenvironment that includes a combination of temperature (37°C), humidity (45–75%), osmolality (275–290 mmol/kg), and pH (7.2–7.4). A mixture of three gases; (1) carbon dioxide (6%), (2) oxygen (5%), and (3) nitrogen (89%) is preferentially used for the proper growth and development of the embryo up to the blastocyst stage.

NEWER CULTURE MEDIA OPTIONS

The two media conventionally used for embryo culture in human IVF usually contain the protein human serum albumin (HSA) or in some cases bovine serum albumin (BSA). However, it has been hypothesized that the presence of protein in media may increase the risk of disease transmission and has long-term adverse consequences. Moreover, since there are high chances of variability in protein composition between different media lots; it may affect embryo development and pose difficulties in maintaining quality control in the laboratory. Thus, efforts have been on the device of a completely chemically defined culture medium that is devoid of any human or animal sources of protein, i.e., a protein-free media option. The formulation of such a media that do not contain any biological derivatives is still in the research stage. But the combinations of chemicals used in preparing a protein-free medium may help us better understand the nutrient requirements and metabolism of human eggs and embryos.

NEW ADVANCES IN FERTILIZATION TECHNIQUES

Modern fertilization techniques have advanced beyond conventional IVF and intracytoplasmic sperm injection (ICSI) to further include intracytoplasmic morphologically selected sperm injection (IMSI) and PICSI as novel approaches.

In physiological intracytoplasmic sperm injection, sperm selection is done based on physiological conditions, i.e., the ability of sperm to bind to hyaluronic acid (HA). HA is a natural compound found in the oocyte cumulus complex. The mature sperm that has completed the process of spermatogenesis has specific receptors for HA and is responsible for remodeling of the plasma membrane, cytoplasmic extrusions, and nuclear maturation.[2]

Indications of PICSI are high sperm DNA fragmentation index (DFI), history of poor embryo development, recurrent pregnancy loss (RPL), high abortion rate, and poor sperm morphology and motility. PICSI reportedly leads to objective sperm selection, low embryo fragmentation, reduced genetic abnormality, increased pregnancy rate, and reduction in abortion rate.[3] However, multicentric studies and systematic randomized controlled trials (RCTs) are needed to confirm the usability of this technique.

TIME-LAPSE TECHNOLOGY

To improve the outcome of assisted reproductive technology (ART) laboratory, different new technologies such as instrumentation, techniques based on computer utilization, and analysis are being used these days. Time-lapse technology (TLT) is a great tool for understanding landmark events of embryo development.

Time-lapse imaging (TLI) uses specialized cameras to capture serial images of embryos at regular intervals. These images can be run as a film to provide us with unlimited possibilities to evaluate embryos, without the stress of handling and overexposure. TLI can function either as a closed system where the camera is fitted in a bench-top incubator which in turn is integrated with the microscope or as an open system where the camera is placed separately inside a routine CO_2 box incubator.

Different Time-lapse Technology Tools Available in ART

Currently, there are several commercially available TLT systems. The choice of the system can be based on practical considerations, such as the laboratory workload, dimensions, and budget, or on the specifications of the individual systems. The key features of systems currently commercially available are summarized in **Table 1**.

Basis of Embryo Assessment in Time-lapse Imaging

Predictive parameters on which embryo assessment by TLI is based are the time of 2nd PB ejection, the time between appearance and fading of pronuclei, time of appearance of nucleation after the first division, and time intervals for cleavage cycles, etc. TLI has revealed that fragmentation in cleavage stage embryos may be either short-lived or permanent and that the smaller temporary fragments may be reabsorbed.[4,5]

Significance of Time-lapse Technology

The biggest advantage of TLT is that it allows for an uninterrupted culture of embryos till the blastocyst stage and facilitates objective assessment of embryos in real-time. However, cost-effectiveness could be a barrier to the widespread use of this technique.

TABLE 1: Key features of systems currently commercially available.

	Embryoscope	Primo vision	EEVA
Illumination	Bright field, low intensity red LED	Bright field, low intensity green LED	Dark field
Microscope/incubator	Incubator with integrated time-lapse system	Microscope that can be placed in standard incubator	Microscope that can be placed in standard incubator
Cultured dish	Embryoslide	9–16 well Primo vision embryo culture dish	EEVA dish
Embryo culture	Single culture	Group culture	Group culture
Plan of view	7 focal planes	11 focal planes	Single plain
Maximum number of embryo monitored	72	96	Depends on dish
Accessories	Comes with software	Comes with software	Automated software scores blastocyst formation potential

(EEVA: early embryonic viability assessment)

ASSISTED EMBRYO HATCHING

Assisted zona hatching was introduced in ART programs to breach the zona pellucida and promote the natural process of hatching. Mechanical,[6] chemical drilling with acid Tyrode's solution, or laser manipulation[7] are the various assisted-hatching techniques that have evolved over the years. Mechanical and laser-assisted hatching methods are followed routinely in IVF laboratories owing to ease of use, efficiency, and reproducibility **(Table 2)**.

Uses of Assisted Hatching

The assisted hatching can be used (1) in recurrent IVF failure to enable blastocyst hatching thereby increasing implantation potential, (2) in elderly women to help overcome zona pellucida hardening due to age-related endocrine disruption and/or the absence of lysis, (3) in frozen-thawed cycles where the vitrification procedure may cause hardening/thickening (>15 μm) of the zona pellucida, and (4) in retrieving the trophectoderm during embryo biopsy for PGT.

SAFETY CONCERNS ASSOCIATED WITH LASER APPLICATION

Since the laser beam is used at such a delicate and important stage of embryo development, it has its share of safety concerns. The most important

TABLE 2: Different types commercially lasers available in market.

Name	Company	Wavelength	Power	Objective
Saturn 5	Research Instruments, UK	1,480 nm	400 mW	40 ×
Saturn 5 Active	Research Instruments, UK	1,480 nm	400 mW	20 ×, 40 ×
LYKOS	Hamilton Thorne, USA	1,460 nm	300 mW	40 ×
ZILOS-tk	Hamilton Thorne, USA	1,460 nm	300 mW	40 ×
XYRCOS	Hamilton Thorne, USA	1,460 nm	300 mW	20 ×, 40 ×
XYClone		1,460 nm	300 Mw	40 ×
Octax Laser and imaging systems	Vitrolife			25 ×

perceivable adverse effect can be anticipated on the DNA integrity which may manifest as chromosomal abnormalities and congenital defects and there may also be a risk of development arrest. The wavelength and pulse length of lasers can harm embryos or gametes. There remains a lack of sufficient evidence to support the use of laser-assisted hatching methods. However, laser-assisted zona thinning could be less detrimental than a complete breach.

PREIMPLANTATION GENETIC TESTING

Preimplantation genetic testing is predominantly used to identify the aneuploidy (PGT-A) status of developing embryos to select the euploid embryo for transfer. It is an invasive method of embryo selection.[8] Embryo biopsy is carried out either at the cleavage stage or blastocyst stage for chromosomal screening of the biopsied cells. Before the advancements in blastocyst culture and the trophectoderm biopsy technique, several studies involved biopsy of the extruded polar body.

The indications for PGT include recurrent implantation failure (RIF), RPL, advanced maternal age, and a history of inherited genetic disorders in parents and/or close family.

Several numerical aberrations like Down's syndrome and Turner's syndrome, trisomies, monosomies, and single gene disorders like cystic fibrosis, sickle cell disease, thalassemia, etc., can be identified by PGT.

Technically, therefore, PGT should supposedly increase the overall pregnancy rates. However, the test is limited in its ability to screen only a few chromosomal defects. Also, it is only the trophectodermal cells (which form the placenta) that are screened whereas the cells of inner cell mass (ICM) (which forms the fetus) are not evaluated. The procedure also suffers from the huge occurrence of false-positive or false-negative results. The test is inconclusive for mosaic embryos.

Therefore, in recent times, a newer technique of preimplantation testing is becoming more popular, which is the noninvasive PGT for aneuploidy or night-A. This method uses the leftover/spent embryo CM in which the embryos are cultured, to sequence the DNA, instead of using the biopsied cells. Since this method is noninvasive and evaluates DNA released in spent media from both the trophectoderm and ICM cells, it is supposed to be more sensitive and reliable in comparison to PGT-A.

A lot of research is still going on in this field but niPGT-A promises to be a more comprehensive, conclusive, and cost-effective technique of aneuploidy testing for futuristic use.

REFERENCES

1. Chronopoulou E, Harper JC. IVF culture media: past, present and future. Hum Reprod Update. 2015;21(1):39-55.
2. Mokanszki A, Tóthné EV, Bodnár B, Tándor Z, Molnár Z, Jakab A, et al. Is sperm hyaluronic acid binding ability predictive for clinical success of intracytoplasmic sperm injection: PICSI vs. ICSI? Syst Biol Reprod Med. 2014;60(6):348-54.
3. Castillo-Baso J, Garcia-Villafaña G, Santos-Haliscak R, Diaz P, Sepulveda-Gonzalez J, Hernandez-Ayup S. Embryo quality and reproductive outcomes of spermatozoa selected by physiologic-ICSI or conventional ICSI in patients with Kruger <4% and >4% normo-morphology. Fertil Steril. 2011;96(S159).
4. Hardarson T, Löfman C, Coull G, Sjögren A, Hamberger L, Edwards RG. Internalization of cellular fragments in a human embryo: time-lapse recordings. Reprod Biomed Online. 2002;5(1):36-8
5. Van Blerkom J. Translocation of the subplasmalemmal cytoplasm in human blastomeres: possible effects on the distribution and inheritance of regulatory domains. Reprod Biomed Online. 2007;14(2):191-200.
6. Cohen J, Alikani M, Trowbridge J, Rosenwaks Z. Implantation enhancement by selective assisted hatching using zona drilling of human embryos with poor prognosis. Hum Reprod. 1992;7:685-91.
7. Antinori S, Panci C, Selman HA, Caffa B, Dani G, Versaci C. Zona thinning with the use of laser: a new approach to assisted hatching in humans. Hum Reprod. 1996;11:590-4.
8. Parikh FR, Athalye AS, Naik NJ, Naik DJ, Sanap RR, Madon PF. Preimplantation Genetic Testing: Its Evolution, Where Are We Today? J Hum Reprod Sci. 2018;11(4):306-14.

CHAPTER 42: Anesthesia for Laparoscopy

Manisha Shembekar, Hemangi Abhyankar

INTRODUCTION

Diagnostic hysterolaparoscopic surgery is the most common, minimally invasive more or less daycare procedure done in otherwise healthy young females to diagnose and treat various gynecological disorders. It is a safe and effective tool to detect correctable abnormalities and also to treat them.

Gynecologic laparoscopic procedures routinely done are shown in **Table 1**.

Laparoscopy involves insertion of a scope, camera, surgical instruments, and insufflator into the abdominal cavity to have a better view and working condition. With the evolution of laparoscopy, various gases such as air, oxygen, nitrous oxide, nitrogen, carbon dioxide, argon, and helium have been tried for insufflation. Ideal insufflating gas should be nontoxic, inexpensive, colorless, noninflammable, readily soluble, and easily ventilated through lungs. Carbon dioxide is widely used now. This insufflation or pneumoperitoneum results in significant physiopathological repercussions related to venous return, circulation, and diaphragmatic kinetics due to raised intra-abdominal pressure.

TABLE 1: Gynecologic laparoscopic procedures.

Nonoperative laparoscopy	Operative laparoscopy
Diagnostic laparoscopy	Total laparoscopic hysterectomy
Fulguration of endometriosis	Laparoscopically-assisted vaginal hysterectomy
Fibroid	Tubal recanalization
Ovarian cyst aspiration	Myomectomy
Fallopian tube patency	Ectopic pregnancy
To obtain biopsies	Oophorectomy
Aspiration of hematoma	Wertheim's procedure
Mini laparoscopic tubal ligation	Adhesiolysis

PHYSIOLOGICAL EFFECTS OF PNEUMOPERITONEUM

Box 1 shows the physiological effects of pneumoperitoneum.

Gynecological laparoscopies are generally performed in Trendelenburg position with added lithotomy position. So, pneumoperitoneum and this position lead to decrease in patients' lung compliance and functional resistance capacity (FRC) thereby resulting in increased airway pressure and basal atelectasis. Thus, there occurs increased ventilation-perfusion (V/Q) mismatch and increase in $paCO_2$.

PHYSIOLOGICAL EFFECTS OF POSITIONING

Effects of Trendelenburg Position

Box 2 shows the physiological effects of positioning.

MANAGEMENT OF ANESTHESIA

Conventionally, all laparoscopic procedures are performed under general anesthesia (GA) with controlled ventilation and secured airway but for

BOX 1: Effects of cardiovascular, respiratory, renal, gastrointestinal, and neurological system.	
Cardiovascular system: IAP <10 mm Hg IAP 10–20 mm Hg As BP = CO × SVR Thus, IAP >20 mm Hg	↑ VR → ↑ CO ↓ VR → ↓ CO → ↑ SVR ↑ BP ↓↓ VR ↓↓↓ CO ↓ BP
Respiratory system: • Lung volumes especially FRC • Airway resistance • Pulmonary compliance • Airway pressure • Risk of barotrauma • V/Q mismatch	↓ ↑ ↓ ↑ ↑ ↑
Renal: • Renal function	↓
Gastrointestinal: • Risk of regurgitation	↑
Neurological: • ICP • CPP	↑ ↓
(BP: blood pressure; CO: cardiac output; CPP: cerebral perfusion pressure; FRC: functional resistance capacity; IAP: intra-abdominal pressure; ICP: intracranial pressure; SVR: systemic vascular resistance; VR: venous return)	

BOX 2: Effects of cardiovascular and respiratory system.	
Cardiovascular:	
• VR	↑
• CO	↑
• BP	↑
Respiratory:	
• Lung volumes	↓
• V/Q mismatch	↑
• Atelectasis	↑

(CO: cardiac output; V/Q: ventilation-perfusion; VR: venous return)

short daycare procedures, various alternatives have been tried, such as laryngeal mask airways, regional anesthesia with intravenous (IV) sedation, total intravenous anesthesia (TIVA), and local anesthetic infiltration. As the daycare patients are expected to return to preoperative state soon after surgery, the anesthetic techniques need to be modified accordingly. The aim is to have less postoperative nausea and vomiting (PONV), less postoperative pain, less patient discomfort, short length of stay in hospital, and the earliest return to routine activities.

Preoperative Evaluation and Patient Preparation

Preoperative evaluation for any comorbidities, previous history of anesthesia exposure, allergies, and current medication are done. Patient is instructed to remain nil orally a night before the surgery. Premedication includes aspiration prophylaxis [preanesthetic oral (PO) ranitidine and metoclopramide] and anxiolysis (alprazolam).

Monitoring

Basic monitor routinely used, ECG, SpO_2, noninvasive blood pressure (NIBP), and temperature are must. End-tidal carbon dioxide ($EtCO_2$) is essential where CO_2 insufflation is used and patient is given GA.

Anesthesia Technique

- *Sedation/anxiolysis:* Midazolam 10–50 µg/kg
- *Analgesia:* Fentanyl 1–2 µg/kg
- *Induction:* Propofol 2–2.5 mg/kg
- *Airway:* Endotracheal tube, laryngeal mask airway
- *Muscle relaxants:* Suxamethonium/Atracurium/Vecuronium
- *Reversal:* Neostigmine/Atropine/Glyco-P

Total intravenous anesthesia results in more rapid and clear recovery and less PONV. Propofol-based TIVA-atracurium relaxation technique seems to suffice for gynecolaparoscopy. Volatile anesthetics are convenient in short daycare procedures and sevoflurane or desflurane can be used. Inhalational agents provide rapid and clear headed recovery. Nitrous oxide should be avoided as it causes postoperative emesis, decreased intestinal motility, and bowel distention.

Regional Anesthesia

It has been used successfully for minor procedures and gained wide popularity. A block from T4 to L5 is necessary for gynecological laparoscopy. It offers many benefits over general anesthesia. Epidural anesthesia is another option. It retains the ability to keep the respiratory control mechanism intact. It allows the patient to adjust the minute ventilation and maintain near normal $EtCO_2$. CSE, i.e., combined spinal epidural anesthesia has an edge over epidural anesthesia for rapid onset of action.

Local Anesthetic Infiltration

It is safe, effective, and less costly alternative as compared to general anesthesia. Good for office micro-laparoscopy, mini-laparoscopy, but also has its limitations.

Regional and local anesthesia techniques become important if there are a genetic problem, patient refusal, and failed difficult airway precludes a general anesthetic.

Anesthesia Techniques

See **Table 2**.

Complications (Table 3)

Reported incidence of complications in gynecological laparoscopy is very low ranging between 1 and 4% minor and 0.3–2.8% major almost similar to other laparoscopic procedures.

TABLE 2: Anesthesia techniques.

Anesthesia technique	Advantages	Disadvantages
Local anesthesia	• Rapid recovery • Can be combined with sedation • Cost effective	• Requires patient co-operation • Uncomfortable for patient
Regional anesthesia	• Awake patient • Less recovery time • Less peristalsis • Less drugs • Problems of GA prevented	• Breathing difficulty • Shoulder tip pain • Patient movement • Patient apprehension
General anesthesia	• Rapid onset • Good analgesia, airway control, muscle relaxation • Quiet surgical field • Adequate carboperitoneum	• Adverse effects of various drugs • Polypharmacy • More recovery time • Costly

TABLE 3: Complications.

Complication	Pathophysiological	Prevention
Cardiac arrhythmias	Hypercarbia and acidemia	IAP <12 mm Hg
Bradycardia	Vagal stimulus to peritoneal stretching	Slow insufflation
Hypotension	• High IAP • Volume depleted patient	Slow insufflation preloading
Gastric reflux	• Trendelenburg position • Obesity	• Aspiration prophylaxis • Airway security • Low IAP
Hemorrhage	Trauma to blood vessels	Careful trocar insertion
Elevation of diaphragm	• Basal atelectasis • V/Q mismatch • R-L shunt	• Ventilatory adjustment • Increased FiO_2
Trendelenburg position	Hypoventilation regurgitation, aspiration	Cuffed tracheal tube
CO_2 embolism	• Intravascular needle placement • CO_2 macroemboli in CNS	Aspiration of needle

(CNS: central nervous system; FiO_2: fraction of inspired oxygen; IAP: intra-abdominal pressure; V/Q: ventilation-perfusion)

REFERENCES

1. McDermott JP, Regan MC, Page R, Stokes MA. Cardiovascular effects of laparoscopy with and without gas insufflation. Arch Surg. 1995;130:984-8.
2. Carry PY, Gallet D, François Y, Perdrix JP, Sayag A, Gilly F, et al. Respiratory mechanics during laparoscopic cholecystectomy: the effect of abdominal wall lift. Anesth Analg. 1998;87:1393-7.
3. Brantly JC, Riley PM. Cardiovascular collapse during laparoscopy: A report of two cases. Am J Obstet Gynecol. 1998;159:735-7.
4. Claeys MA, Gepts E, Camu F. Haemodynamic changes during anesthesia induced and maintained with propofol. Br J Anesth. 1983;60:3-9.
5. Barker P, Langton JA, Murphy PJ. Regurgitation of gastric contents during general anesthesia using laryngeal mask airway. Br J Anaesth. 1992;69(3):314-5.
6. Poindexter AN, Abdul Malak M, Fast JE. Laparoscopic tubal sterilisation under local anesthesia. Obstet Gynecol. 1990;75(1):5-8.
7. Brain AIJ. The laryngeal mask: A new concept in airway management. Br J Anaesth. 1983;55:801-5.
8. Joshi GP, Inagaki Y, White PF, Taylor-Kennedy L, Wat LI, Gevirtz C, et al. Use of the laryngeal mask airway as an alternative to the tracheal tube during ambulatory anesthesia. Anaesth Analg. 1997;85:573-7.
9. Rauh R, Hemmerling TM, Rist M, Jacobi KE. Influence of pneumoperitoneum and patient positioning on respiratory system compliance. J Clin Anesth. 2001;13:361-5.
10. Collins LM, Vaghadia H. Regional anesthesia for laparoscopy. Anesthesiol Clin North Am. 2001;19:43-55.
11. Stewart AV, Vaghadi H, Collins L, Mitchell GW. Small-dose selective spinal anaesthesia for short-duration outpatient gynaecological laparoscopy: Recovery characteristics compared with propofol anaesthesia. Br J Anaesth. 2001;86:570-2.

CHAPTER 43 | Anesthesia for Oocyte Retrieval

Manisha Shembekar

INTRODUCTION

In vitro fertilization, which started in 1970, has become a routine procedure today in couples seeking conception. More often than not, the patient is elderly. There are few health considerations that should be taken into account.

Coexisting conditions:
- Tuberculosis is a leading cause of infertility in our country, hence, patients may be taking anti-Koch's regimen [Ak strain transforming (AKT)].
- Thyroid disorders coexist with infertility.
- Some of them are taking anticoagulants like aspirin and heparin. Aspirin should be stopped 3 days prior to ovum pickup. If patient is on heparin, activated prothrombin time should be done and heparin stopped prior to the procedure.
- Psychomotor illness is common among infertile patients and drug interactions with antidepressants should be considered.
- Diabetes mellitus and hypertension have to be taken into account as comorbidities.

Pain during oocyte pickup is due to piercing of vagina and ovarian capsule by the needle. It is essential to provide adequate pain relief so that the patient remains immobile during the procedure and danger of injuring adjacent vessels is minimized.

The ideal anesthetic agent should be safe, effective with minimum duration of exposure, and should have minimal concentration in follicular fluid.

TYPES OF ANESTHESIA
- Monitored anesthesia care
- Regional anesthesia
- General anesthesia

Monitored Anesthesia Care

Monitored anesthesia care is quite popular in western countries, where conscious sedation is used. Drugs commonly used are midazolam and fentanyl or fentanyl and propofol.

Regional Anesthesia

- Paracervical block with lignocaine and conscious sedation with midazolam and fentanyl is a good option for day-care procedure and results in early recovery.
- Spinal anesthesia using bupivacaine can be given along with fentanyl. However, recovery will take longer.
- Epidural anesthesia can be tried but has no added advantage.

General Anesthesia

Drugs which can be safely used are:

- *Propofol:* It is extensively studied and was found to have no adverse effects on oocytes and cleavage of embryos. It has antiemetic property and provides early recovery.
- Midazolam, a benzodiazepine, is most commonly used and is found to have no adverse effect on oocytes.
- Narcotics—fentanyl and alfentanil are commonly used along with midazolam and propofol. They provide excellent analgesia and have short duration of action.
- Ketamine is a good option along with midazolam.
- Nitrous oxide inactivates methionine synthetase and thus decreases thymidine available for DNA synthesis of dividing cell. However, the process occurs slowly in the liver and it was found that the brief duration of exposure to N_2O does not harm the fertilization process.
- Inhalational agents such as halothane, isoflurane, and sevoflurane are best avoided.

SUGGESTED READING

1. Ben-Shlomo I, Moskovich R, Katz Y, Shaley E. Midazolam/ketamine sedative combination compared with fentanyl/propofol/isoflurane anesthesia for oocyte retrieval. Hum Repord. 1999;14:1757-9.
2. Botta G, D'Angelo A, D'Ari G, Merlino G, Chapman M, Grudzinskas G. Epidural anesthesia in an in vitro fertilization and embryo transfer program. J Assist Reprod Genet. 1995;12:187-90.
3. Gonen O, Shulman A, Ghetler Y, Shapiro A, Judeiken R, Beyth Y, et al. The impact of different types of anesthesia on in vitro fertilization-embryo transfer treatment outcome. J Assist Repord Genet. 1995;12:678-82.
4. Ng EH, Chui DK, Tang OS, Ho PC. Paracervical block with and without conscious sedation: a comparison of the pain levels during egg collection and the postoperative side effects. Fertil Steril. 2001;75:711-7.
5. Rosen MA, Roizen MF, Eger EI 2nd, Glass RH, Martin M, Dandekar PV, et al. The effect of nitrous oxide on in vitro fertilization success rate. Anesthesiology. 1987;67:42-4.
6. Trout SW, Vallenand AH, Kemmann E. Conscious sedation for in vitro fertilization. Fertil Steril. 1998;69:799-808.

7. Tsen LC, Schultz R, Martin R, Datta S, Bader AM. Intrathecal low dose bupivacaine versus lidocaine for in vitro fertilization procedures. Reg Anesth Pain Med. 2001;26:52-6.
8. Wikland M, Evers H, Jacobsson AH, Sandqvist U, Sjoblom P. The concentration of lidocaine in follicular fluid when used for paracervical block in a human IVF-ET programme. Hum Reprod. 1990;5:920-3.
9. Wilhelm W, Hammadeh ME, White PF, Georg T, Fleser R, Biedler A. General anesthesia versus monitored anesthesia care with remifentanil for assisted reproductive technologies: effect on pregnancy rate. J Clin Anesth. 2002;14:1-5.

CHAPTER 44

Anesthetic Considerations for Operative Hysteroscopy

Manisha Shembekar

INTRODUCTION

Hysteroscopy involves visualization of uterine cavity for diagnostic or therapeutic purposes.

Diagnostic procedures are required:
- To find the cause of abnormal uterine bleeding and obtain a biopsy
- To investigate the cause of primary or secondary infertility
- In recurrent miscarriages.

Therapeutic procedures are:
- Removal of submucous fibroids
- Removal of polyps
- Resection of intrauterine septum
- Targeted biopsy
- Adhesiolysis of intrauterine synechiae.

Hysteroscopic procedures require distention of the uterine cavity. The most common distending media that have been used are:
- Carbon dioxide gas
- Glycine and mannitol or sorbitol that are hypotonic
- Normal saline, which is isotonic.

Carbon dioxide is no longer used as distention medium as vision is obscured due to bleeding during the procedure. Hence, fluid media are preferred.

The equipment used for distention is called hysteromat or endomat. The maximum pressure should be 70–100 mm Hg or pressure just adequate to visualize uterine cavity. Resection of the endometrium or fibroids requires use of large diameter hysteroscopes with continuous flow of irrigating medium. They involve a working element with electrically active loop using monopolar current with nonelectrolyte distending media like glycine or sorbitol. However, these solutions are hypotonic and utmost vigilance is required to prevent excessive absorption, which may cause life-threatening hyponatremia. Isotonic electrolyte containing fluids like normal saline cannot be used with monopolar energy as it leads to activation of ions and dispersal of electric current and hence reduces power density, which may be ineffective to destroy the tissue. Newer resectoscopes have been developed to use bipolar current and they are compatible with electrolyte containing distention media such as ringer lactate or normal saline. These solutions have reduced the incidence of hyponatremia considerably.

ANESTHESIA FOR HYSTEROSCOPIC PROCEDURES

Regional anesthesia either spinal or epidural is preferred over general anesthesia for early recognition of symptoms of fluid overload.

Short procedures like diagnostic hysteroscopy can be done under total intravenous anesthesia (TIVA).

General anesthesia is given if the patient is anxious or if laparoscopy may be done along with hysteroscopy where either laryngeal mask airway or endotracheal tube is inserted.

Hysteroscopy may also be performed as an office procedure using miniature (1.9 mm) hysteroscope. Oral administration of nonsteroidal anti-inflammatory drugs (NSAIDs) should be done to reduce pain during procedure, opiates are not recommended. Intracervical and paracervical infiltration of local anesthetic can be done to alleviate vasovagal response during the procedure.

Complications of Hysteroscopy

Complications of hysteroscopy are:
- Fluid overload or transurethral resection of prostate (TURP) like syndrome
- Air embolism
- Uterine perforation

Fluid Overload

Fluid deficit is defined as difference between the volume of irrigating fluid that goes inside the uterine cavity and that flushes out of the uterine cavity during the procedure.

Fluid deficit of 1,000 mL results in fluid overload while using hypotonic solution like glycine. Fluid deficit of 2,500 mL while using isotonic solution like normal saline may cause fluid overload in a healthy woman of reproductive age group. However, for women with cardiorespiratory compromise or renal impairment, threshold should be reduced to 750 mL for hypotonic solution and 1,500 mL for isotonic solution.

Absorption of distention medium from open sinuses of the uterine cavity can cause fluid overload. It can occur with both isotonic and hypotonic solutions; however, incidence is higher with hypotonic solutions.

Factors which lead to fluid overload are: High intrauterine distention pressure, duration of procedure, depth of myometrial penetration, size of myoma, and volume of medium used.

Flowchart 1: Intravasation of irrigant (glycine).

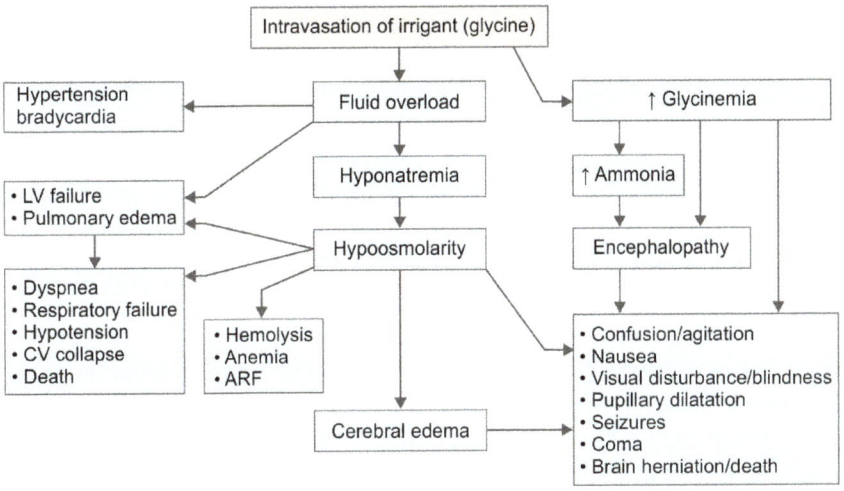

(ARF: acute renal failure)

Signs and symptoms of fluid overload are due to hyponatremia, which is common with glycine or any hypotonic medium. Patient will have:
- Nausea and vomiting
- Confusion and disorientation
- Focal weakness and convulsions
- Pulmonary edema and cardiac failure
- Coma, respiratory arrest, brainstem herniation, and death.

Input and output should be meticulously calculated using calibrated drapes and reservoirs and must be assessed at every 10-minute interval. A closed loop system should be employed for exact estimation of input and output of the distention medium. A decrease in serum sodium of 10 mmol/L corresponds to 1,000 mL of fluid absorbed if the solution is 1.5% glycine **(Flowchart 1)**.

Management of suspected hypervolemic hyponatremia due to fluid overload (Table 1): Moderate fluid overload causes hypervolemia and dilutional hyponatremia. If serum Na^+ concentration falls below 120 mmol/L, symptoms develop. Patient complains of headache, nausea, vomiting, and weakness. If intravasation continues, water moves into intracellular and interstitial space leading to brain edema and rise in intracranial pressure. Patient may have symptoms such as agitation, confusion, nausea, vomiting, headache, and visual disturbances. If continued, this can lead to brainstem herniation, coma, and death.

Asymptomatic hyponatremia can be treated with fluid restriction and frusemide.

Symptomatic hyponatremia requires multidisciplinary approach and high dependency care. 100 mL bolus of 3% saline over 10 minutes to be repeated

TABLE 1: Management of suspected hypervolemic hyponatremia due to fluid overload.

Acute hypervolemic hyponatremia	Management
Asymptomatic hyponatremia (Na^+ >120 mmol/L)	Fluid restriction <1 L/day and 40 mg frusemide
Symptomatic hypoosmolar (Na^+ <120 mmol/L)	• Hypertonic saline (3%) (1 L = 513 mmol, normal saline 1 L = 154 mmol) • Supplemental oxygen, indwelling urinary catheter, high dependency unit, multidisciplinary involvement

three times followed by intravenous (IV) infusion of 3% hypertonic saline 1–2 mmol/L/h is indicated. The target is to increase serum sodium 6 mmol/L over 24 hours until 130 mmol/L is achieved. Rapid correction of hyponatremia may cause pontine myelinolysis or osmotic demyelination syndrome. After recovery from hyponatremia, a biphasic reaction occurs and patient suffers from swallowing difficulty, gait changes, and other neurological symptoms.

Normal sodium levels are between 135 and 145 mmol/L.

Air or Gas Embolism during Hysteroscopy

Air or gas embolism is rare but can occur during hysteroscopic procedure. Air can enter the uterine cavity if the tube is not primed with fluid or appearance of bubbles in the solution. If the patient develops sudden desaturation, air embolism should be suspected.

TIPS AND TRICKS TO REDUCE FLUID ABSORPTION

- Use of gonadotropin-releasing hormone (GnRH) agonist before resection of myoma, which can reduce the volume of fibroid.
- Intracervical injection of dilute vasopressin reduces absorption of fluid.
- Intrauterine pressure should be kept below mean arterial pressure. A pressure between 70 and 100 mm Hg is considered safe.
- Use of automated fluid administering systems which maintain a constant pressure and accurate calculation of fluid deficit.

SUGGESTED READING

1. AAGL Practice Report: practical Guidelines for the Management of hysteroscopic distension media. J Minim Invasive Gynecol. 2013;20:137-48.
2. Aschopoulos M, Polyzos NP, Lavasidis LG, Vrekoussis T, Dalkalitsis N, Paraskevaidis E. Safety issues of hysteroscopic surgery. Ann N Y Acad Sci. 2006;1092:229-34.
3. Aydeniz B, Gruber IV, Schauf B, Kurek R, Meyer A, Wallwiener D. A multicenter survey of complications associated with 21676 operative hysteroscopies. Eur J Obstet Gynecol Reprod Biol. 2002;104:160-4.
4. Cicinelli E, Didonna T, Ambrosi G, Schönauer LM, Fiore G, Matteo MG. Topical anaesthesia for diagnostic hysteroscopy and endometrial biopsy in postmenopausal

women: a randomised placebo-controlled double-blind study. Br J Obstet Gynaecol. 1997;104:316-9.
5. Cooper NAM, Smith P, Khan KS, Clark TJ. Analgesia and conscious sedation for pain control during outpatient hysteroscopy: a systematic review and meta-analysis. Personal communication; 2009.
6. Lau WC, Tam WH, Lo WK, Yuen PM. A randomized double-blind placebo-controlled trial of transcervical intrauterine local anaesthesia in outpatient hysteroscopy. BJOG. 2000;107:610-3.
7. Propst A, Liberman RF, Harlow BL, Ginsburg ES. Complications of hysteroscopic surgery: predicting patients at risk. Obstet Gynecol. 2000;96:517-20.
8. Varol N, Maher P, Vancaillie T, Cooper M, Carter J, Kwok A, et al. A literature review and update on the prevention and management of fluid overload in endometrial resection and hysteroscopic surgery. Gynaecol Endosc. 2002;11(1):19-26.

Index

Page numbers followed by *b* refer to box, *f* refer to figure, *fc* refer to flowchart, and *t* refer to table.

A

Abdomen 142
Abortion 317
Acid Tyrode's solution 378
Acid-fast bacilli 146
Acne 249
Adenoma, prostatic 74
Adenomyoma 43, 43*f*
Adenomyosis 43, 43*f*, 69, 70, 129, 132, 381
    treatment of 311
Adhesiolysis, hysteroscopic 72
Adhesions 59
Adnexa 310, 311, 312*fc*
Adnexal diseases, ultrasound of 43, 43*t*
Adnexal torsion 246
Agonist protocol 103*f*, 234, 269
Agonist trigger, advantages of 266*f*
Air 392
    embolism 390
Airway 383
    pressure 382
    resistance 382
Albumin, role of 297
Amenorrhea, hypothalamic 161
Amino acid 308, 375
Amniotic fluid stem cells 338
Analgesia 383
Anastrozole 219
Androgens 10
    excess 91, 191
Androstenedione 200, 201
Anejaculation 86, 87
    evaluation of 88*fc*
    management of 87
    situational 87
    treatment of 88*fc*
Anesthesia 381, 386, 390
    epidural 387
    general 382, 384, 386, 387, 390
    local 384
    management of 382
    regional 384, 386, 387, 390
    spinal 387
    technique 383, 384, 384*t*
    total intravenous 383, 390
    types of 386
Aneuploidy 373
Anovulation
    chronic 218
    classification of 182*t*
Anovulatory disorders 190
Antagonist
    injection, addition of 177
    protocol 103*f*, 269
Anti-β2-glycoprotein 327
Antibiotics 10, 145, 147
    therapy 71
Anticardiolipin 326
    antibodies 327
Anticoagulation doses 328*t*
Antiemetics 300
Antiestrogens 219
Anti-Koch's regimen 386
Anti-Müllerian hormone 5, 26, 28, 48, 58, 100, 101, 109, 150, 158, 159, 198, 204, 209, 214, 218, 257, 258, 260, 306, 341
    receptor 347
Antioxidants 194, 224, 227
    administration 96
    therapy 215
Antiphosphatidylserine 327
Antiphospholipid
    antibodies 310
    evaluation for 334
    syndrome 326, 327
Antisperm antibody 21, 160
    tests for 165
Anti-thyroperoxidase antibodies 106
Antituberculous therapy 146
Antral follicle count 5, 26, 29, 34, 35, 100, 101, 158, 159, 198, 204, 209, 214, 257, 258, 341

Anxiety 87
Anxiolysis 383
Aplasia 38, 38*f*
Apoptotic sperm detection 306
Applebaum uterine scoring system 318*t*
Arcuate uterus 40, 40*f*, 332
Arm deformities 168
Aromatase inhibitors 96, 185, 219, 251
Arrhythmias, cardiac 385
Artificial intelligence 345, 354, 372
  role of 345, 346*f*
  workflow of 346, 347*fc*
Asherman's syndrome 71, 142, 310, 316, 339
Aspermia 21
Aspirin 224, 228, 275, 314, 319
  low-dose 255, 320, 328
Assisted hatching, use of 378
Assisted reproductive techniques 20, 34*fc*, 87, 109, 110, 119, 124*b*, 134, 204, 209, 236, 262, 272, 274, 279, 280*f*, 281*f*, 304, 345, 355, 364
  quality management principle protocols 279*f*
  sections of 287*f*
Atracurium 383
Atropine 383
Autoimmune
  ovarian damage 341
  syndrome 326
Autologous bone marrow-derived stem cells 341
Autologous peripheral blood mononuclear cells, intrauterine infusion of 313
Azoospermia 11, 16, 18, 21, 23, 24*fc*, 78, 80, 83, 84, 90, 92*fc*, 93, 160, 167, 339, 361
  causes of 83
  classification of 90*fc*
  diagnosis of 83
  differential diagnosis of 94*fc*
  evaluation of 84*fc*, 85*f*, 90
  factor 13, 167
  histopathological types of 86
  management of 90, 94, 94*fc*
  nonobstructive 23, 96, 167, 168, 170
  obstructive 23, 94
  prevalence of 90
  treatment of 84*fc*, 85*t*
Azoospermic male 91
  evaluation of 91

B

Barotrauma, risk for 382
Basal hormone levels 163*t*

B-cell lymphoma 338
Bedaquiline 145
Biopsy, endometrial 144, 168, 308, 309*fc*
Blastocyst 308, 369*f*
  assessment 308*fc*
  grading 370*t*
  spent culture media 373*t*
  transfer 311
    policy 365
Blood
  borne infection 141
  flow 309
    endometrial 319
  group rhesus type 213
  investigations 4
  pressure 382
    noninvasive 383
Body mass index 3, 101, 219
  measurement 310
Bologna criteria 208
Bone marrow 337
  stem cells 339, 340
  stromal cells 338
Bovine serum albumin 376
Bradycardia 385
Brainstem herniation 391
Bromocriptine 113, 114, 179

C

Cabergoline 113, 114, 179, 255
Cancer 247
  cervical 247
Candida albicans 140
Carbon dioxide 381, 389
  gas 389
Cardiac failure 391
Cardiac output 382, 383
Cardiovascular system 382
  effect of 382*b*, 383*b*
Cartridge-based nucleic acid amplification test 60
Cellular criteria 367*f*
Central nervous system 385
Cerebral perfusion pressure 382
Cervical
  canal, evaluation of 49
  cerclage 332
  incompetence 329, 332
  lesions 43
Cervicitis, mild cases of 145
Cetrorelix 233
Chemotherapy 219, 317
Chlamydia
  antibody test 59
  trachomatis 140, 142

Chlamydial infections 143
Chromopertubation 59
Chromosomal number, abnormal 326
Cilia 142
Cleavage stage embryo grading 368*t*
Clofazimine 146
Clomiphene
   citrate 45, 101, 104, 133, 151, 153, 175,
       175*t*, 184, 184*f*, 219, 220, 247, 250,
       259, 316
      challenge test 26, 28, 216
      dose protocol 176*f*
      failure 176
      resistance 176
Coital factors 149
Coma 391
Combined oral contraceptive pills 134, 235
Comparative genomic hybridization 334
Complete blood count 143, 216
Computer-assisted sperm analysis 287
Conception, products of 71
Confusion 391
Congenital uterine
   anomalies 65, 330
      investigations for 63
   factors
      evaluation of 63
      management of 63
Conjunction regimen step-up protocol
       102*f*
Controlled ovarian
   hyperstimulation 199, 234, 236, 249,
       257
   stimulation 199, 221, 222, 261, 293, 341
Conventional multidose antagonist
       protocol 237*f*
Conventional therapy 177, 178*f*
Convulsions 391
Copy number variants 334
Corpus luteum 36, 36*f*
Corticosteroids 195, 224, 229
C-reactive protein 143
Cryopreservation 297
Cumulative pregnancy rate 72, 201*f*, 218
Cumulus-oocyte complexes 282, 283
Cycle cancellation 297
Cycloserine 146
Cystic fibrosis 13
   gene mutations 166
      transmembrane conductance regulator
       24, 93, 293
       gene mutation 23
Cysts 37*t*
Cytokine factors 130
Cytoplasmic fragmentation 306
Cytoplasmic vacuoles, number of 306

D

D-chiro-inositol 193
Death 391
   causes of 298
Decision tree algorithm 346, 347*fc*
Deep vein thrombosis 245
Dehydroepiandrosterone 200, 201*f*, 202,
       226, 259
   sulphate 202
Delivery, preterm 67
Density-gradient technique 356, 356*f*
   advantages of 357*t*
   disadvantages of 357*t*
Deoxynucleotidyl 150
Deoxyribonucleic acid 283, 358, 359
   breakage detection fluorescence in situ
       hybridization 306
   fragmentation index 19, 215, 334, 377
Dermoid cysts 48
Dexamethasone 179
Diabetes mellitus 3, 158, 310
Diaphragm, elevation of 385
Diarrhea 185
Diet 300
Diethylstilbestrol 64*f*
Dimeric glycoprotein 28
Diminished ovarian reserve 27, 158, 198,
       200, 205, 208
   diagnosis of 208
   management of 199
Disorientation 391
Distal tubal disease, management of 61
Diuretics, role of 301
Donor sperm treatment 97
Dopamine 114
   agonist 114, 255, 297
Doppler ultrasound 318
Double intrauterine insemination, role
       of 177
Douglas pouch 36
Dual stimulation protocol 236, 237*f*
Dual trigger 266, 297

E

Echogenicity 309
Edema, pulmonary 391
Edessy stem cells score 341
Eight-cell stage 369*f*
Ejaculatory duct
   obstruction 86
   transurethral resection of 95
Ejaculatory dysfunction 174
Embryo 165, 310, 311, 312*fc*
   assessment 305, 306, 308*fc*
      basis of 377

cryopreservation of 253, 253*f*
growth pattern of 368*t*
implantation failure 304
morphology 365
selection of 311, 348*fc*, 364, 365
transfer 123, 267
  number of 304
Embryogenesis, critical evaluation of 373
Embryoscope 308
Empty follicle syndrome 267, 270, 270*t*
Endocervical canal 49
Endocrine 21, 106
  disorders 333
  disturbances 15
  etiologies 333
  evaluation 22*t*, 75, 163
  tests 18, 83
Endometrial aspirates 144
Endometrial motion 318
Endometrial receptivity 309
  analysis 322
  assays 314
Endometrial recurrent implantation failure 305
Endometrial scratch 313, 319, 322
Endometrial thickness 42, 309, 316, 316*t*, 318, 339
Endometrioma 124, 209
  removal of 125
  surgical treatment of 124*b*
  treatment for 46
Endometriosis 45, 46, 59, 69, 99, 117-120, 122, 124, 158, 161
  displays 46
  effect of 120
  etiopathogenesis of 117
  fertility index 47, 124
  fulguration of 381
  lesions of 122
  mild-moderate 102
  sever 125
  treatment of 120, 125
Endometritis 41, 41*f*, 142, 310, 311, 313*fc*, 316
  chronic 71, 168, 314
  postpartum 317
Endometrium 119
  assessment of 305, 308
  hysteroscopic instillation 51
Endomyometrial junction 48, 131
Endotracheal tube 383
End-tidal carbon dioxide 383
Enzyme 119
  linked immunosorbent assay 58
Epididymis 83
  examination of 10

Epididymitis 147
Erectile dysfunction 174
Estradiol 214, 258
  hemihydrates 319
  valerate 319
Estrogen 224, 229, 319
  production 119
Ethambutol 60, 146
Ethionamide 146

F

Factor V Leiden 327, 334
Fallopian tube 49
  evaluation of 6
  patency 381
  ultrasound evaluation of 59
Fast track and standard treatment 153, 177
Febrile morbidity 136
Female anovulatory infertility, causes of 190
Female genital tuberculosis 60, 146*fc*
  treatment of 145
Female infertility 106, 107, 108*f*, 109, 150*t*
  causes of 33
  investigations for 150
  management 169*fc*
Female partner, evaluation of 159*fc*
Female reproductive system 338*t*
Female unexplained infertility, causes of 149, 149*t*
Fentanyl 383
Fertility 50, 127, 159
Fertilization 109*fc*
  defects 149
Fetal karyotyping 326
Fibroids 42, 42*f*, 48, 127, 131, 132, 137, 317, 381
  evaluation of 69
  management of 134
  mapping 132
  multiple 127
  perfusion of 130
  physical impact of 130
  size of 134
Fibrotic intrauterine 142
Fimbrial agglutination 55
Fimbrial phimosis 55
First polar body morphology 306
Fitz-Hugh-Curtis syndrome 142
Flow index 100
Fluid
  absorption 392
  overload 390, 391, 392*t*
  therapy 300

Fluorescence in situ hybridization 22
  analysis 326
Folic acid 224, 228
Follicle
  number per ovary 100
  stimulating hormone 12, 14, 24, 26, 27,
      75, 92, 94, 100, 106, 133, 150, 158-
      160, 176, 183, 187*f*, 200, 203, 204,
      214, 218, 258, 262, 264, 266, 267
    recombinant 234
    synchronization of 104
Follicular cohort synchronization 233
Follicular fluid 371
  biochemical marker 306
Follicular monitoring 34, 176
Follicular number 198*f*
Folliculogenesis 118
Four-cell stage 369*f*
Free androgen index 183
Frozen
  embryo transfer 195, 304
  thawed donor sample cycles 177

G

Galactorrhea 156
Gametes 305, 310, 311, 312*fc*
Ganirelix 233
Gas embolism 392
Gastric reflux 385
Gastrointestinal system, effect of 382*b*
Genes, endometrial expression of 119
Genetic disease, sever 24
Genital tract infection 140
  lower 140
  male 147*t*
Genital tuberculosis, female 60, 146*fc*
Giant oocyte 305
Glass wool filtration technique 357, 357*f*
  advantages of 357*t*
  disadvantages of 357*t*
Globozoospermia 18
Glucocorticoids 314
Glucose 308, 375, 389, 391*fc*
Gonadotropin 100, 152, 177, 178*f*, 185, 186,
    220, 235, 237*f*, 247, 251
  administration 96
  dosage 235
  exogenous 104
  protocol 186
  releasing hormone 70, 82, 103, 106,
      120, 183, 187, 188, 200, 232, 264,
      266, 267*t*, 272, 274
    agonist 204, 219, 222, 233*f*, 237, 252,
        265, 267, 275

antagonist protocol 219, 221, 232,
    233*f*, 253
  use of 392
  therapy 177
  types of 251
Gonococcal infection 142
Granulocyte colony-stimulating factor
    312, 314, 319, 321
Granulosa cells 338
Granulosus, central 305
Growth
  endometrial 318*t*, 322
  hormone 200, 202, 204, 227
Gynecologic laparoscopic procedures 381,
    381*t*, 382

H

Hashimoto's thyroiditis 310
Healthy sperms, facilitates selection of 306
Heart disease, congenital 99
Hematoma, aspiration of 381
Hemiuterus 332
Hemoglobin 213
Hemolysis, elevated liver enzymes, and
    low platelets 327
Hemorrhage 385
Heparin 275
Hirsutism 249
Human chorionic gonadotropin 83, 106,
    175, 200, 204, 234, 262, 272, 274,
    275, 294, 304, 319, 339
  low-dose 320
  supplementation 96
  trigger 265*t*
Human endometrium 339
Human follicle stimulating hormone 203
Human immunodeficiency virus 213
Human menopausal gonadotropin 83,
    133, 185, 203, 234, 237, 259
Human serum albumin 376
Hyaluronic acid 358, 376
  binding test 358
Hybrid leiomyomas 129
Hydration 300
Hydrogenase isoenzymes 202
Hydrosalpinx 60, 310
  evidence of 144
  presence of 214
Hydroxychloroquine 328
Hydroxyethyl starch 245, 255
Hydroxysteroid dehydrogenase
    isoenzymes 202
Hyperandrogenemia 249, 317
Hyperandrogenism 91, 191

Hyperinsulinemia 249
Hyperplasia 129
    congenital adrenal 249
    endometrial 41, 41*f*, 69
Hyperprolactinemia 99, 106, 111, 112,
        113*fc*, 181
    causes of 112*f*
    clinical presentations of 111
    diagnosis of 183*fc*
    management of 114
    mild 114
    treatment of 183*fc*
Hyperthyroidism 108*f*, 310
Hypervolemic hyponatremia 392*t*
    management of 391
Hypocaloric diet 181
Hypogonadism
    hypergonadotropic 83
    hypothalamic 317
    male 81, 81*fc*
    primary 81
    secondary 82, 83
Hypogonadotropic hypogonadism 83, 86,
        97, 269
    causes of 85*b*
Hyponatremia
    acute hypervolemic 392
    hypervolemic 392*t*
Hypospadias 174
Hypotension 385
Hypothalamic-pituitary
    testicular axis 163
    thyroid axis 107*f*
Hypothyroidism 99, 108*f*, 110, 310, 333
    subclinical 107, 110
Hysterolaparoscopy 45, 310
Hysterosalpingo contrast sonography 57,
        58, 133
Hysterosalpingogram 57, 58, 150
Hysterosalpingography 6, 7, 56, 63, 128,
        133, 159, 216, 310, 329
Hysteroscopic procedures 389, 390
Hysteroscopic septal incision 65
Hysteroscopy 7, 49, 51, 314, 330, 389, 390,
        392
    complications of 390
    operative 389

I

Immunoglobulin, intravenous 312
Immunotherapy 312, 314
Impaired endocrine function 118
Implantation 119
In utero diethylstilbestrol 317

In vitro fertilization 46, 58, 61, 70, 78, 87,
        101, 102, 118, 123, 152, 153, 166,
        169, 170, 200, 208, 213, 217, 234,
        249, 252, 262, 279, 282, 283, 289,
        304, 322, 345, 356, 364, 375, 386
    cycles 29
    technique 375
In vitro maturation 255, 298
Infections 140, 142
    chronic 144
    control 285
    degree of 141
Infertile couple 156, 157*t*, 157*t*, 168
    evaluation of 1
    management of 133*fc*
Infertile female 2, 117
Infertile males 17, 165
Infertility 15, 45, 47, 49, 63, 72, 106, 114,
        117, 130, 140, 166, 249, 337, 338
    anovulatory 217
    causes of 149, 155*f*
    diagnostic of 18
    endometriosis associated 121*t*, 123, 130
    epidemiology of 155
    etiology of 161*t*
    evaluation 156, 161*t*, 216*fc*
    general causes of 1
    male 15, 34, 147, 150*t*
    management of 45, 134, 169
    mechanism of 129
    step by step management of 99, 155
    ultrasound in 33
Inguinal surgeries 159
Injury, endometrial 314
Inner cell mass 379
Inositol 193
Inspired oxygen, fraction of 385
Insulin
    resistance 184, 249
    sensitizing agents 184, 192
Interferon gamma released assays 144
Interleukin-1 receptor-associated kinase
        1 338
Intra-abdominal pressure 382, 385
Intracranial pressure 382
Intracytoplasmic anomalies 305
Intracytoplasmic morphologically selected
        sperm injection 306, 360, 376
    technique 360*f*
Intracytoplasmic sperm injection 13, 79,
        94, 165, 169, 170, 282, 283, 348,
        355, 357-359, 365, 376
Intralipid 312
Intraovarian autologous platelet-rich
        plasma therapy 260

Intrauterine adhesions 49, 50, 71, 134, 329, 332
 removal of 311
Intrauterine contraceptive device 55
Intrauterine death 67
Intrauterine growth restriction 67
Intrauterine insemination 30, 78, 100, 101, 122, 141, 152, 153, 169, 170, 174, 176, 177, 217, 221, 276, 282, 321, 355
 cycle, superovulation for 220
 indications of 102, 174
 protocol for 175
 timing of 176
Intrauterine septum, resection of 389
Intrauterine synechiae 55
 adhesiolysis of 389
Intravenous fluid therapy 302
Invasive imaging technique 14
Irregular cycles 1
Irreversible primary testicular failure 82
Isoniazid 60, 146

K

Kallmann syndrome 9, 83
Karyotype 326
 analysis 23
 testing 314
Ketamine 387
Key performance indicators 279, 280f, 283
Kidney disease, chronic 3
Kisspeptins 268
Klinefelter syndrome 9, 84, 162, 167

L

Lactate 375
Laparoscopic conservative adenomyomectomy 70
Laparoscopic microsurgical techniques 48
Laparoscopic ovarian
 drilling 45, 46, 188, 251
 surgery 104
Laparoscopically-assisted vaginal hysterectomy 381
Laparoscopy 8, 45, 59, 134, 144, 330, 381
 indications for 45
 nonoperative 381
 operative 122, 381
Laparotomy 134
L-arginine 312, 320
Laryngeal mask airway 383
L-carnitine 195
Leiomyoma 127, 129, 329
 subclassification system 129
 submucous 50

Letrozole 101, 104, 151, 175, 175t, 185, 203, 219, 220, 237, 251
 dose protocol 176f
 step-up protocol 176
 therapy 176
Leukemia inhibitory factor 347
Leukocytes, quantification of 165
Levofloxacin 145
Levonorgestrel-releasing intrauterine system 134
Levothyroxine 110
 treatment 110
Linezolid 146
Liquefaction time 78
Live birth rates 132, 258, 368
L-methylfolate 194
Low molecular weight heparin 314
Lowenstein-Jensen medium 144
Low-molecular-weight heparin 224, 228, 345
Lung volumes 382
Lupus anticoagulant 326, 327
Luteal phase defect 275, 333
 mechanism 272, 273fc
Luteal phase support 267, 272, 274f, 276
 drugs used in 273, 274fc
 duration of 272
Luteinized unruptured follicle 36
Luteinizing hormone 12, 46, 100, 106, 150, 160, 200, 219, 234, 250, 259, 262, 264, 265t, 266, 266f, 272, 311, 320, 339
 addition of 235
 multiple 118
 recombinant 203, 234
Lymphocyte immunization therapy 312
Lymphocytosis 60

M

Machine learning 345
 use of 353f
Magnetic activated cell sorting 358
 separation technique 357, 358f
Magnetic assisted cell sorter 365
 technique
  advantages of 358t
  disadvantages of 358t
Magnetic resonance
 guided focused ultrasound surgery 135
 imaging 7, 65, 66f, 128, 146, 330
Male infertility 15, 24, 34, 147, 150t, 159
 diagnosis of 10
 evaluation of 8, 9fc, 13, 74, 89, 159
 field of 90
 investigations for 150
 management 170fc

Male partner
  assessment of 20
  evaluation of 15, 16, 160*fc*
Male subfertility 1
Male unexplained infertility, causes of 149, 149*t*
Malignancy 129
Mannitol 389
Mantoux test 144
Masturbatory anejaculation 87
Matrix metalloproteinases 119
Mature follicle, features of 36*b*
Mature oocyte 367*f*
Medroxyprogesterone acetate 237
Melatonin 194, 203
Menstrual cycle 220, 221, 314
  luteal phase of 272
  natural 262
  pattern 27
Menstrual irregularities 249
Mesenchymal stem cell 337, 338
  characteristics of 337
Metabolic syndrome 249
Metabolomics 371
  study 309
Metformin 179, 184, 192, 224, 225, 250, 297
  effect of 193*f*
Methylene 50
Microfluidics sperm sorting
  advantages of 363*t*
  disadvantages of 363*t*
Micronutrients, multiple 195
Midazolam 383
Midtubal diseases 55
Mild stimulation in vitro fertilization 232
Minerals 195
Mini laparoscopic tubal ligation 381
Minimal ovarian stimulation protocol 104*f*
Miscarriage 334
Mitochondrial deoxyribonucleic acid 203
Mitochondrial replacement therapy 203
Mitotic spindle 306
Monosomy X 326
Motile sperm organelle morphology examination 360
  spermatogram, classification of 361*t*
Motility 80
Mouse embryo assay 288
Moxifloxacin 146
Müllerian anomalies, complex 68
Müllerian anomaly 63, 317, 329
  classification of 64*f*
Müllerian ducts 65
Müllerian hormone 120
Multiple gestation 242, 245*t*, 253, 255

Muscle relaxants 383
Mycobacteria growth indicator tube 60, 144
Mycobacterium
  bovis 141
  tuberculosis 60, 141
Myoinositol 179, 224, 225
Myoma 45, 310
Myomectomy 131, 132, 137, 311, 381
  hysteroscopic 134
  laparoscopic 48
Myometrial blood flow 319
Myometrial lesions 42, 42*t*

N

N-acetyl cysteine 194
Naïve Bayes classifier algorithm 349, 350*fc*
  use of 350*t*
Narcotics 387
Nausea 383, 391
Neisseria gonorrhoeae 140
Neoplasia 74, 168
Neosalpingostomy 61
Neostigmine 383
Neurological system, effect of 382*b*
Nitric oxide 320
Nitrous oxide 387
Noninvasive chromosomal screening 372, 373
Nonliquefaction 78
Nonobstructive azoospermia 23, 96, 167, 168, 170
  causes of 85*t*
Nonseptate clear cysts 36*t*
Nonsteroidal anti-inflammatory drugs 3, 390
Normal thin endometrium, development of 317*f*
Normogonadotropic anovulation, treatment of 183*t*
Normozoospermia 78
Nuclear
  criteria 367*f*
  maturity 305

O

Obstruction, reversal of 94
Obstructive azoospermia 23, 94
  treatment of 86
Oligoasthenoteratozoospermia 11, 21
Oligomenorrhea 1, 156
Oligo-ovulation 218
Oligospermia 78, 160
  sever 80, 361

Oligozoospermia, sever 23, 167, 168, 170
Omega 3 fatty acids 195
Oocyte 106, 119, 218, 305
   cryopreservation 260
   donation 235
   in vitro maturation of 298
   maturation, physiology of 263*f*
   maturity 305
   morphology 306*fc*, 365
   number of 26, 210
   pickup 237*f*
   quantity 26, 208
      assessment of 214
   retrieval 62, 386
   stages of 367*f*
Oopheritis 219
Oophorectomy 381
Oral contraceptive 195, 234
   pill
      pretreatment 195
      short priming of 234
Oral ovulogens 101*fc*, 219
   combination of 178
Orchitis 147
Ovarian biopsy 29
Ovarian cyst 36, 47
   aspiration 381
Ovarian Doppler 29
Ovarian failure 161
Ovarian follicle pool 27*f*
Ovarian hyperstimulation syndrome 100,
        218, 224, 231, 241, 243*t*, 253, 264,
        266, 267, 293, 302
   management of 242, 245*t*, 299*f*
   pathophysiology of 294*fc*
   prevention of 254
   risk for 46
   sever 192
   severity of 241*t*
Ovarian induction, letrozole for 186*f*
Ovarian lesions 43
Ovarian reserve 26, 120, 199, 200*t*, 208, 218
   markers 210
   evaluation of 34, 35*f*, 198
   low 49
   test 4, 5, 26, 26*fc*, 198, 209, 214
Ovarian stimulation 30, 151, 153, 217, 222
   complications of 241
   drugs for 219
   protocol 231, 232, 234
Ovarian surface epithelium 106
Ovarian surgery 1, 209
Ovarian torsion 246
Ovarian volume 29

Ovary
   evaluation of 4
   morphophysiology of 107*f*
   ultrasound of 34
Ovulation
   disorders of 181
   induction 58, 101, 101*fc*, 179, 181
      cycle 276
      drugs, use of 250
   surgical induction of 188
   trigger 221
Ovulatory cycles 156
Ovulatory disorder 162
Ovulatory dysfunction 129, 191
Ovulatory functions 118
Ovum pick-up 237, 269, 274
   day of 87

P

Pain relief 300
Paracentesis, indications for 302
Peak systolic velocity 35, 36
Pelvic
   adhesions 45, 47, 161
      detection of 47
      diagnosis of 47
   anatomical disruption 117
   anatomy distortion 117, 121
   infection 140, 209, 219
   inflammatory disease 3, 45, 55, 57, 58,
        141, 158
   radiation 317
Pelvis 142
Penile vibratory stimulation 87
Pentoxifylline 319
Percutaneous epididymal sperm aspiration
        79, 94, 96, 170
Pergolide 113
Peritubal disease, management of 59
Perivitelline space granularity 306
Phenotypes 190
Phosphatase and tensin homolog 338
Phosphatidylserine 358
Phospholipids 358
Physiological intracytoplasmic sperm
        injection 375
   technique 360*f*
Pipelle 322
Pituitary gland 97
Placenta mesenchymal stem cells 338
Placenta, morphophysiology of 107*f*
Plasma exchange 328
Plasminogen activation inhibitor 306
Platelet rich plasma 260, 313, 321, 341

Pneumoperitoneum, physiological effects of 382
Polar body 282
Polycystic morphology 35, 35*f*
Polycystic ovarian morphology 35, 191
Polycystic ovarian syndrome 5, 45, 91, 99-101, 159, 175, 176, 183*t*, 190, 191*t*, 218, 249, 252*f*, 267, 333
  management of 100
  pathogenesis of 99*fc*
  phenotypes, classification of 191*t*
  sonomorphology of 100*t*
Polycystic ovary
  management of 249
  ultrasound features of 35*f*
Polyfollicular growth 247
Polymerase chain reaction 146, 327
Polypectomy 311
  hysteroscopic 70
Polyploidy 368*f*
Polyps 41, 41*f*, 50, 129, 310, 329
  endometrial 70, 332
  removal of 389
Polyzoospermia 78
Poor ovarian
  reserve 35, 35*f*, 257
  response, Bologna criteria for 209*fc*
Poor responders 237*f*
  Bologna criteria for 257*b*
POSEIDON
  classification 210
  criteria 199*f*
Positron emission tomography scan 144
Postadhesiolysis adhesion 47
Postejaculatory urinalysis 163
Post-trigger check points 269
Power Doppler 43
Preconception 327
Pregnancy 302
  ectopic 46, 245, 381
  loss 325
    early 120, 234
    recurrent 325, 329, 377
  molar 326
  number of 316*t*
  rate 281, 320
    spontaneous 150
Preimplantation genetic
  diagnosis 334
  testing 326, 373, 375, 379
  thrombophilia workup 314
Pre-in vitro fertilization
  evaluation 213
  priming 234
Premature luteinizing hormone 231

Premature ovarian
  failure 340
  insufficiency 317
Prenatal genetic testing 308
Progesterone 273
  plus estrogen 275
  premature elevation of 231
  support 177
Programmed cell death protein 4 338
Proinflammatory immune function 200
Propofol 383, 387
Prostate
  examination of 10
  transurethral resection of 94, 390
Protein
  C activity 327
  S activity 327
Prothrombin 334
Proximal tubal disease, management of 61
Pulsatile administration 97
Pulsatility index 35
Pyosalpinx 60
  evidence of 144
Pyrazinamide 60
Pyruvate 308, 375

Q

Quality assurance 279
Quality control 279
Quality management 279, 282
Quinagolide 113

R

Radioactive iodine treatment 109
Random forest algorithm 348
  experimental results of 349*t*
  use of 349*t*
Random stimulation protocol 237
Randomized controlled trials 62, 132, 377
Rapid plasma regain 216
Reactive oxygen species 355, 357
  estimation hormonal evaluation 12
Rectal probe electroejaculation 87
Recurrent implantation failure 304
Refractory endometrium 339
Regurgitation, risk for 382
Renal anomalies 329
Renal failure, acute 391
Renal function 382
Renal system, effect of 382*b*
Reproductive autoimmune syndrome 327, 327*t*
Reproductive medicine 91, 345, 346, 346*f*, 347*fc*, 348*t*

Reproductive system evaluation 214
Reproductive tract 95
Resistance index 36, 38, 100
Respiratory arrest 391
Respiratory system, effect of 382b, 383b
Retractile bodies 305
Retrograde ejaculation, evaluation of 12
Rheumatoid arthritis 310
Rifampicin 60, 146
Rifampin 60
Robertsonian translocation 326
Rotterdam criteria 99fc

S

Saline
   infusion
      sonography 56, 329, 329f
      sonohysterography 216
   normal 389
Salpingitis 141t
   isthmica nodosa 55
   types of 141
Sedation 383
Selective estrogen receptor 184
Semen 87, 164, 165, 309
   analyses 10, 11, 16, 17, 20, 74, 79fc, 160, 161t, 164, 215
      interpretation of 76, 78
   characteristics 76
   examination 91
   fructose in 93
   macroscopic analysis of 20t
   microscopic analysis of 20t
   pH 93
   sample 96
   specimen 16
   volume 21, 91
Seminal vesicles 74
Seminal vesiculitis 147
Septum 310
   resection 311
Serum prolactin level, assessment of 82
Sex chromosomal aneuploidy 167
Sex chromosome 326
Sex hormone binding globulin 106, 250
Sexual dysfunction, male 21
Sildenafil 276, 312, 320
   citrate 87
Simple cyst paraovarian cyst 36, 36f
Single cell gel electrophoresis assay 306
Single embryo transfer 371
Sion's test 56
Smooth endoplasmic reticulum 367f
   clusters 306

Somatic cell nuclear transfer 342
Sonohysterography 7, 42
Sonohysterosalpingography 56
Sperm 119, 164, 311
   assessment 306, 307fc
   chromatin
      dispersion 150, 306
      structure assay 150, 165, 306
   chromosome aneuploidy 168
   concentration 78
      normal 167
   deoxyribonucleic acid fragmentation 11
      index 22
      tests 165
   fluorescent in situ hybridization 22
   function 119
      tests 19, 20
   morphology 364, 366f
      abnormal 168
   preparation
      need of 355
      techniques 355
   sample 174
   scoring 361t
   selection technique 355, 362f
   sorting, microfluidics for 362
   viability tests 165
Spermatogenesis, endogenous 82
Spermatozoa 80
   abnormal 80
Spermiogenesis, completion of 96
Spindle transfer 203
Standard operating procedures 279, 337
Stem cell 337, 338
   application of 337
   endometrial 322
   research 342
   role of 338
   therapy 322, 342
Sterility 285
Sterilization reversal, management of 61
Steroids 10
Stimulate angiogenesis 340
Stimulation 252f
   protocols 296
Strassmann's laparoscopic metroplasty 68
Streptomycin 146
Stroma, endometrial 71
Submucous fibroid 42, 42f, 69, 128, 136, 137
   removal of 128, 389
Submucous myomas, classification of 130t
Subserosal fibroids, removal of 48, 137
Support vector machines 349, 351f
   use of 352t

Surgery
  hysterolaparoscopic 381
  laparoscopic 125, 150
Suxamethonium 383
Swim-up technique 355, 356*f*
  advantages of 356*t*
  disadvantages of 356*t*
Synchrony, loss of 311
Synechiae 42, 42*f*
Systemic lupus erythematosus 310

T

Tamoxifen 219
Teratozoospermia 360, 361
Teratozoospermic index 80
Test tubal patency 132
Testicular biopsy 14, 19, 93
  histopathological types of 86*b*
Testicular sperm 215
  aspiration 94, 96, 170
  extraction 13, 79, 93, 170, 311
Testosterone 200, 201, 226
  deficiency 82
  gel 202
    preparations 82
  replacement therapy 82
  supplementation 201
  transdermal 200
Tetraploidy 326
Thalassemia major 326
Thin endometrium 311, 316
  sonographic finding of 317*f*
Three-dimensional ultrasound 7
  sonography 66*f*
Thrombophilia panel 334
Thyroid
  autoimmunity 106, 109
    mechanism of 109*fc*
  cancer treatment 109
  disorders 106, 111*fc*, 310, 386
  dysfunction 107, 114
  hormone 333
  stimulating hormone 106, 150, 159, 183, 216
Thyroxine 179
Time-lapse
  imaging 372*f*, 377
  technology 377
    significance of 377
Total laparoscopic hysterectomy 381
Total motile count 355
Transabdominal metroplasty 68
Transabdominal sonography 34
Transrectal ultrasonography 14, 94, 164

Transrectal ultrasound 14
  scan 24
Transvaginal sonography 34, 318
Transvaginal ultrasound 63, 128
Trendelenburg position 385
  effect of 382
Trichomonas vaginalis 140
Trigger
  choice of 269
  modifications 297
  physiology of 262
  prerequisites of 268
  types of 262, 264*t*
Triploidy 326
Trisomy 326
Trophic activity 340
True follicular density 29
Tubal abnormalities 214
Tubal assessment tests 56, 57*t*
Tubal block 48
  unilateral 174
Tubal cells 142
Tubal cornual occlusion 50
Tubal damage, classification of 56
Tubal delinking 61
Tubal factor 55, 141, 169*fc*
  evaluation of 55
  infertility 60
    management of 60
  management of 55
Tubal illness 119
Tubal infertility
  causes of 55
  evaluation of 58*fc*
Tubal lesions 43
Tubal pregnancies 245
Tubal recanalization 381
Tuberculin test 144
Tuberculosis 45, 60, 140, 141, 386
  genital 141
Tubo-ovarian masses 60
Tubular epithelium, destruction of 79
Tumors
  necrosis factor-alpha 118
  benign 127
Two-cell stage 369*f*

U

Ultrasonography 57, 144, 164, 304, 309, 310
  scrotal 164
Ultrasound
  abdominal 13
  criteria 268
  evaluation 59-76

monitoring 33*fc*
scrotal 13
Unexplained infertility 131, 149, 150, 152, 168, 174
   treatment of 152*t*
Upper genital tract infection 140, 141
   treatment of 145
Urethritis 147
Urinary tract infection 77
Urine color 300
Urogenital abnormalities
   acquired 15
   congenital 15
Uterine
   abnormalities 162
      acquired 41, 41*t*, 332
      congenital causes of 38, 38*t*
   anomalies 310
      classification of 330*f*
      congenital 65, 330
   artery
      Doppler flow 319
      embolization 135, 137
   cavity 49, 215
   contractions 130
   didelphys 68
   factors 63, 169*fc*
      congenital 63
      evaluation of 63
      management of 63
   fibroids 68, 69, 131, 332
   fluid proteome 309
   pathology 158
      acquired 68
   perforation 390
   peristalsis 125
   septa 50
   septum 65
   tube, morphophysiology of 107*f*
   unification 68
Uterus 63, 127, 310, 311, 312*fc*
   baseline scan of 38, 38*f*
   bicornuate 39, 39*f*, 40, 40*f*, 40*t*, 67, 68, 331
   complete
      bicorporeal 331
      septate 66*f*
   didelphys 39, 39*f*
   evaluation of 7
   hypoplasia of 38, 38*f*
   investigations for 305
   morphophysiology of 107*f*
   partial
      bicorporeal 331
      subseptate 331

septate 39, 39*f*, 40, 40*f*, 40*t*, 65, 329*f*, 331
subseptate 66*f*
ultrasound of 38, 38*b*
unicornuate 38, 38*f*, 67

V

Vacuolization 305
Vaginal fluid 309
Vaginismus 174
Vaginosis, bacterial 140
Varicoceles
   detection of 13
   examination of 10
   management of 96
Vas deferens 83
   congenital bilateral absence of 14, 24, 77, 160
Vasal aplasia 86
Vascular endothelial growth factor 294, 318, 334
Vasoepididymostomy 95, 95*f*
Vasovasostomy 94, 95*f*
Vecuronium 383
Viagra 87
Viscosity 78
Vitality 80
Vitamin
   D 194, 214
   D_3 194
   E 319
Vomiting 383, 391

W

Weight loss 181
Wertheim's procedure 381
Wrist deformities 168

X

X chromosomes 167
X-ray chest 144

Y

Y chromosome 167, 168
   microdeletions 9, 23, 84, 166-168
Y deletions 162

Z

Zeta potential technique 358, 359*f*
   advantages of 359*t*
   disadvantages of 359*t*
Zona pellucida 378
Zygote morphology 365

EU GSPR Authorised Reprsentative
Logos Europe, 9 rue Nicolas Poussin
1700, La Rochelle, France
Phone: +33 (0) 6 67 93 73 78
E-mail: contact@logoseurope.eu

www.ingramcontent.com/pod-product-compliance
Ingram Content Group UK Ltd.
Pitfield, Milton Keynes, MK11 3LW, UK
UKHW050427150426
5217IPUK00019B/1281